IET HEALTHCARE TECHNOLOGIES SERIES 39

Digital Methods and Tools to Support Healthy Ageing

Other volumes in this series:

Volume 1 **Nanobiosensors for Personalized and Onsite Biomedical Diagnosis** P. Chandra (Editor)
Volume 2 **Machine Learning for Healthcare Technologies** D.A. Clifton (Editor)
Volume 3 **Portable Biosensors and Point-of-Care Systems** S.E. Kintzios (Editor)
Volume 4 **Biomedical Nanomaterials: From Design To Implementation** T.J Webster and H. Yazici (Editors)
Volume 6 **Active and Assisted Living: Technologies and Applications** F. Florez-Revuelta and A.A Chaaraoui (Editors)
Volume 7 **Semiconductor Lasers and Diode-based Light Sources for Biophotonics** P.E Andersen and
          P.M Petersen (Editors)
Volume 9 **Human Monitoring, Smart Health and Assisted Living: Techniques and Technologies** S. Longhi,
          A. Monteriù and A. Freddi (Editors)
Volume 13 **Handbook of Speckle Filtering and Tracking in Cardiovascular Ultrasound Imaging and Video**
          C.P. Loizou, C.S. Pattichis and J. D'hooge (Editors)
Volume 14 **Soft Robots for Healthcare Applications: Design, Modelling, and Control** S. Xie, M. Zhang and W. Meng
Volume 16 **EEG Signal Processing: Feature extraction, selection and classification methods** W. Leong
Volume 17 **Patient-Centered Digital Healthcare Technology: Novel applications for next generation healthcare
          systems** L Goldschmidt and R. M. Relova (Editors)
Volume 19 **Neurotechnology: Methods, advances and applications** V. de Albuquerque, A. Athanasiou and
          S. Ribeiro (Editors)
Volume 20 **Security and Privacy of Electronic Healthcare Records: Concepts, paradigms and solutions** S. Tanwar,
          S. Tyagi and N. Kumar (Editors)
Volume 23 **Advances in Telemedicine for Health Monitoring: Technologies, design and applications** T.A. Rashid,
          C. Chakraborty and K. Fraser
Volume 24 **Mobile Technologies for Delivering Healthcare in Remote, Rural or Developing Regions** P. Ray,
          N. Nakashima, A. Ahmed, S. Ro and Y. Soshino (Editors)
Volume 26 **Wireless Medical Sensor Networks for IoT-based eHealth** F. Al-Turjman (Editor)
Volume 29 **Blockchain and Machine Learning for e-Healthcare Systems** B. Balusamy, N. Chilamkurti, L.A. Beena
          and P. Thangamuthu (Editors)

Digital Methods and Tools to Support Healthy Ageing

Edited by
Pradeep Kumar Ray, Siaw-Teng Liaw and
J. Artur Serrano

The Institution of Engineering and Technology

Published by The Institution of Engineering and Technology, London, United Kingdom

The Institution of Engineering and Technology is registered as a Charity in England & Wales (no. 211014) and Scotland (no. SC038698).

The Institution of Engineering and Technology
Michael Faraday House
Six Hills Way, Stevenage
Herts, SG1 2AY, United Kingdom

www.theiet.org

British Library Cataloguing in Publication Data
A catalogue record for this product is available from the British Library

ISBN 978-1-83953-462-1 (hardback)
ISBN 978-1-83953-463-8 (PDF)

Typeset in India by Exeter Premedia Services Private Limited
Printed in the UK by CPI Group (UK) Ltd, Croydon

Contents

Acknowledgements   xv
About the editors   xvii

1 Book overview: digital health for ageing population   1
   1.1 Introduction   1
   1.2 Section 1 – "Underpinning Principles"   2
   1.3 Section 2 – "Digital Services for Healthy Ageing" 4
   1.4 Section 3 – "Digital Tools for Healthy Ageing"   5
   1.5 Summary   7
   References   8

PART I Underpinning principles of Digital Health

2 Digital health maturity – a foundational principle   11
Siaw-Teng Liaw

   2.1 Introduction   11
   2.2 Conceptual framework   12
      2.2.1 Digital health   12
      2.2.2 Digital health maturity   13
      2.2.3 Digital health profile: indicators of digital health
           maturity 13
   2.3 Digital health maturity assessment   16
   2.4 Exercises   21
   2.5 Conclusion   21
   References   22

3 Global demographic changes and ageing population:
an overview   25
Sam Ro, Willy Huang, and Karpurika Raychaudhuri

   3.1 Introduction   25
   3.2 Global trend in population ageing: a reality check 27
   3.3 Challenges and issues of population ageing   36
      3.3.1 Challenges to the healthcare system 36
      3.3.2 Challenges to economy   42
   3.4 Analysis and policy implications   44
   3.5 Concluding remarks   48
   References   49

4   Digital health and elderly care in low- and middle-income countries: opportunities and challenges   **53**
Fatema Khatun, Sabrina Rasheed, Sifat Parveen Sheikh,
Kazi Nazmus Saqeeb, and Daniel D. Reidpath

4.1   Introduction   53
4.2   Context of elderly care in LMIC   54
4.3   The digital divide   54
4.4   Use of digital tools for elderly care   56
4.5   Framework for caregiver-mediated digital health support for
      elderlies in LMICs   56
4.6   Ethics and policy implications   59
      4.6.1   Policy implications   61
4.7   Conclusion   63
References   64

5   Health co-benefits in climate action policies for healthy ageing   **71**
Sardar Masud Karim, Siaw-Teng Liaw, and Pradeep Ray

5.1   Introduction   71
5.2   Co-benefits of climate action   72
5.3   Defining co-benefits   73
5.4   Co-benefits: applications, frameworks, methods and assessment
      tools   75
      5.4.1   Applications of co-benefits concept   75
      5.4.2   Identifying, quantifying and incorporating co-benefits
              into policy-decision-making   76
      5.4.3   Impact assessment tools of climate action policies   82
5.5   HIA as a framework to integrate health dimension in all policies 83
      5.5.1   Case study: HIA in phases IV and V of the WHO
              European Healthy Cities Network   84
      5.5.2   Methods   84
      5.5.3   Results   84
5.6   Health co-benefits in the context of UN SDG   87
      5.6.1   Co-benefits as potent motivator for local climate action 88
      5.6.2   The Australian perspective   89
5.7   Health co-benefits in policy process: Australian case study   90
      5.7.1   Background   90
      5.7.2   Methods   90
      5.7.3   Results   90
      5.7.4   Discussion   91
5.8   Conclusion   91
References   91

6   Health data privacy for aged population in Australia   **97**
Koel Ghorai, Guneet Randhawa, and Jan M. Smits

6.1   Introduction   97

6.2 Regulations dealing with Australian online health data 99
  6.2.1 General regulations 99
  6.2.2 Specific to health records 101
6.3 Identifying and mapping legal actors to corresponding roles
  and regulations: legal framework 107
  6.3.1 Identifying legal actors and resources (data) 107
  6.3.2 Data types and assurance levels 108
  6.3.3 Mapping actors to their rights and responsibilities
    (as per GDPR) 108
  6.3.4 Identification of appropriate regulations 108
6.4 Use case 1: My Health Record for aged care and the
  legal framework 111
  6.4.1 Overview of My Health Record for aged care 111
  6.4.2 Health record registration process and upload 113
  6.4.3 Identification of legal actors 114
  6.4.4 Legal analysis 114
6.5 Use case 2: legal analysis of online health record of dementia
  patient in aged care 115
  6.5.1 Overview of online health record of Australian
    dementia patient in aged care 115
  6.5.2 Identification of legal actors 117
  6.5.3 Legal analysis 117
6.6 Conclusion 118
References 122

PART II Digital Health Services for Healthy Ageing

7 Silvercare: a model for supporting healthy ageing services 127
Kasturi Bakshi, Jacqueline Blake, and Pradeep Ray

7.1 Introduction 127
7.2 Background of care for the elderly around the world 128
  7.2.1 Japan 128
  7.2.2 Scotland 129
  7.2.3 Netherlands 130
  7.2.4 Germany 130
  7.2.5 Singapore 131
7.3 Silvercare model 131
  7.3.1 Beneficiaries 132
  7.3.2 Coordinators 132
  7.3.3 Support group 132
  7.3.4 Service providers 132
  7.3.5 Tablet-based well-being project 133
7.4 Case study in India: Silvercare model of KINSPARC 134
  7.4.1 Local background 134
  7.4.2 Structure and function of the Silvercare team 135
  7.4.3 Operations 136

	7.4.4	Silvercare activities in Kalyani	136
	7.4.5	Project outcomes	138
7.5	Case study in Australia		138
	7.5.1	Local background	139
	7.5.2	Structure and organisation	139
	7.5.3	Operations	139
	7.5.4	Outcomes	140
7.6	Discussion		140
	7.6.1	Performance expectancy	140
	7.6.2	Attitude towards using the system	141
	7.6.3	Social influence	141
	7.6.4	Facilitating conditions	141
	7.6.5	Self-efficacy	141
	7.6.6	Anxiety	142
	7.6.7	Intention to use the system	142
7.7	Conclusion		142
References			143

8   Safeguarding the elderly in a pandemic: role of lockdown policies and digital health technologies   **147**
Nazia Akter, Yan Hanrunyu, and Pradeep Kumar Ray

8.1	Introduction		147
8.2	Research context		148
	8.2.1	Digital services and technologies for outbreak tracing	149
	8.2.2	Use of mobile applications for safe reopening	149
	8.2.3	Use of wearables with digital health services	149
	8.2.4	Contact tracing tools and services	149
	8.2.5	Use of AI and big data in digital health services	150
8.3	Research questions		151
8.4	Research design		151
	8.4.1	Database and keywords	151
	8.4.2	Criteria for inclusion and exclusion	152
	8.4.3	Limitations	152
	8.4.4	Screening results	152
8.5	Findings		153
	8.5.1	Actions taken by different countries to implement lockdown	153
	8.5.2	Impacts of such actions on the health of the elderly and how much they are affected	153
	8.5.3	Digital health and other approaches to strict lockdown and their effectiveness	154
8.6	Discussion		155
8.7	Conclusion		158
References			159

9 **Digital mental health in Bangladesh "MonerDaktar":**
caring seniors during COVID-19   **163**
Tanjir Rashid Soron, Md Moshiur Rahman, and Zaid Farzan Chowdhury

9.1   Introduction   163
9.2   Aging and mental health problems   164
9.3   COVID-19 and mental health crisis of elderly people   165
9.4   Digital mental health services in Bangladesh   165
9.5   DMHI for senior citizens   170
9.6   The development and testing of "MonerDaktar"   171
      9.6.1   Design of "MonerDaktar"   171
      9.6.2   Testing and assessment of "MonerDaktar"   172
9.7   "MonerDaktar" as a DMHI   173
      9.7.1   A real case example   173
9.8   Evaluation and challenges   174
9.9   Conclusion   176
References   176

10 **Digital health for aged care from a service perspective**   **183**
Yuan You, Yan Hanrunyu, and Pradeep Kumar Ray

10.1 Introduction   183
10.2 Aged care services and providers   185
      10.2.1 Asia   185
      10.2.2 Australia   185
      10.2.3 Europe   187
10.3 Service workflows   188
      10.3.1 Drug request and delivery process   189
      10.3.2 Participants   190
      10.3.3 Scenarios   190
      10.3.4 Sub-processes   190
10.4 Supply chain model: Jidoka   192
      10.4.1 Medication adherence as a supply chain management
              problem   193
      10.4.2 Measuring quality using RFID   193
10.5 Tools for medication adherence monitoring   194
10.6 Discussion   196
10.7 Conclusion and future work   198
References   199

11 **Role of digital technology in aged care in China**   **203**
Zhiyu Hao, Chao Xu, Lina Li, and Pradeep K Ray

11.1 Introduction   203
11.2 Methodology   205
      11.2.1 Identification of resources and search strategy   205

11.2.2 Selection of relevant articles   206
11.2.3 Data extraction and analysis   206
11.3 Results   206
    11.3.1 Plans and promotions of the government and the industry 206
    11.3.2 Case of technology in aged care in China   209
    11.3.3 Existing digital technology in aged care in China   214
    11.3.4 Development prospect   214
11.4 Case study of Haiyang Group   217
    11.4.1 Description of business   217
    11.4.2 Description of industry   218
    11.4.3 Technology   219
    11.4.4 Description of market   219
11.5 Discussion   222
11.6 Study limitations   223
11.7 Conclusion   223
Acknowledgement   224
References   224

PART III   Digital Tools for Healthy Ageing

12 Using powered exoskeletons for rehabilitation in healthy ageing – a societal perspective   231
J. Artur Serrano, Eduard Fosch-Villaronga, and Roger A. Søraa

12.1 Introduction   231
12.2 Powered exoskeletons and their function – a summary of
      current technologies   233
12.3 A symbiosis between powered exoskeletons and social robots 236
    12.3.1 Can a social enhanced exoskeleton help in healthy
            aging?   236
    12.3.2 From a rehabilitation device to a companion   237
    12.3.3 Assessing social exoskeletons using Robot Impact
            Assessment (ROBIA)   238
12.4 RRI and societal considerations for exoskeletons'
      implementation   238
    12.4.1 Accessibility considerations   239
    12.4.2 Economic considerations   239
    12.4.3 Inclusivity considerations   240
    12.4.4 Environmental considerations   240
    12.4.5 Cultural considerations   240
    12.4.6 Legal considerations   240
    12.4.7 Ethical considerations   241
12.5 Conclusion   241
    12.5.1 Acknowledgments   242
    12.5.2 Disclosure statement   242
    12.5.3 Funding   242
References   242

13 SENSE-GARDEN – A concept and technology for care and well-being in dementia treatment **247**
J. Artur Serrano

13.1   Introduction 247
    13.1.1 The concept 248
    13.1.2 Primary users of SENSE-GARDEN: persons living with dementia 250
13.2   History of SENSE-GARDEN 251
13.3   Design and development of SENSE-GARDEN technology and method 253
    13.3.1 User-centered design process 254
    13.3.2 SENSE-GARDEN system architecture 255
    13.3.3 Building a SENSE-GARDEN room 257
    13.3.4 The final technology: a SENSE-GARDEN room and system 258
13.4   The existing SENSE-GARDENs 259
    13.4.1 Bokkotunet care home, Odda (Norway) 260
    13.4.2 Aan de Beverdijk care home, Hamont-Achel (Belgium) 260
    13.4.3 Lar Santa Joana Princesa care home, Lisbon (Portugal) 260
    13.4.4 ELIAS Emergency University Hospital in Bucharest (Romania) 260
13.5   Dissemination in the media 260
13.6   Testing the SENSE-GARDEN technology 261
    13.6.1 Qualitative impact studies 261
    13.6.2 Quantitative impact studies 262
    13.6.3 Ethical concerns 263
13.7   SENSE-GARDEN resources 263
13.8   The future SENSE-GARDENs 263
13.9   Conclusion 264
13.10 Acknowledgments 265
13.11 Disclosure statement 265
13.12 Funding 265
References 265

14 Challenges and opportunities in the adoption of IoT for the elderly's health and well-being: a systematic review **269**
Dr Golam Sorwar and Md. Rakibul Hoque

14.1   Introduction 270
14.2   Methodology 271
14.3   Use cases of IoT 271
    14.3.1 Use cases of wearables 271
    14.3.2 Use cases of smart homes 272
14.4   Barriers in IoT adoption 279
    14.4.1 Barriers in the adoption of wearables 279
    14.4.2 Barriers in the adoption of smart homes 280

14.5 Future directions of IoTs study	281
14.5.1 Future directions for wearable studies	281
14.5.2 Future directions for smart home studies	281
14.6 Conclusions	282
References	283

15 Designing mobile healthcare applications for elderly users 287
Alan Yang

15.1 Introduction	287
15.2 Technology trends for elderly populations in academic literature	288
15.3 Design trends for elderly populations in practice	291
15.4 Suggestions for designers	291
15.5 Conclusion	296
References	296

16 Telepresence robots for healthy ageing 301
Chongdan Pan, Mingzhong Wang, and Pradeep Ray

16.1 Introduction	302
16.2 Research method	303
16.2.1 Design principles	303
16.2.2 Requirements and specifications	304
16.2.3 Design processing using QFD	305
16.2.4 Evaluation methodology	308
16.3 Results	309
16.3.1 FLEXTRA	309
16.3.2 Functionality test	314
16.3.4 Suitability for pandemics like COVID-19	315
16.4 Discussion	320
16.5 Limitations	320
16.6 Conclusion	321
16.7 Acknowledgment	321
References	321

17 Conclusion and future work 323
17.1 Underpinning principles of healthy ageing	324
17.1.1 Digital health maturity	324
17.1.2 Ageing population in the world	324
17.1.3 Geriatric care	324
17.1.4 Healthy ageing and climate change	325
17.1.5 Privacy protection of ageing population in digital services	325
17.2 Digital services for healthy ageing	325
17.2.1 Human resource management	325
17.2.2 Government and business policies	326
17.2.3 Digital mental health services	326

    17.2.4 Supply chain management in digital health   327
    17.2.5 Country case studies   `327
17.3 Digital technologies for healthy ageing   327
    17.3.1 Exoskeletons for rehabilitation   327
    17.3.2 Innovative digital care technology for the mental
           health of the elderly   328
    17.3.3 IoT and smart home technologies for healthy ageing   328
    17.3.4 Designing mobile applications for the aged population   328
    17.3.5 Robots for healthy ageing   329
17.4 Summary   329
References   329

Index   333

Acknowledgements

This book is a result of collaborative research on Digital health for Healthy Ageing involving more than 30 researchers from Australia, Bangladesh, China, India, Japan, Netherlands, Norway and USA. The book brings together research from multi-disciplinary perspectives of digital health, such as technologies, services and common principles (e.g., maturity, geriatrics, privacy, demographics and environment) based on a number of projects all over the world. These include the work led by the three editors; Prof Pradeep Ray at Centre For Entrepreneurship at University of Michigan-Shanghai Jiao Tong University-China, Prof Siaw-Teng Liaw at the WHO Collaborating Centre on eHealth at UNSW-Australia and several European Union (EU) projects led by Prof Artur Serrano at NTNU-Norway. The editors would like to acknowledge related grants and institutions.

It would be quite impossible to name all the individuals and institutions that helped the projects here and the list will be tedious. Authors would like to acknowledge related grants and institutions in their chapters. We would like to show our special gratitude to Mr. Hanrunyu Yan, who provided vital support in carefully collecting manuscripts from the authors, screening and standardizing them in preparation for this book

About the editors

Prof Pradeep Ray is currently the Director of the Centre For Entrepreneurship (http://umji.sjtu.edu.cn/entrepreneurship/index.html) and has led to completion in 2020 the mHBR (mHealth for Belt and Road region involving more than 12 countries) initiative that led to the IET book "Mobile Technologies For Delivering Healthcare In Remote, Rural Or Developing Regions **(2020)**" **edited by** *Pradeep Kumar Ray, Naoki Nakashima, Ashir Ahmed, Soong-Chul Ro, Yasuhiro Soshino.* Previously, Pradeep was the founder and Director for ten years at the Asia Pacific ubiquitous Healthcare research Centre (APuHC) University of New South Wales (UNSW), Australia that was designated as a WHO Collaborating Centre on eHealth (in 2013) with a focus on mHealth for the Seniors. In APuHC, Pradeep has been working on a range of innovative projects on eHealth and mHealth (jointly with the industry, country governments and global bodies like WHO, ITU and IEEE) in eHealth (using Information and Communication Technologies in Healthcare) and mHealth (healthcare using mobile phone technologies) across the Asia Pacific region. He has represented Australia in two European Union (EU) projects involving information technologies for seniors. He has been the founder of IEEE Healthcom, the premier international conference on eHealth technologies and services that has been held annually since 1999.

Siaw-Teng Liaw is a clinical informatician and directs the WHO Collaborating Centre on eHealth. Teng educates information, computer and health science students. His research focuses on telehealth/virtual care, digital health maturity and quality and utility of real-world data from information systems, apps and sensors. He chairs the IMIA Primary Care Informatics Working Group and RACGP Ethics Committee. He is Fellow of the International Academy of Health Sciences Informatics and American College of Medical Informatics.

J. Artur Serrano is a professor in Care Technology and Well-being at the Department of Neuromedicine and Movement Science (INB), Faculty of Medicine and Health Sciences, NTNU/Norwegian University of Science and Technology. Scientific coordinator of several EU projects, such as SENSE-GARDEN and VictoryaHome (www.victoryahome.eu). Artur was co-editor of the Journal for Telemedicine and Telecare and guest editor of the International Journal of E-Health and Medical Communications. He is interested in e-Health, dementia care, immersive technologies, and social robotics.

Chapter 1

Book overview: digital health for ageing population

1.1 Introduction

To celebrate age, the health and well-being of the seniors need to be nurtured. The older generation needs to be empowered and protected from the adversities of ageing such as social isolation and a system that will enable them to live with dignity in the society needs to evolve. Instead of seeing the seniors as a burden to society, there is a need to appreciate that elderly people are a storehouse of knowledge, wisdom, experience and skill. The older generation, which includes people from all spheres of life, represents a growing reservoir of talents that can be tapped to reap a 'longevity dividend'. There is a need to leverage the positive aspects of ageing to counter the concerns like increase in public pensions, declining workforce, declining productivity and economic growth, increasing demand for healthcare and need for personal assistance.

Although there has been an increase in life expectancy of the population all over the world, the SARS-COV-2 pandemic(Covid-19) has highlighted the vulnerability of this population group to pandemics caused by communicable and non-communicable diseases, unhealthy lifestyle/behaviour and adverse environmental impacts, such as climate change. 'As healthcare systems around the world are learning to cope with growing ageing populations, many are looking towards digital healthcare technology to help with improving care for the elderly' [1]. The strong uptake of digital technology, e.g. telehealth to prevent virus transmission between patients and health professionals during Covid-19, can be leveraged for the post-pandemic future to improve access and equity to safe and high-quality integrated person-centred healthcare at lower cost through a combination of the benefits of telehealth, eHealth, personalised healthcare and evidence-based care. That would result in better quality of life for the elderly with increasing comorbidities and frailty as life expectancy increases, particularly in developing countries. This book presents a discussion of evolving digital technologies (e.g., smartphones) and innovative services that are now helping to improve the quality and cost of healthcare for the elderly.

As the life expectancy of people has increased, the focus is on how to enhance the quality of life for the ageing population. While digital transformations are happening in all walks of society and the business, there are potentials for improving the quality of life of the elderly using digital methods and tools. Many countries in the world, particularly Europe and East Asia (e.g., Japan and China), may find this digital paradigm really useful as observed with the strong growth in telehealth during the pandemic. This book evolved from a new multi-country and multi-disciplinary initiative called *Digital Health for the Ageing Population*. This project (2019–2021) aims to promote the general awareness of digital health for the ageing population with collaborative research across several countries (developed and developing) including Australia, Bangladesh, China, India, Japan, Norway, the Netherlands and the USA. This project follows from the recently completed project *mHealth for Belt and Road* region (2018–2020) involving more than 50 investigators from 14 countries. The outcome of the project was published in the recent IET book *Mobile Technologies for Delivering Healthcare in Remote, Rural or Developing Regions* [2].

This book is organized into three sections:

1. "Underpinning Principles" – This section examines digital health maturity as a foundational principle of successful development, deployment and use of digital tools to improve population health and integrated person-centred health services in the context of the individual, carers, communities, health facilities and national health systems. It promotes a collaborative, multi-disciplinary quality improvement approach to address the bio-psycho-socio-technical aspects of healthy ageing and care for citizens in age-friendly environments. This approach encompasses standard-based development and implementation of interoperable digital health interventions aimed at individuals, populations, health system and the environment. Good quality data is essential to support evidence-based decisions for and by the individual, health professional, health organisation, health system, governments and community. Empowered citizens through meaningful community engagement are important to address the ethical, legal and social issues associated with digital health.
2. "Digital Health Services for Healthy Ageing" – This section investigates digital health services from a multi-disciplinary entrepreneurship/business perspective including, e.g. *Silvercare*, an innovative new model for human resource management, public health policies during pandemic (a business strategy issue), supply chain management (service operations management) and case studies of evolving new digital mental health services for the elderly in Bangladesh (entrepreneurship) and China (marketing).
3. "Digital Tools for Healthy Ageing" – This section investigates the use of exoskeletons for rehabilitation, multimedia tools for dementia, use of Internet of Things (IoT) for smart aged-care homes, mobile applications for various aged-care services and telepresence robots.

These are described in Sections 1.2–1.4.

1.2   Section 1 – "Underpinning Principles"

The WHO defines healthy ageing as 'the process of developing and maintaining the functional ability that enables well-being in older age', where 'functional ability comprises the health-related attributes that enable people to be and to do what they have reason to value' [3]. The 2015 WHO World Report on Ageing and Health [3] also describes eight domains of age-friendly environments: housing, social participation, respect and social inclusion, civic participation and employment, communication and information, community support and health services, outdoor spaces and built environment, and transportation. Achieving these require political, managerial, clinical and technical leadership, along with a trained workforce, at all levels of society and its institutions.

Chapter 2 describes digital health maturity as a multi-dimensional construct with five essential digital health foundations: (a) information and communication technology (ICT) infrastructure, (b) essential digital health tools, (c) readiness for health information sharing, (d) factors to promote health system adoption and (e) a cross-cutting quality improvement program [4] to monitor progress towards a robust interoperable health information system delivering high-quality data over the data lifecycle [5]. Digital health maturity assessment is a collaborative quality improvement process by individuals, health professionals, health organisations and health systems to harness digital tools to achieve national strategic health priorities. This co-assessment will guide the co-creation and co-implementation of maturity-guided digital health programs and roadmaps. The application of a digital health profile and maturity assessment toolkit (DHPMAT) is also described. The author invites you to try out the DHPMAT on the cases reported in the rest of the book.

Chapter 3 describes the current state of global ageing and the international variations in issues and challenges faced. It also discusses the impacts of these trends on digital technology and policy. Europe (24%) will have the largest proportion of citizens older than 65 years, whereas Africa (6%) will have the lowest. Using a projected median age for 2050, the oldest countries will be South Korea, Japan, Italy and Singapore (>50 years) with sub-Saharan countries the youngest (<30 years). In parallel, the main health concerns are transitioning from communicable to non-communicable diseases, with dementia providing particular challenges to digital health. A corresponding shift to general practice and primary care, with an emphasis on long-term care, is also occurring. The digital divide and associated economic and other impacts are reflected in the international variations of age-friendly environments and digital health developments.

Chapter 4 examines the opportunities and challenges of implementing digital health solutions to aged care in low- and middle-income countries (LMICs), comparing with higher income countries (HICs) from a digital divide perspective. Individual ability to use digital health is affected by physical, material, mental, social, temporal and cultural factors. A number of case studies of digitally supported aged care are described to introduce a socio-ecological model for caregiver-mediated digital health support for the elderly in LMICs. Finally, the ethics and policy implications are described.

Chapter 5 examines how climate action policies can have benefits for health. This is important as ageing homeostatic mechanisms do not respond well to extreme weather changes or degradation of the environment. In 2001, the Intergovernmental Panel on Climate Change described 'health co-benefits' as the range of intended non-climate-related benefits from climate change mitigation policies, strategies and actions. Domains of research into health co-benefits include development, greenhouse gas emissions, climate and air pollution, and rising sea levels. The Paris Climate Agreement has accelerated sustainable development policies on the broader economic, social, health and environmental benefits of low-carbon policies. However, despite substantial evidence for co-benefits, the policy impact remains limited and under-developed. This chapter describes the 'co-benefits approach' in planning for climate change with a focus on local governments and health impact assessments with a focus on the elderly.

Chapter 6 examines Australian health data privacy, with a focus on the 16% of the population aged >65 years. Healthcare providers are increasingly working with patient health records online for improved access. This has been accelerated by Covid-19, where telehealth has been crucial in preventing client–clinician transmission of the virus. The pandemic has also affected the mental health of many citizens, which will persist into the post-pandemic era, along with 'long Covid'. This has raised greater awareness and concerns about the privacy and security of online health data. Australian health data privacy regulations and policy is analysed in the context of the Australian My Health Record system and an Aged-Care Facility that cares for patients with dementia.

1.3   Section 2 – "Digital Services for Healthy Ageing"

As summarized in Section 1.1, this section provides a collection of five chapters (7–11) to discuss digital health from a multi-disciplinary perspective of entrepreneurship. This is important because it is best to use a service perspective in the application of technology in a sector where users (e.g., elderly clients and health professionals) are not conversant with the technology [1]. This section lays the foundation for a more in-depth discussion of digital tools from a technological perspective in Section 1.4.

Chapter 7 investigates the problem of the development and implementation of aged-care services cost-effectively worldwide. This is a challenging problem, considering the rapid ageing of the population in many parts of the world as discussed in Section 1.2 of this book. This chapter presents an innovative solution using a model called *Silvercare,* being used in some countries where younger pensioners (<70 years) called coordinators provide support to older seniors (>70 years) called beneficiaries, in their neighbourhood on issues such as new technology adoption and evolving e-government initiatives in different countries. These coordinators are unpaid volunteers and hence the support is cost-effective. So *Silvercare* provides an innovative human resource management model for evolving aged-care services. This chapter presents the *Silvercare* model and its applications through case studies in India and Australia.

Chapter 8 discusses aged-care services from digital health governance perspective, in the context of pandemic management, as the primary victims of Covid-19 have been the elderly. Governments all over the world manage a pandemic (e.g. Covid-19) using a framework of 4Ts (Testing, Tracing, Tracking and Treating) and various forms of lockdown, which have their own limitations especially for the older generation. Moreover, there is a strong requirement for integrated ICT services, technologies, management strategies during a pandemic, especially to protect the elderly population. This chapter represents a systematic literature review and analysis of the lockdown approaches and their limitations and possible strategy improvements with the use of digital technologies and services to better manage a pandemic in the context of a developing country.

Chapter 9 discusses the role of digital health to address mental health disorders that are prevalent all over the world irrespective of age, sex, education, financial status and socio-demographic features. However, the mental health of the elderly is becoming more and more important as people live longer. The healthcare and well-being of the elderly people are under immense threat during the Covid-19 pandemic with the fear of being infected by the Covid-19, bereavement, social isolation, etc. The scenario is worst in the LMICs, likewise in Bangladesh. More than 92% of the population is deprived of any sort of mental healthcare. There is a severe scarcity of mental health professionals, widespread stigma, cultural barrier and financial constraints, fear of being infected and dependency on others to travel made their mental healthcare access almost restricted. With the explosive growth of digital technology, a new window has been opened in Bangladesh to explore and implement digital healthcare. 'MonerDaktar' is the first and largest online mental healthcare platform to address this long-standing problem by connecting psychiatrists and clinical psychologists with clients from anywhere at their convenient . During the Covid-19 crisis, this platform has been working as the lifeline for mental healthcare in Bangladesh. 'MonerDaktar' connected more than 2 500 clients with our 109 mental health professionals so far. This online service stood to be more helpful for the 357 enlisted senior citizens as they were more vulnerable to the infection.

Chapter 10 presents the operations management of aged-care services. This chapter tackles the problem from a supply chain management perspective, widely used in operations management in many businesses, such as manufacturing, services and healthcare. According to research data, more people die of medication problems than in road accidents. Hence this chapter discusses supply chain management with a case study in medication management of the elderly, a common context in aged-care services. Chapter 16 of Section 3 will discuss a technological implementation of this medication management service of the elderly, using telepresence robots in the context of a collaborative study across Europe and Australia.

The study in Chapter 11 aimed to explore the role of digital technology in aged care in China. A systematic literature review was undertaken and involved three steps. The first two steps focused on identifying and selecting relevant papers, followed by extracting and analyzing data from selected papers. With the background of ageing population in China, the analysis revealed the promotions and potential popularity of using digital technology in aged care. Various emerging technologies as well as a case study of Haiyang Group (the largest private-sector aged-care provider in China) were introduced to demonstrate the important role of digital technology for aged care in China. The specific roles and generalized roles were summarized to include the help for the elderly, the involvement of relatives, the role of elderly care institutions and the evolving changes in the aged-care industry.

1.4   Section 3 – "Digital Tools for Healthy Ageing"

Chapter 12 explores how powered exoskeletons may be used in rehabilitation for the elderly population. It argues that combining characteristics of social robots with state-of-the-art exoskeletons to create a social exoskeleton will promote a disruptive innovation in the use of this technology for care. In order to implement technology into existing societal infrastructures, careful attention has to be given to the potential impacts. The chapter draws attention to these in the light of the concept of Responsible Research and Innovation as advocated by the European Commission. Seven specific societal considerations for technologists, regarding, namely accessibility, economy, inclusivity, environment, culture, law and ethics, are analysed and discussed.

Chapter 13 presents SENSE-GARDEN, a virtual and memory-adaptable space helping in creating stimuli for the senses in ageing people with dementia. It is a novel, technological solution for dementia care, which was developed as part of an interdisciplinary EU project funded by Ambient Assisted Living (AAL) Programme in collaboration with the funding agencies in the implementation countries Norway, Belgium, Romania and Portugal [6]. The project's funding period started in June 2017 and ran until November 2020. The SENSE-GARDEN project created four individualized, immersive spaces for people living with dementia. A SENSE-GARDEN is a room built inside of a dementia care environment (i.e. care home or hospital) that combines immersive technologies, digital media and multi-sensory stimuli to create environments personalized to the life story of the person with dementia. Four of these SENSE-GARDEN spaces have been created and are currently in operation in each of the intervening countries. A SENSE-GARDEN uses techniques from reminiscence therapy, in which the individual is encouraged to remember, reflect upon and share past moments from their lives including people, places and events that are relevant and meaningful. By using digital technologies to present familiar music, photographs, films and scents within an immersive environment, it is hoped that the SENSE-GARDEN can provide residents living with dementia, their relatives and members of staff the opportunity to engage with the life story of the individual in a new and exciting way. These spaces can increase the awareness of people with dementia by providing stimuli to the different senses, such as sight, touch, hearing, balance and smell, leading to a re-connection with the reality around them. The SENSE-GARDEN, with the help of a caregiver, encourages people with dementia to exercise at both the mental and physical level and takes them back into places they feel connected to. They can, for example, cycle or stroll in a well-known space and feel like they are going home. Such experiences may have an effect on invigorating their identity and helping to recover the sense of self.

Chapter 14 discusses the role of an emerging, popular technology called the IoT as a means for the development of new digital tools for healthy ageing. IoT technologies like wearables and smart homes are now being employed to offer innovative ways to enable the elderly population for an independent living and improve healthcare and well-being. While IoT is meant to ease the life and care of the elderly, the adoption of IoT-based devices is reported very low in aged-care sector unlike in other sectors of the economy, such as manufacturing, that are witnessing a major growth of IoT solutions. Therefore, new studies should be conducted periodically to gain updated knowledge in terms of use cases and efficiency. Consequently, the authors have conducted an integrative review of the existing literature on the use of IoT for older people. A total of 26 review studies were reviewed as the sources of secondary data. Broadly three themes were identified: (1) use cases, (2) adoption barriers and (3) future research directions. The review identified that the use cases of IoT solutions fall into different categories such as physiological monitoring, emergency detection, safety monitoring, social interaction and cognitive assistance at various levels. On the other hand, the most frequently reported barriers were privacy, security, cost, perceived usefulness and interoperability. The most common future research directions suggested about the inclusion of users' perspectives and use of artificial intelligence in future research. The authors conclude that lack of formal clinical studies and contradictions in existing study findings are frequently reported. Hence, the authors suggest gathering more empirical evidence as a strong basis for large-scale adoption of IoTs by the aged population.

Chapter 15 addresses the important aspect of how digital tools can be developed systematically for elderly consumers, while most digital applications are developed for young user. Individuals over the age of 60, categorized as elderly, pose a unique challenge to mobile health application designers. Effective application design for this demographic recognizes and accounts for the average physical and mental obstacles that impair adoption and continued usage of healthcare applications for the older population. Application designers must also acknowledge the aesthetic and content preferences of the elderly and how they may differ from mobile phone users in other age groups. This chapter will present the challenges associated with designing mobile healthcare applications for the elderly followed by a series of recommendations for developers interested in designing an app for this demographic.

Chapter 16 discusses the role of telepresence robots that have become critically important to perform remote healthcare operations, complying with social distancing measures. Researchers have been investigating the use of robots in the world for the elderly in various types of applications, such as communication with relatives and friends at a distance, transportation of medical supplies and equipment across healthcare/aged-care facilities and surgical procedures. In China, ground zero of the Covid-19 outbreak, robots are being used in hospitals to deliver food and medication and take patients' temperatures. Drones are deployed to transport supplies, spray disinfectants and do thermal imaging. The project 'Robots for Elderly' (involving Australia, China, Bangladesh and EU) was aimed at better emotional health of the elderly and their security at home. The aim of this project was to design, implement and test a low-cost telepresence robot for healthcare. The focus has been on implementing a low-cost telepresence robot for healthcare management for the elderly during pandemics like Covid-19. This project used an innovative, multi-disciplinary collaboration across disciplines (software, electronics engineering, mechatronics and public health) involving young university talents from these fields. The project addressed the needs for the healthcare of the elderly, most affected by the Covid-19, and came up with a simple low-cost design of telepresence robot that can be deployed widely in hospitals and aged-care establishments.

1.5 Summary

The chapters of the book have been summarized above. Section 1 – "Underpinning Principles" (Chapters 2–6) will be next, followed by Section 2 – "Digital Services for Healthy Ageing" (Chapters 7–11). The book ends with Section 3 – "Digital Tools for Healthy Ageing" (Chapters 12–16), followed by the conclusion in Chapter 17.

References

[1]   Health Europa. *Improving care for the elderly with digital healthcare technology* [online]. 2020. Available from https://www.healtheuropa.eu/improving-care-for-the-elderly-with-digital-healthcare-technology/98553/ [Accessed Jul 2021].

[2]   Ray P.K., Nakashima N., Ahmed A., Ro S.-C., Soshino Y. (eds.). *Mobile Technologies for Delivering Healthcare in Remote, Rural or Developing Regions*. UK: IET Press; 2020. Available from https://shop.theiet.org/mobile-technologies-for-delivering-healthcare-in-remote-rural-or-developing-regions.

[3]   World Health Organization. *World report on ageing and health* [online]. 2015. Available from https://www.who.int/ageing/publications/world-report-2015/en/ [Accessed Jul 2021].

[4]   Liaw S.-T., Zhou R., Ansari S., Gao J. 'A digital health profile & maturity assessment toolkit: cocreation and testing in the Pacific Islands'. *Journal of the American Medical Informatics Association*. 2021, vol. 1, pp. 494–503.

[5]   Liaw S.-T., Guo J.G.N., Ansari S., *et al*. 'Quality assessment of real-world data repositories across the data life cycle: a literature review'. *Journal of the American Medical Informatics Association*. 2021 26 Jan 2021.

[6]   SENSE-GARDEN. 2018. Available from www.sense-garden.eu [Accessed Jun 2021].

Part I

Underpinning principles of Digital Health

Chapter 2

Digital health maturity – a foundational principle

Siaw-Teng Liaw[1]

2.1 Introduction

In May 2018, the 71st World Health Assembly (WHA) passed Resolution WHA71.7 on Digital Health requesting the Director General "to develop in close consultation with the Member States and with inputs from stakeholders, a global strategy on digital health, identifying priority areas including where the World Health Organisation (WHO) should focus its efforts." In addition, it urged the Member States:

> To assess their use of digital technologies for health, including in health information systems at the national and subnational levels, in order to identify areas of improvement, and to prioritize, as appropriate, the development, evaluation, implementation, scale-up and greater utilization of digital technologies, as a means of promoting equitable, affordable and universal access to health for all, including the special needs of groups that are vulnerable in the context of digital health [1].

The 2016 WHO Global Observatory on eHealth 3rd survey highlighted the rapid growth of digital health initiatives, especially mHealth (83% respondent countries reported at least one project) [2]. It also reported that 17% of countries have a national policy or strategy regulating the use of "big data" in the health sector and discussed the poor data quality, fragmentation, duplication and negative impacts of unreasonable data collection burdens on staff morale [2].

Regardless of their digital health infrastructure and organisational maturity for information sharing, all countries need to harness digital health to make the best use of their available information assets to strengthen their health systems. The data required for Universal Health Coverage need to be developed as part of a country-driven, integrated approach to information management. However, the diverse formats and quality

[1]WHO Collaborating Centre on eHealth, UNSW Sydney, Australia

of available census and survey data are often not compliant to international standards or benchmarks, preventing objective comparisons across the health system. In this context, the 2016 survey emphasised that very few countries reported evaluations of government-sponsored digital health programmes. In contrast to the numerous digital health pilot projects in all countries, there have been very few monitoring and systematic evaluations of these digital interventions. This limits the global sharing of knowledge of what worked well and what mistakes could be avoided [3].

Successful implementation and realisation of benefits of digital health rely on strategies and solutions that are well aligned with the government's priorities, needs and context. Countries' digital health strategies must determine how digital solutions best reflect the needs of health professionals and citizens for information as well as management and health system data requirements. Countries need to determine their level of maturity in digital health development. These concerns are consistent with the development and implementation of digital health strategies globally.

As a step toward adapting the global agenda to the national context, eHealth (digital health) country profiles are proposed to provide summarised insights for governments, policymakers, administrators and other stakeholders on harnessing digital health solutions to address their countries' health priorities in the context of their stage of digital development [2]. They need the knowledge and skills to systematically and logically shift emphasis from small pilot programmes to large-scale deployments. Standardised and interoperable systems are the goal, moving away from *information silos*.

2.2 Conceptual framework

This section defines and describes the concepts and relationships in a conceptual framework for creating digital health profiles and assessing digital health maturity.

2.2.1   Digital health

Digital health is understood to mean "the field of knowledge and practice associated with any aspect of adopting digital technologies to improve health, from inception to operation." This definition is in line with WHO EB142/20 of 2017, which stated that "… the term 'digital health' is often used as a broad umbrella term encompassing eHealth as well as developing areas such as the use of advanced computing sciences in the fields of 'big data', genomics and artificial intelligence, for example."

Digital health encompasses eHealth, which was defined as the "cost-effective and secure use of information and communication technology (ICT) to support health and health-related fields, including health services, health surveillance and health-related literature, education, knowledge and research" (Resolution WHA58.28 on e-health (2005). Digital health puts more emphasis on digital consumers, with a wider range of smart devices and connected equipment being used, together with other innovative and evolving concepts as that of Internet of Things and the increasing use of artificial intelligence, big data and analytics. The terminology used is based on the WHO Classification of Digital Health Interventions [4].

2.2.2   Digital health maturity

A maturity model is a set of structured levels that depict the individual and organisational behaviours, practices and processes that reliably and sustainably produce required outcomes [5]. The aim is to measure the ability of an actor or entity to continuously improve in specific dimensions until the desired level of development or maturity is reached [6]. A maturity model is critical to define an entity's current maturity and where it aims to be in the future, the desired maturity. It describes the processes required to achieve desired outputs and improvements. Inherent in all maturity models is the need for quality improvement, measurement, monitoring and evaluation programmes.

The digital health maturity model serves as a roadmap for the logical improvement from one maturity level to the next by defining relevant concepts and their attributes of each level. In doing so, the factors essential to achieving interoperable and fit-for-purpose digital health systems will be identified and assessed to measure and guide the development of mature digital health systems.
Work done related to digital health maturity models include the:

1.   Global Digital Health Index (GDHI) of countries [7];
2.   Informatics Capability Maturity Model of health organisations [8], including integrated primary care centres [9] and
3.   Community Readiness of citizens and communities to adopt mHealth in a rural developing country setting [10, 11].

More specific and technical models and guides include the:
4.   Health Information Systems Interoperability Maturity Toolkit (HISIMT) [12], which consists of an interoperability maturity model and assessment tool, a user guide and the tool.
5.   Health Information System (HIS) Stages of Continuous Improvement Toolkit (HISSCIT), a maturity model with an explicit emphasis on data quality and continuous improvement [13, 14].

There are significant overlaps in the technical and operational indicators of digital health maturity across the health system continuum from national and health regions to health facilities to the community.

It is important to recognise that the digital health tools used to strengthen health systems at all levels of care are also potential sources of data for the measurement and monitoring of indicators of digital health maturity, including the impacts in care, quality improvement, health professional development and risk management.

2.2.3   Digital health profile: indicators of digital health maturity

Digital health maturity indicators take on different meanings and significance from the perspectives of the patient, health professional, health organisation and health system. For instance, the country profile uses national indicators to guide the dialogue and decision-making at the national health system level. The nature and

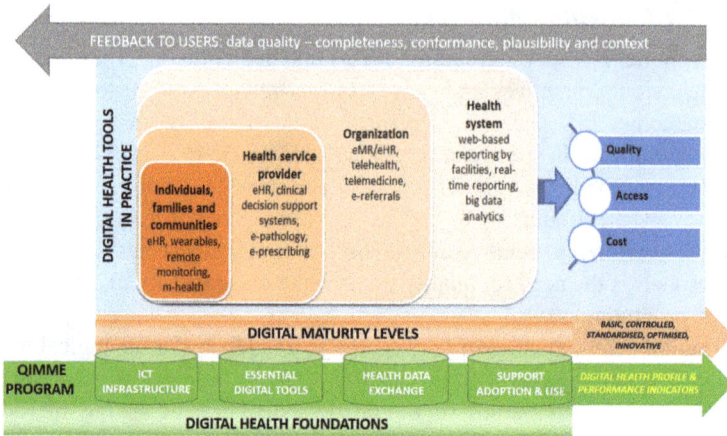

Figure 2.1   Health service-oriented conceptual framework for digital health maturity assessment

granularity of the indicators change as the focus shifts down to the organisational or professional health practitioner level.

Figure 2.1 illustrates a health service-oriented conceptual framework where the health services are underpinned by four essential digital health foundations to improve the access to, quality and cost-effectiveness of care [15].

The two streams in the framework are:

1. the health services as applied to patients (and carers), health professionals, organisations and the health system and
2. the essential digital health foundations to support the services including:
   (a) **Essential ICT infrastructure,** which is assessed by *20 indicators including the ICT development index rank, with a focus on ICT coverage, access, affordability and resilience of* electric power supply, mobile phone signal and internet coverage, conditions of use and user access to hardware and platforms in different settings, and ownership and use of digital tools.
   Key question: What is the extent of distribution of and access to national digital network and services?
   (b) **Essential digital tools** to collect, record, store and exchange personal health information accurately and securely across different service providers and levels of care, which is assessed by 31 indicators of the establishment and use of digital tools including a unique identifier, health information system, electronic medical record (EMR), electronic health record (EHR), patient registries, clinical decision support, telemedicine and mHealth, social media, eLearning and big data analytics.
   Key question: What is the extent of digital health tools deployed, used and maintained?

(c) **Readiness for information sharing**, which is assessed by 25 indicators including an interoperability framework, enterprise architecture, information standards, data quality and legal frameworks to ensure privacy, security and confidentiality to promote safe sharing and use of information, and prevent harm and misuse of information.
Key question: How are personal data collected and managed to a national and global standard?

(d) **Health system adoption**, which is assessed by 28 indicators including leadership and governance, enabling policies and strategies, partnerships, funding and investment in digital health, digital and health literacy, and workforce with competencies for digital health development and deployment, services and applications.
Key question: Can the workforce and community adopt and use complex digital health?

(e) **Quality improvement, measurement, monitoring and evaluation (QIMME)**: This is a cross-cutting foundation to assess the maturity of elements in each essential digital health foundation.
What are the impacts of your current digital health foundations? How do you know if you are achieving your milestones in the roadmap to a robust interoperable digital health system providing good quality data?

The "essential foundations" for digital health drew upon:

1. The GDHI [7], which drew on the World Health Organisation (WHO) and International Telecommunication Union (ITU) national eHealth strategy toolkit [16]. It listed a maturity level based on the following elements: leadership and governance; strategy and investment; legislation, policy and compliance; workforce; standards and interoperability; infrastructure; services and applications;

2. The 2015 Atlas of eHealth country profiles, which listed eHealth foundations, legal frameworks, telehealth, EHRs, eLearning, mHealth, social media, big data [17] and

3. The WHO Practical Guide to conducting research and assessment [3], mHealth Assessment and Planning for Scale Toolkit [18] and Global Monitoring and Evaluation Framework for the UN Decade in Education for Sustainable Development [19].

Seventeen indicators were selected to describe the country's multilingual/multicultural diversity, politics and socioeconomic situation, and general rule of law. A national approach provides an overview that can highlight the inequitable distribution of digital health maturity and associated access to and equity, cost, safety and quality of care. This will assist in digital health services planning in facilities, communities and citizens in low-resource settings such as rural and remote areas and vulnerable population groups such as Indigenous peoples or minorities [20].

There are five maturity levels, with descriptors provided to assess the digital health assets into each level:

Level 1 – BASIC with unpredictable performance: the system processes are ad-hoc with disjointed and uncoordinated processes, knowledge is not shared, and the service is focused on avoiding downtime.

Level 2 – CONTROLLED, where the service is reactive and problem-driven; the system processes are manageable and performance getting predictable, coordinated but inconsistent, knowledge is starting to be shared.

Level 3 – STANDARDISED, where the service is predictable and request-driven; the system is compliant to standards and best practice, performance is coordinated and consistent, knowledge sharing within the organisation promoting collaboration.

Level 4 – OPTIMISED, where the service is optimised and service-driven; there is a focus on efficiencies and continuous quality improvement, service is pro-active and accountable, knowledge sharing and collaboration with other organisations across the enterprise.

Level 5 – INNOVATIVE, where the service is value-driven; the service drives innovation, pioneers new dynamic processes, and there is industry level knowledge-sharing and collaboration.

Figure 2.2 summarises the Digital Health Maturity Model with examples of elements of each essential digital health foundation provided in each cell for each level of maturity. If the model is being used to assess individual or community digital health maturity, one can use relevant indicators for the same elements of the essential foundations.

Co-creation is the core methodology underlying this knowledge-sharing-in-action and capacity-building approach. It uses information and communication technologies and discursive processes around specific tasks or objectives to harness the collective creativity of the participants to share multidisciplinary and multifaceted data and create the information and knowledge. Participants in co-creation play multiple roles in socialising and evolving the nature and quality of the knowledge based on their perceptions and contexts [21]. In this context, the emerging social network will define and develop the digital health profile and assess the maturity to guide the development of a digital health roadmap for the organisation or country. The knowledge resource and social capital that is produced can then be accessed and used for its intended purpose.

2.3   Digital health maturity assessment

Figures 2.2 and 2.3 illustrate how the information from the digital health profile is to be used to assess the digital health maturity. The process of digital health maturity assessment includes:

1. Co-creating the digital health profile
    (a) Collect information on the country's essential digital health foundations from a range of published sources, such as the WHO and International

Digital Health Maturity Levels (with examples)					
Essential digital health foundations	**Level 1: BASIC** ✓ Focus: AVOIDING DOWNTIME ✓ Ad-hoc and chaotic ✓ Unstable environment ✓ Unproven, disjointed & uncoordinated processes ✓ Knowledge not shared **UNPREDICTABLE**	**Level 2: CONTROLLED** ✓ Focus on getting control ✓ Coordinated but inconsistent processes ✓ Processes manageable & getting predictable ✓ Knowledge silos exist **REACTIVE & PROBLEM DRIVEN**	**Level 3: STANDARDISED** ✓ Standards and best practice ✓ Centralised/consistent processes ✓ Organisation level knowledge sharing ✓ Proactive & Predictable **REQUEST DRIVEN**	**Level 4: OPTIMISED** ✓ Continuous improvement ✓ Efficiency ✓ Consolidated 'lean' processes ✓ Cross organisation knowledge sharing & collaboration ✓ Proactive & accountable **SERVICE DRIVEN**	**Level 5: INNOVATIVE** ✓ Catalyst for innovation ✓ Pioneers new dynamic process ✓ Industry level knowledge sharing & collaboration ✓ Drives innovation **VALUE DRIVEN**
ICT & IoMT infrastructure e.g. penetration, affordability, reliability, ICT supply chain	Examples: Accessible (available & affordable) but unreliable Internet and supply chain	Examples: Accessible & somewhat reliable Internet and supply chain	Examples: Support services and ICT hardware (supply chain) mostly accessible	Examples: Fully accessible & timely support services and ICT hardware	Examples: Infrastructure & support services facilitate innovations
Essential tools e.g. unique ID, social media, HIS/eHR/eMR, mHealth, teleHealth	Examples: Local ad hoc adoption & use of digital tools; Telephone = teleHealth	Examples: Regional coordination of adoption & use of digital tools; Asynchronous info sharing	Examples: National benchmarks & standards for digital tools; Synchronous info sharing	Examples: Data analytics & Quality of real-world data; teleHealth integrated with eHR	Examples: Innovations with decision support systems with integrated teleHealth and eHR systems
Readiness for information sharing e.g. standards-based, interoperable, security & privacy protocols, etc	Examples: Standalone datasets; No terminology standards	Examples: Ad-hoc sharing of datasets; Local terminology	Examples: Data sets integrated with HIS; National terminology	Examples: Data shared & interoperable; Data-driven policy & practice	Examples: National Common Data Model driving ethical use of linked health data for innovations
Health system adoption e.g. regulations, policy, strategy, governance, capacity building, funding	Examples: No digital health legislation; No training programs; No governance structures	Examples: Digital health privacy/security legislations; Ad-hoc training programs; Ad-hoc governance	Examples: Other digital health legislations; Accredited training programs; Relevant digital health committees	Examples: Artificial Intelligence legislation; National training programs; National digital health agency	Examples: Legislation facilitate innovations; Multisectoral programs; Digital health ministry

Figure 2.2   Digital health maturity model with examples at each level of maturity

	Digital Health Maturity Levels (with descriptors and examples)				
	Level 1: BASIC	**Level 2: CONTROLLED**	**Level 3: STANDARDISED**	**Level 4: OPTIMISED**	**Level 5: INNOVATIVE**
Essential digital health foundations	✓ Focus on *national downtime* ✓ Ad-hoc and chaotic ✓ Unstable environment ✓ Unproven, disjointed and uncoordinated processes ✓ Knowledge not shared ✓ Unpredictable performance	✓ Focus on getting control ✓ Coordinated but inconsistent processes ✓ Processes manageable & getting predictable ✓ Knowledge silos exist ✓ REACTIVE & PROBLEM-DRIVEN	✓ Standards and best practice ✓ Centralised & consistent processes ✓ Organisation level collaboration and knowledge sharing ✓ Proactive ✓ Predictable performance ✓ REQUEST DRIVEN	✓ Continuous improvement ✓ Efficiency ✓ Consolidated 'lean' processes ✓ Cross organisation knowledge sharing & collaboration ✓ Proactive & accountable ✓ SERVICE DRIVEN	✓ Catalyst for innovation ✓ Pioneers new dynamic processes ✓ Industry level knowledge sharing & collaboration ✓ Drives service innovation ✓ VALUE DRIVEN
ICT infrastructure e.g. ICT penetration, affordability, reliability, ICT supply chain	**Descriptors:** □ Unreliable Internet □ Unreliable 2G, 3G, 4G □ Very low percentage of the population have access to the Internet □ Negligible broadband service subscriptions □ Unreliable supply chain **Examples:** Accessible (available & affordable) but unreliable	**Descriptors:** □ Somewhat reliable Internet □ Somewhat reliable 2G, 3G, 4G □ Less than half of the population have access to the Internet □ Low broadband service subscriptions □ Parts/services available in weeks **Examples:** Accessible & somewhat reliable	**Descriptors:** □ Reliable Internet □ Reliable 2G, 3G, 4G □ Approximately half of the population have access to the Internet □ Moderate broadband service subscriptions □ Parts/services available in-house **Examples:** Support services and ICT hardware (supply chain) mostly accessible	**Descriptors:** □ Approximately all of the population have access to the Internet □ High broadband service subscriptions □ Reliable for critical apps for patient care □ Parts/services available with Quality Improvement in place **Examples:** Fully accessible & timely support services and ICT hardware	**Descriptors:** □ Sufficiently reliable to enable innovations □ Parts/services available and services innovating **Examples:** Infrastructure & support services facilitate innovations
Essential tools e.g. unique ID, social media, HIS/eHR/eMR, mHealth, teleHealth	**Descriptors:** □ Ad-hoc non-unique ID □ Local procurement & implementation of HIS/eHR □ Use of social media □ Telephone consultation **Examples:** Local ad hoc adoption & use of digital tools; Telephone = teleHealth	**Descriptors:** □ Unique ID in Dapt only □ Regional procurement & implementation of HIS/eHR □ Social media for information □ Asynchronous image sharing **Examples:** Regional coordination of adoption & use of digital tools; Asynchronous info sharing	**Descriptors:** □ Unique ID in all of facility □ National benchmarks & standards for HIS/eHR □ Social media for wellbeing □ Synchronous video consult **Examples:** National benchmarks & standards for digital tools; Synchronous info sharing	**Descriptors:** □ National unique ID □ Data driven QI of HIS/eHR & Data Quality assessment □ Social media for personalised health information □ Video consult + eHR **Examples:** Data analytics & Quality of real-world data; teleHealth integrated with eHR	**Descriptors:** □ Linked Data R&D driving policy and practice □ Ethical use of health data □ Social media for interactive personalised care □ Video consult + Electronic Decision Support **Examples:** Innovations with decision support systems with integrated teleHealth and eHR systems
Readiness for information sharing e.g. standards-based, interoperable, hardware, software & protocols to support security & privacy	**Descriptors:** □ Ad-hoc sharing of patient registry info with HIS/eHR □ No terminology standards **Examples:** Standalone clinical & managerial datasets; No terminology standards	**Descriptors:** □ Patient info shared routinely but not integrated with HIS/eHR □ Ad-hoc terminology standards **Examples:** Ad-hoc sharing of standalone datasets; Local terminology	**Descriptors:** □ Patient info integrated in HIS/eHR and shared in facility □ National standard terminology recommended but not embedded **Examples:** Data sets shared and integrated with HIS/eHR; National terminology	**Descriptors:** □ Patient info integrated and shared with other facilities □ National standard terminology implemented and embedded **Examples:** Data shared & interoperable across facilities; National datasets driving policy and practice	**Descriptors:** □ National standardized data asset driving policy and practice □ National Common Data Model **Examples:** National Common Data Model driving ethical use of linked health data for innovative policy & practice
Health system adoption e.g. regulations, policy, strategy, governance, capacity building, funding	**Descriptors:** □ No digital health regulations □ No existing national strategy for digital health or eHealth or health information systems □ No training programs □ No governance structures **Examples:** No legislations for digital health services; No training programs; No governance structures	**Descriptors:** □ Privacy legislation present □ National strategy for digital health/eHealth/health information system is drafted or in process □ Ad-hoc training programs □ Ad-hoc governance structures **Examples:** Digital health privacy/security legislations; Ad-hoc training programs; Ad-hoc governance	**Descriptors:** □ ICT legislation present □ National digital health strategy and/or plan(s) with identified priorities is endorsed and in implementation □ Accredited training programs □ ICT committee within organisation management **Examples:** Other digital health legislations; Accredited programs; Relevant digital health committees	**Descriptors:** □ Big data & Artificial Intelligence legislation present □ National digital health monitoring and evaluation framework present □ National multi-professional training programs □ National digital health agency **Examples:** Big data & Artificial Intelligence legislations; National training programs; National digital health agency	**Descriptors:** □ Artificial Intelligence (AI)legislation present □ Exporting training programs □ Digital health ministry **Examples:** Legislations facilitating innovations; Multisectoral programs; Digital health ministry
Quality improvement, measurement, monitoring & evaluation (QIMME)	**Descriptors:** □ Ad-hoc QIMME arrangements if at all **Examples:** Local ad hoc QIMME arrangements	**Descriptors:** □ QIMME incorporated but uncoordinated **Examples:** QIMME routinely embedded in digital health programs	**Descriptors:** □ Coordinated QIMME for Comparative Effectiveness Research (CER) by regions **Examples:** QIMME coordinated for CER across programs and regions	**Descriptors:** □ Digital Health program scaled up & normalised with CER ongoing nationally **Examples:** National digital health program with embedded QIMME enabling CER	**Descriptors:** □ Innovating with digital health program, including QIMME of new models of care **Examples:** Innovating with novel QIMME methods for new models of care

Figure 2.3   The digital health maturity assessment tool for use in practice

Telecommunication Union, and interviews with the country's key informants;

2. Co-assessing digital health maturity

    (a) Use the Digital Health Profile and Maturity Assessment Toolkit (DHP-MAT) [15] and approach to co-assess the digital health maturity with the country's key informants.

    Figure 2.3 is the maturity assessment template illustrated with more examples in each cell of the matrix.

3. Conduct consultations with clinical, technical, managerial and other relevant professionals, e.g. educators and social-change agents and citizens, using Figure 2.4 as a guide, on

    (a) the evidence-based selection of safe and effective digital health interventions.

Document the priorities and issues with as much details and specificity as possible.

Country context	
Harnessing digital health interventions to benefit health priorities in delivering integrated person-centred services & universal health coverage?	• **Health priorities:** *e.g. universal health coverage through universal health insurance* • **Objectives for digital health development:** *Improve digital health maturity by one level* • **Opportunities:** *e.g. current strengths; Entry points (individual, facility or population); Donor Agencies* • **Challenges:** *e.g. rurality; low digital health literacy; proprietary systems; sustainability*
Mission of digital health development *Co-created user-centred digital health interventions to meet the country's health priorities*	• **Practical goal:** e.g. Develop a strategy with simple, measurable, achievable, realistic and time limited (SMART) objectives that are aligned with the digital health maturity to ensure that interventions are implementable and sustainable.

Essential digital health foundations	Example of a practical goal based on maturity level assessed	Examples of activities (resources) to achieve identified practical goal
ICT infrastructure	*(Current maturity level: Basic)* *A mobile phone network that is fit-for-purpose and affordable for all citizens in all settings e.g. urban-rural, rich-poor, young-old, male-female, etc.*	**Desired Maturity level: Standardised** • Identify evidence-based, reliable, cost-effective and sustainable options. • Apply for national ICT infrastructure and strategic funding (global aid agencies).
Essential tools	*(Current maturity level: Controlled)* *Up to date & well-maintained digital health assets with affordable, usable & useful evidence-based digital tools.*	**Desired Maturity level: Standardised** • Establish and ensure compliance to standards for reasonably-priced digital health tools; • Identify systems for a national unique person (patient/clinician) and facility identifier.
Readiness for information sharing	*(Current maturity level: Controlled)* *Data/information fit to be shared in terms of data quality and interoperability.*	**Desired Maturity level: Standardised** • Identify relevant national/international standards for data, data models, architecture, and data analytics software; • Establish data and information governance and stewardship structures.
Health system adoption	*(Current maturity level: Controlled)* *Training programs for a digital health workforce to achieve the above.*	**Desired Maturity level: Standardised** • Pre-service & in-service training of workforce in digital health tools, e-learning, etc.; • Digital literacy programs in schools, colleges and work places.
QIMME	*(Current maturity level: Controlled)* *A program logic model to measure reach, effectiveness, adoption, implementation & maintenance (RE-AIM) of the digital health intervention and related to outputs and impacts.*	**Desired Maturity level: Standardised** • Develop and obtain support for a QIMME program for a regional digital health intervention, emphasizing measurable process, outputs and impact indicators along with realistic deliverables and milestones.

Figure 2.4   A guide to using the DHPMAT to develop a digital health programme and roadmap

  i.   The WHO guideline: recommendations on digital interven-
       tions for health system strengthening stressed that invest-
       ments into digital health interventions must be evidence-
       based and include an assessment of risks against comparative
       options [22];

(b) the implementation, adoption, use, maintenance and sustainability of the
     selected digital health interventions with guidance from:
  i.   The WPRO *eHealth Regional Action Agenda* document [20],
  ii. The WHO endorsed tools on the development of national
       digital health strategic plans [16],
  iii. Technical guides, such as the HISIMT [12] and
  iv. The non-adoption, abandonment, scale-up, spread, and sus-
       tainability framework to understand cascading users, organ-
       isations, technology and health system challenges [23]; and
(c) the safety and quality improvement and evaluation plan with guidance
     from:
  i.   The WHO endorsed tools on implementation, quality im-
       provement and evaluation [3, 22]
  ii. Publications on the Reach, Effectiveness, Adoption, Imple-
       mentation and Maintenance framework to evaluate the imple-
       mentation of digital health [24].

The WHO-endorsed document – *Monitoring and Evaluating Digital Health Interventions: A Practical Guide to Conducting Research and Assessment* – empha-sises a common quality improvement framework for evaluating digital health inter-ventions to generate the evidence required for decisions on approaches to harnessing interventions to strengthen national health systems. The desired maturity is achieved when a country has a systematic and coordinated monitoring and quality improve-ment programme across the enterprise.

The end-product of this exercise is a digital health profile and a maturity assessment which will guide the development of a digital health programme and roadmap appropriate to the maturity. The roadmap will guide the activities for each milestone of the journey up the maturity scale. This all-of-government and com-munity discussion and planning will be informed by the digital health maturity and considering the country's health priorities, opportunities and threats. By adopting a maturity model and quality improvement approach, this co-creation approach to developing a digital health profile and co-assess the digital health maturity will facilitate ownership by the key leadership and stakeholders to ensure the suc-cessful development, implementation, quality improvement and sustainability of digital health interventions and programmes. The University of New South Wales (UNSW) WHO Collaborating Centre on eHealth, Western Pacific Regional Office and collaborators from Pacific Island Countries have co-created countries' digital health profiles and co-assessed their digital health maturity using the DHPMAT [15] to support a quality improvement and monitoring approach to digital health developments.

The embedded cross-cutting Quality Improvement, Measurement, Monitoring and Evaluation (QIMME) foundation will ensure an iterative process based on the evaluation of each step in the journey to achieve an innovative, flexible and nimble digital health system that complies with data quality and interoperability standards. This will address the poor data quality, fragmentation, duplication and negative impacts of unreasonable data collection burdens on staff morale identified in the 2016 survey undertaken by the WHO Global Observatory on eHealth [2]. Only then can we begin to achieve the aspirations expressed by the 2018 WHA [1].

2.4 Exercises

1. Consider the following statement adapted from Chapter 3: "Technology should also aim at providing cheaper, more accessible healthcare services to the citizens, i.e. Universal Health Coverage (UHC)." Compare and contrast a Low and Middle Income Country (LMIC) and High Income Country (HIC).

    What is the digital health maturity level required to achieve this technically, ethically, legally and socially? What are the social, human, technical and financial resources required? Consider the essential digital health foundations separately. Is it possible to have a global measure of digital health maturity?
2. Consider case study 2 from Chapter 4: the role of digital health in supporting the informal caregiver and elderly patient in rural Thailand. Use the DHPMAT to assess the strengths, weaknesses, opportunities and threats to a successful rollout and maintenance of the programme for the whole population of the rural province.
3. Consider the case from Chapter 6: the use of online health records to manage patients with dementia in the aged care – at home or in residential aged care facilities. What is the digital health maturity required to successfully implement this?

You can use this same approach to other cases reported in Parts 2 and 3.

2.5 Conclusion

Digital health maturity is a foundational principle and a multidimensional construct comprising four essential digital health foundations and a cross-cutting quality improvement and evaluation foundation. Digital health maturity assessment is a quality improvement process from a personal, professional, organisational and system perspective, within the context of harnessing digital tools to achieve a country's strategic health priorities. The co-creation approach is an essential element with a capacity of development emphasis, beginning with the co-creation of the digital health profile and co-assessment of the maturity status, using a well-tested DHPMAT. This information from the DHPMAT is used to co-develop an achievable and sustainable digital health roadmap and operational plan with a realistic budget. The DHPMAT enables an overview and roadmap for the multisectoral co-implementation, co-monitoring and co-evaluation of digital health programmes and progress in achieving milestones in the roadmap.

References

[1] World Health Organisation Secretariat. *Resolution 7: Digital Health*. WHO, (ed.). WHA717; Geneva: WHO; 2018.

[2] World Health Organisation Global eHealth Observatory. *Global Diffusion of Ehealth: Making Universal Health Coverage Achievable*. Report of the third global survey on eHealth; Geneva: World Health Organization; 2016.

[3] World Health Organization. *Monitoring and Evaluating Digital Health Interventions: a Practical Guide to Conducting Research and Assessment*. Licence: CC BY-NC-SA 3.0 IGO; Geneva: World Health Organization; 2016.

[4] World Health Organization. *Classification of Digital Health Interventions V1.0: a Shared Language to Describe the Uses of Digital Technology for Health*. License: CC BY-NC-SA 3.0 IGO; Geneva: WHO; 2018.

[5] Hammond W.E., Bailey C., Boucher P., Spohr M., Whitaker P. 'Connecting information to improve health'. *Health Affairs*. 2010, vol. 29(2), pp. 284–8.

[6] Carvalho J.V., Rocha Álvaro., Abreu A. 'Maturity models of healthcare information systems and technologies: a literature review'. *Journal of Medical Systems*. 2016, vol. 40(6), p. 131.

[7] Global Digital Health Index Consortium. 'Global digital health index indicator guide'. Global Digital Health Index consortium; 2016.

[8] UK Department of Health Informatics Directorate. *Informatics capability maturity model*. in Division ICD, (ed); UK: NHS; 2018.

[9] Liaw S.-T., Kearns R., Taggart J., *et al.* 'The informatics capability maturity of integrated primary care centres in Australia'. *International Journal of Medical Informatics*. 2017, vol. 105, pp. 89–97.

[10] Khatun F., Heywood A.E., Ray P.K., Hanifi S.M.A., Bhuiya A., Liaw S.-T. 'Determinants of readiness to adopt mHealth in a rural community of Bangladesh'. *International Journal of Medical Informatics*. 2015, vol. 84(10), pp. 847–56.

[11] Khatun F., Heywood A.E., Ray P.K., Bhuiya A., Liaw S.-T. 'Community readiness for adopting mHealth in rural Bangladesh: a qualitative exploration'. *International Journal of Medical Informatics*. 2016, vol. 93, pp. 49–56.

[12] MEASURE Evaluation and Health Data Collaborative. *Health Information Systems Interoperability Maturity Toolkit: Users' Guide*. North Carolina: University of North Carolina at Chapel Hill; 2017.

[13] MEASURE Evaluation and Health Data Collaborative. *Global Digital Health Resources and Maturity Models: a Summary Overview*. Washington, DC: United States Agency for International Development (USAID); 2017.

[14] MEASURE Evaluation and Health Data Collaborative. *His Stages of Continuous Improvement Toolkit*. Washington, DC: USAID; 2017.

[15] Liaw S.-T., Zhou R., Ansari S., Gao J., *et al.* 'A digital health profile & maturity assessment toolkit: cocreation and testing in the Pacific Islands'. *Journal of the American Medical Informatics Association.* 2021, vol. 28(3), pp. 494–503.

[16] World Health Organisation & International Telecommunication Union. *WHO-ITU: National eHealth Strategy Toolkit.* Geneva: WHO & ITU; 2012.

[17] World Health Organisation GOfe. 'Atlas of eHealth country profiles: the use of eHealth in support of universal health coverage'. *Based on the findings of the third global survey on eHealth 2015.* 2015.

[18] World Health Organisation. *The MAPS Toolkit: mHealth Assessment and Planning for Scale.* Geneva: WHO; 2015.

[19] Tilbury D. 'Tracking our progress: a global monitoring and evaluation framework for the un DESD'. *Journal of Education for Sustainable Development.* 2009, vol. 3, pp. 189–93.

[20] World Health Organization W. *Regional Action Agenda on Harnessing E-Health for Improved Health Service Delivery in the Western Pacific.* Manila: WHO Western Pacific Regional Office; 2017.

[21] Langley J., Wolstenholme D., Cooke J. '"Collective making" as knowledge mobilisation: the contribution of participatory design in the co-creation of knowledge in healthcare'. *BMC health services research.* 2018, vol. 18(1), p. 585.

[22] Organisatin W.H. *WHO Guideline: Recommendations on Digital Interventions for Health System Strengthening.* Licence: CC BY-NC-SA 3.0 IGO; Geneva: World Health Organization; 2018.

[23] Greenhalgh T., Wherton J., Papoutsi C., *et al.* 'Beyond adoption: a new framework for theorizing and evaluating Nonadoption, abandonment, and challenges to the scale-up, spread, and sustainability of health and care technologies'. *Journal of Medical Internet Research.* 2017, vol. 19(11), p. e367.

[24] Gaglio B., Shoup J.A., Glasgow R.E. 'The RE-AIM framework: a systematic review of use over time'. *American Journal of Public Health.* 2013, vol. 103(6), pp. e38–46.

Chapter 3

Global demographic changes and ageing population: an overview

Sam Ro¹, Willy Huang², and Karpurika Raychaudhuri¹

Grow old along with me! The best is yet to be, the last of life, for which the first was made. – Robert Browning

3.1 Introduction

Population ageing, or the increase in the relative number of older persons in a society, has been recognized as a major global issue for decades. In 1982, the United Nations held the first World Assembly on Ageing in Vienna, then in 2002, the Second World Assembly on Ageing was held in Madrid, producing a landmark declaration called 'Political Declaration on the Madrid International Plan of Action on Ageing (MIPAA)' setting out three priority areas of '(i) older persons and development', '(ii) advancing health and well-being into old age' and '(iii) ensuring enabling and supportive environments' [1]. Various UN agencies worked together to promote this agenda. Notably, the World Health Organization (WHO) has been avidly promoting active and healthy ageing since the turn of the century, and in 2016, the 69th World Health Assembly adopted a resolution for 'Global Strategy and Action Plan on Ageing and Health 2016-2020' [2], which led to an UN-wide initiative 'The Decade of Healthy Ageing' from 2021 to 2030 [3].

At the start of this new initiative, it is worth giving the issue a closer examination and providing an overview of the issue at the global level. Two things need to be considered for this. First, population ageing is happening in most of the countries in the world, but the extent and speed differ from country to country. Second, the challenges brought by population ageing make it a major global issue; however, the exact nature of the challenge depends on the particular

¹Center for Entrepreneurship, UM-SJTU Joint Institute, Shanghai Jiao Tong University, Shanghai, China
²SJTU-Paris Tech Elite Institute of Technology, Shanghai Jiao Tong University, Shanghai, China

Table 3.1   List of selected countries in SDGs Regions

SDG Region	Selected countries
Australia/New Zealand	Australia
Europe and Northern America	Germany, Italy, Sweden, United States of America
Eastern and South-Eastern Asia	China, Japan, South Korea, Singapore, Thailand
Central and Southern Asia	Bangladesh, India, Iran, Kazakhstan, Pakistan
Latin America and the Caribbean	Brazil, Chile, Mexico, Peru
Northern Africa and Western Asia	Israel, Saudi Arabia
Oceania	Fiji
Sub-Saharan Africa	Angola, Chad, Ethiopia, Niger

context. The first item, different speed and extent of population ageing, certainly is a major factor that shapes the challenges to society. These are the main tasks of this chapter: providing an overview of the global population ageing by (i) describing the speed and extent of population ageing in different parts of the world and (ii) providing a summary of the discussions concerning the challenges it brings to societies.

The next section illustrates global trends in population ageing using indicators such as the proportion of the population by age groups, life expectancy, fertility rates and dependency ratio. We will use the statistical data compiled by international organizations such as the UN and WHO for this purpose. To highlight diversity in different regions and countries of the world, we have adopted the UN's Sustainable Development Goals (SDGs) Regions, which divide the world into eight regions [4, p. 59]. There are different ways of classifying countries in the world into regions such as geographic regions, WHO regions, World Bank income groups and so on, but we opted for the SDG Regions because of the close relationship between the issues of population ageing. In addition, we chose 27 countries as in Table 3.1 to examine the trends at the country level.

Next, in Section 3.3, we will discuss the challenges of population ageing in two areas of healthcare for the elderly and economic impacts on society. These two topics derived from the priority areas identified by MIPAA. If we regard the third priority area as an enabling factor for the first two, those first two areas can be paraphrased as (i) ensuring sustainable development of the society in the context of population ageing and (ii) bringing sustainability (health and well-being) to the people at old age. These are closely intertwined with the challenges of sustainable development. Indeed, from the very start, the UN's SDGs included the empowerment of the older persons as one of the key agenda [5, p. 23] and the population ageing constitute one of the important contexts in which the promotion of the SDGs takes place. Each country will have more specific challenges but instead of discussing those, we will limit our discussions to these two broad areas of challenges and discuss implications of policy in Section 3.4.

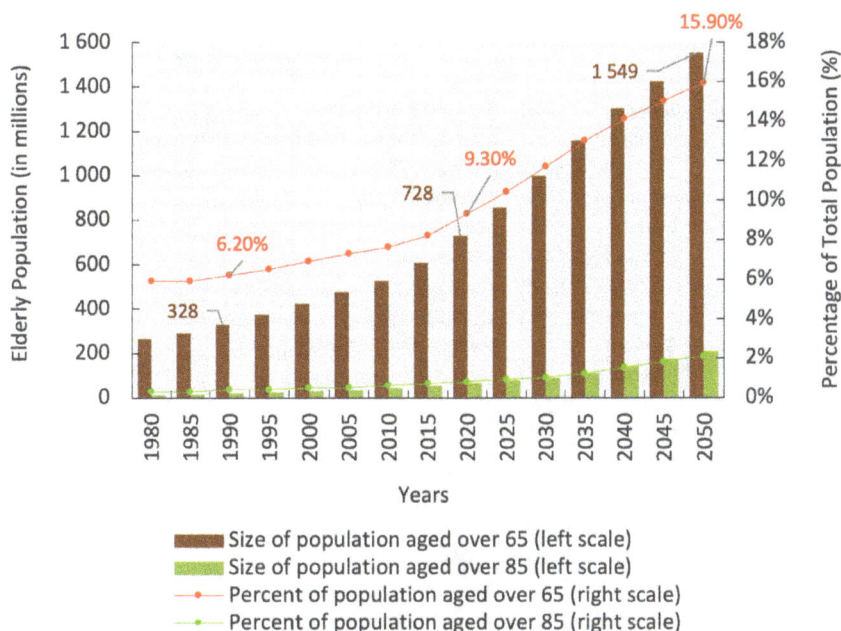

Figure 3.1   *World population growth and ageing. Data source: United nations department of economic and social affairs, population division. World population prospects 2019. (https://population.un.org/wpp/ DataQuery/).*

3.2 Global trend in population ageing: a reality check

According to the projection by the UN, the world population will grow from 7.8 bil-lion in 2020 to 9.7 billion in 2050 and that of the population 65 of age or above will increase from 727 million (9.3%) in 2020 to 1.5 billion (16%) by 2050. At the same time, the proportion of the oldest old (85+) as a percentage of the total population will more than double from 0.8% in 2020 to 2.1% in 2050 (Figure 3.1).

Among the selected countries, Japan has the highest proportion of population above 65 in age, amounting to 28.4% of the total population in 2020, followed by Italy (23.3%), Germany (21.7%), Sweden (20.3%) and the US (16.6%), but the ranking is expected to change in 2050 when South Korea will have the highest pro-portion of the elderly population (38.1%), followed by Japan (37.7%), Italy (36.0%), Singapore (33.3%) and Germany (32.3%) (Figure 3.2).

The highest rates of growth, however, will be experienced in developing coun-tries, led by Saudi Arabia growing from 1.2 million to 7.7 million, or growth by 531.0%. Iran (277%), Angola (261%), Bangladesh (254%) and Ethiopia (206%) are also expected to experience very high rates of growth, whereas the growth would have slowed down significantly in Japan (11.0%), Germany (32%), Italy (39.0%) and the US (54.1%) and moderately in Australia (80.8%) and Israel (96.3%).

% of population aged 65+

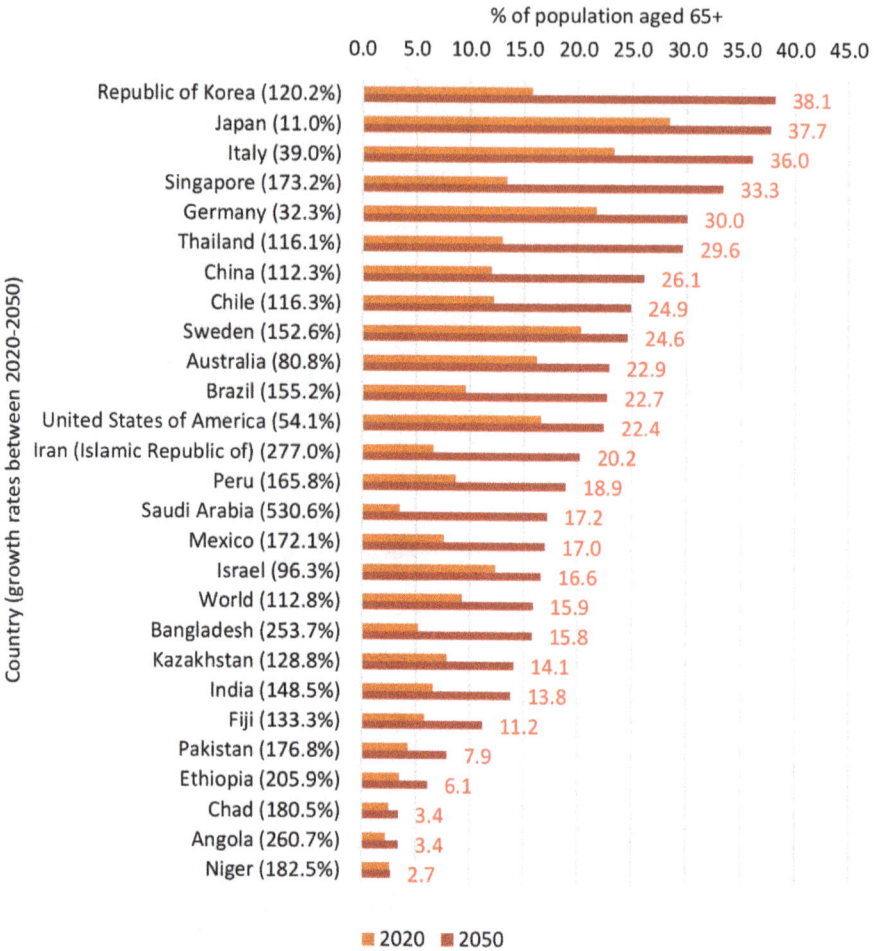

Figure 3.2   *Proportion of population aged 65+ as a percentage of all population, selected countries, 2020 and 2050. Note: Growth rates in brackets are calculated based on the estimated size, not proportion, of the population above 65 in age, in 2020 and in 2050. Data Source: United Nations Department of Economic and Social Affairs, Population Division. World Population Prospects 2019 (https://population.un.org/wpp/DataQuery/).*

These are very closely related to increasing life expectancy and decreasing birth rates around the world (Figure 3.3). Globally, life expectancy has increased from 64.5 in 1995 to 72.3 in 2020 and then expected to increase to 76.7 in 2050. Growth is expected to continue but at a slower rate. The gender gap, with the female outliving male for about 5 years globally, is also expected to continue although the gap will narrow down a little [4, 6].

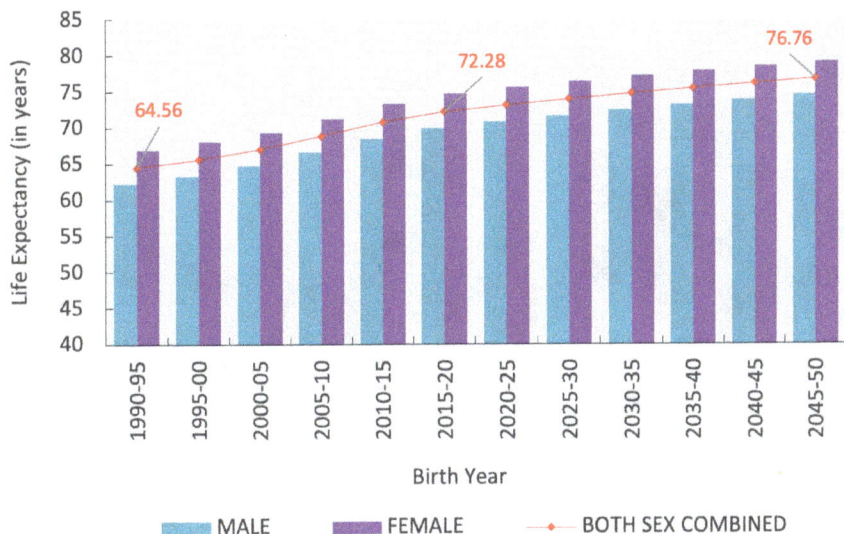

Figure 3.3   *Life expectancy of the world 1990–2050. Data source: United nations department of economic and social affairs, population division. World population prospects 2019. (https://population. un.org/wpp/DataQuery/).*

There is a gap of more than twenty years in life expectancy between the highest (Australia/New Zealand) and the lowest region (sub-Saharan Africa) currently. This gap will reduce slightly by 2020 with sub-Saharan Africa expected to make the largest gain of almost 8 years in life expectancy by that year. Australia/New Zealand, Europe and Northern America, Eastern and South-Eastern Asia, and Latin America and the Caribbean regions will all have a life expectancy above 80 and Central and Southern Asia, Oceania and sub-Saharan Africa will have lower than the world average (Figure 3.4).

The discrepancy gets more pronounced when we look at the data from selected countries (Figure 3.4). The gap between Japan and Chad is currently 34 years which will narrow to 27 years by 2050. Life expectancy in most of the selected countries will exceed 80 by 2020 with Japan, Singapore, Italy, Australia, Korea, Israel and Sweden leading with 86 years or longer, while Mexico, Saudi Arabia, Bangladesh and Kazakhstan will increase to be between 77 and 80, India, Pakistan, Ethiopia and Fiji between 70 and 75, and Niger, Angola and Chad below 70. The last three countries will experience the largest gain of about 8 years. The growth rate overall, however, has already significantly slowed down since the 1970s and is expected to continue to drop till 2050. Outside the selected countries, Russia and South Africa are experiencing particularly slow growth in life expectancy due to risky health behaviours among men in Russia and HIV/AIDS in South Africa [7].

The other side of population ageing is the reducing fertility rate.(Figure 3.5) The world fertility rate has been dropping fast from a peak of 5.06 in 1964 to 3.56

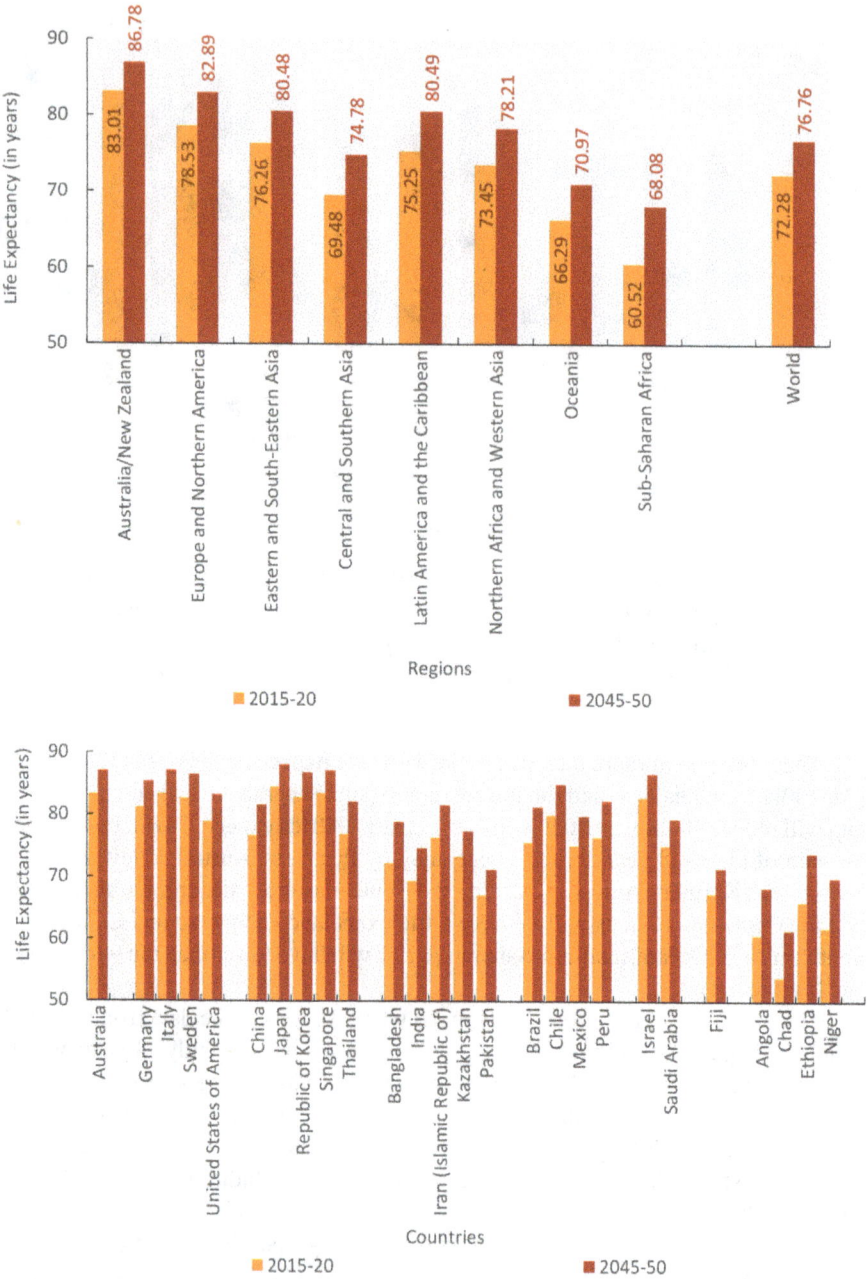

Figure 3.4   *Life expectancy by SDG regions and selected countries. Data
source: United nations department of economic and social affairs,
population division. World population prospects 2019. (https://
population.un.org/wpp/DataQuery/).*

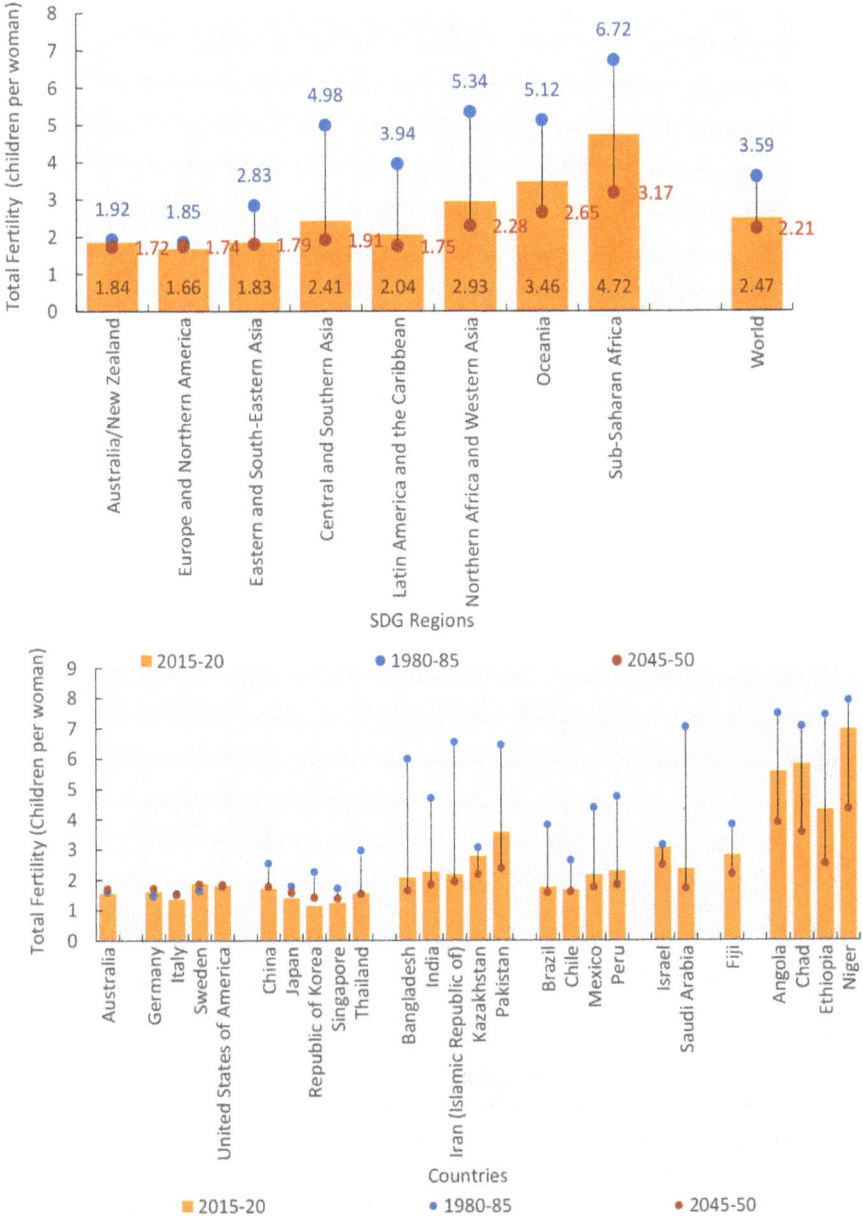

Figure 3.5   *Fertility rate by geographical and SDG regions and by selected countries from 1980–85 to 2045–50. Data Source: United Nations Department of Economic and Social Affairs, Population Division. World Population Prospects 2019. (https://population.un.org/wpp/ DataQuery/).*

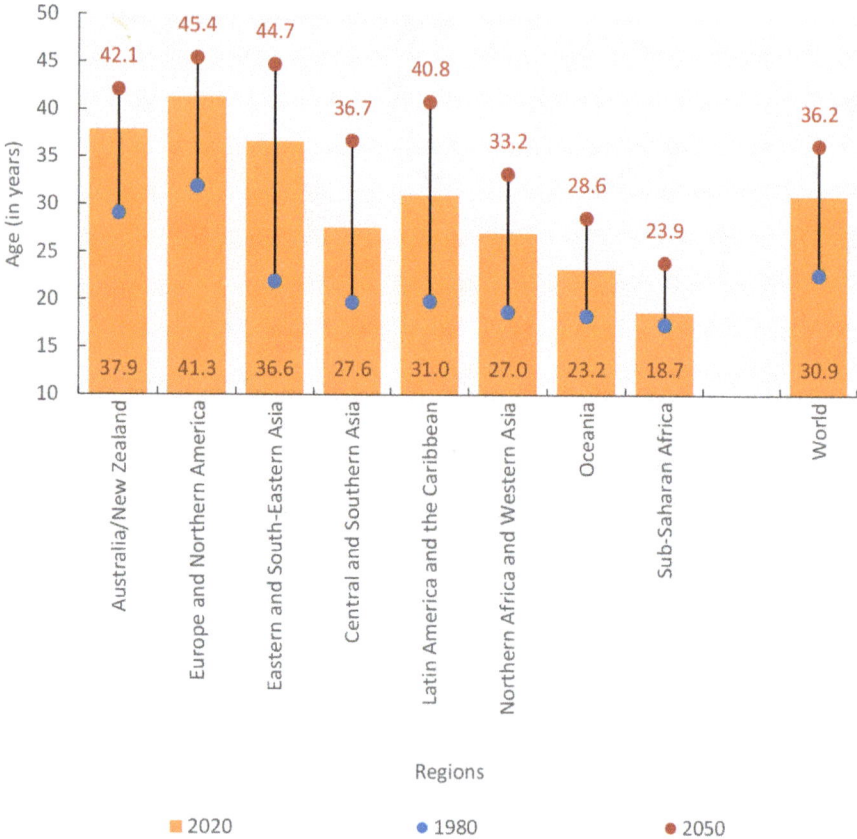

Figure 3.6   Median age projection by SDG regions. Data source: United nations department of economic and social affairs, Ppopulation division. World population prospects 2019. (https://population.un.org/wpp/ DataQuery/).

in 1985 then to 2.45 in 2015. This is projected to come down to around 2.2 by 2050. Both regional and country-specific trends are projected to show a tendency towards convergence: countries with low fertility rates will experience either stagnating or slightly increasing rates, while countries with high fertility rates will experience significant drops. Korea currently has the lowest fertility rate of 1.1 followed by Singapore (1.2), Italy (1.33) and Japan (1.37). These countries, together with Germany, Australia, China and the US are expected to make small increases in fertility rates by 2050. Among developed countries, Israel is the only country that has a higher fertility rate than the world and expected to stay above the world rate in 2050 despite a slight drop.

The increasing life expectancy and decreasing fertility rate will raise the median age of the world population from 30.9 in 2020 to 36.2 in 2050.(Figure 3.6) There are, however, regional differences: Europe and Northern America will have the highest

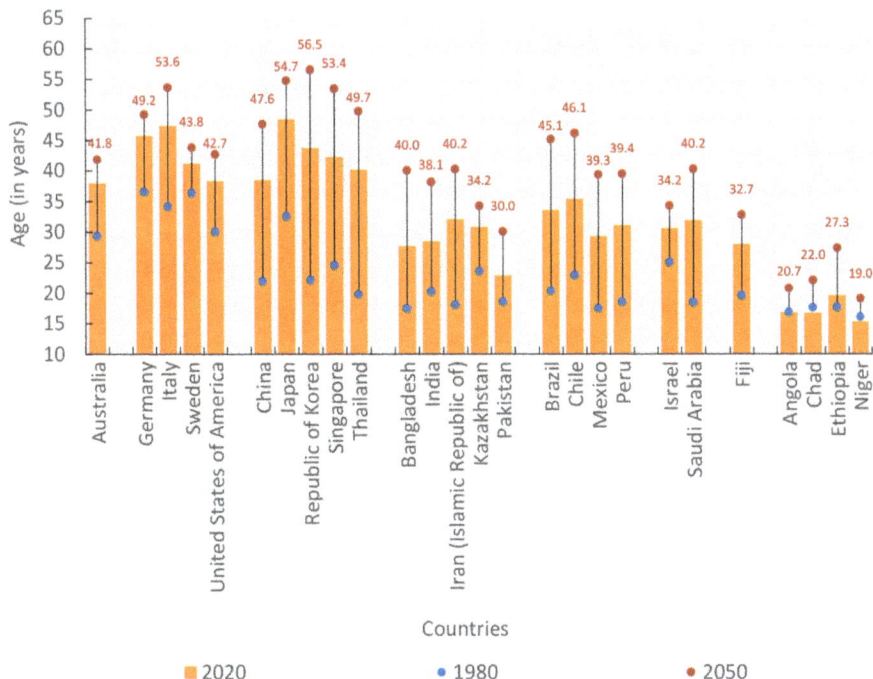

Figure 3.7 *Median age of selected countries. Data source: United nations department of economic and social affairs, population division. World population prospects 2019. (https://population.un.org/wpp/ DataQuery/).*

median age (45.4), while sub-Saharan Africa remains the youngest with 23.9. The largest gain is expected in Latin America and Caribbean countries (9.8) and Eastern and South-Eastern Asia (8.1).

All selected countries will experience growth in median age albeit unevenly. (Figure 3.7) Japan currently has the highest median age but that of South Korea will be the highest by 2050 increasing from 43.7 in 2020 to 56.5 in 2050. Four countries including South Korea, Japan, Italy and Singapore will record median ages of over 50, while Ethiopia and sub-Saharan African countries will have median ages under 30. The growth will be particularly high in Eastern and South-Eastern Asian countries but there is also noticeable diversity. Bangladesh is expected to experience an increase of more than 12 years, together with Korea and Brazil. Among developed countries, Australia, the US and Sweden will have relatively low median age, and Israel will continue to have a younger population than the world.

More revealing of the concern of the population ageing, however, is the old-age dependency ratio (OADR). It is the ratio of population aged 65 or above per 100 working population aged between 15 and 64. As in Figure 3.8, the total dependency ratio, which includes child dependency ratio of the proportion of people age 0–14 per 100 working-age population, had been declining from 75.4% in 1965 to

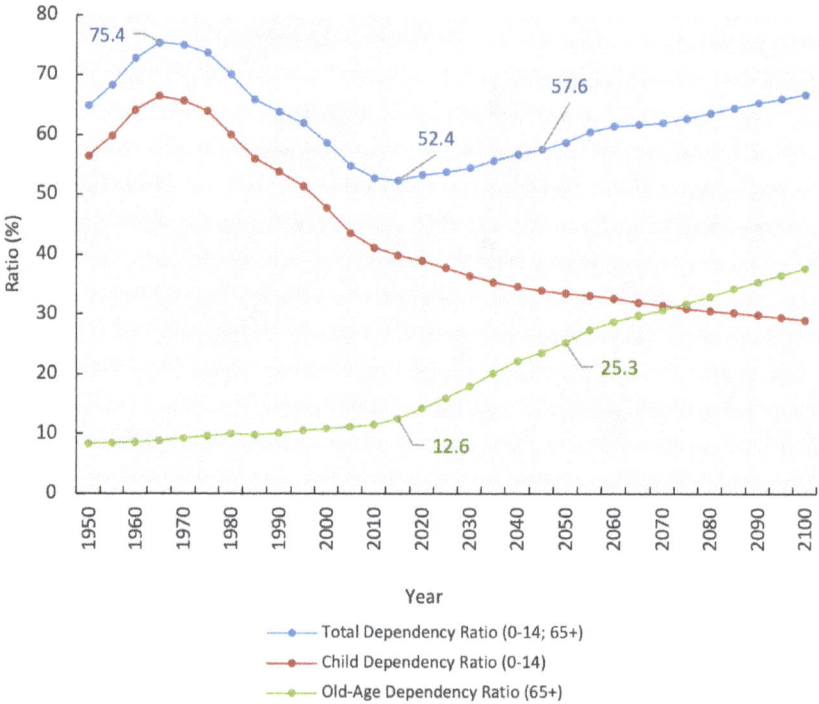

Figure 3.8   Dependency ratio, World, 1950–2100. Data source: United nations department of economic and social affairs, population division. World population prospects 2019. (https://population.un.org/wpp/ DataQuery/).

52.4% in 2015 due to the rapidly decreasing child dependency ratio; but it started to increase again, pushed by the rapidly increasing OADR, which is expected to reach 25.3% by 2050 doubling from the level in 2015.

Europe, Northern Americaand Australia/New Zealand have the highest OADR currently, but Eastern and South-Eastern Asia will catch up fast and these three regions are expected to have OADR above 40% by 2050. All other regions will double the current level except sub-Saharan Africa, where it will increase from 6.8% to 9.2% in the next 30 years. Among the selected countries, Japan, South Korea, Italy and Singapore are going to experience the highest ratio by 2050 with the OADR of 70% above, followed by Singapore, Germany and Thailand recording between 50% and 69%, then by China, Sweden, Chile, Australia, the US, Brazil and Israel, 30–49%. Other countries will have below 30% with sub-Saharan African countries recording 10% or lower (Figure 3.9).

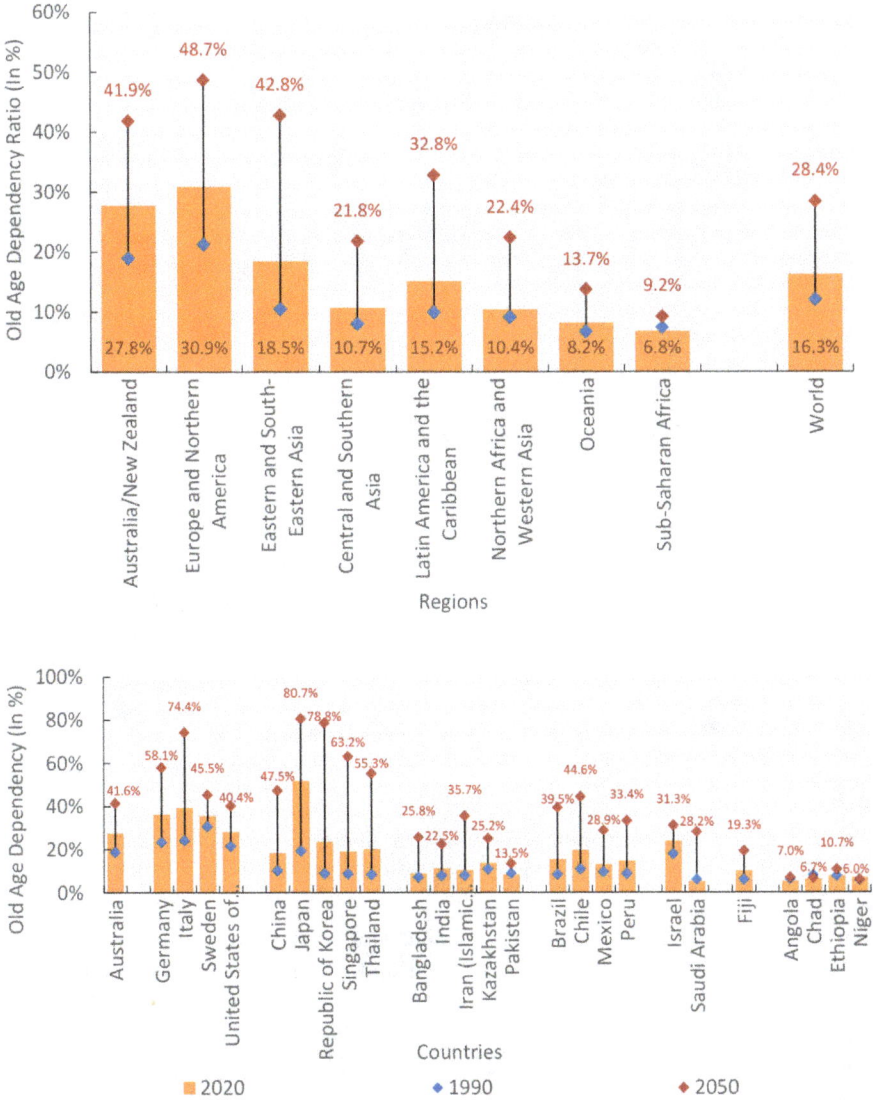

Figure 3.9   *Old-age dependency ratio for SDG region and selected countries1990, 2020 and 2050. Data source: United nations department of economic and social affairs, population division. World population prospects 2019. (https://population.un.org/wpp/ DataQuery/).*

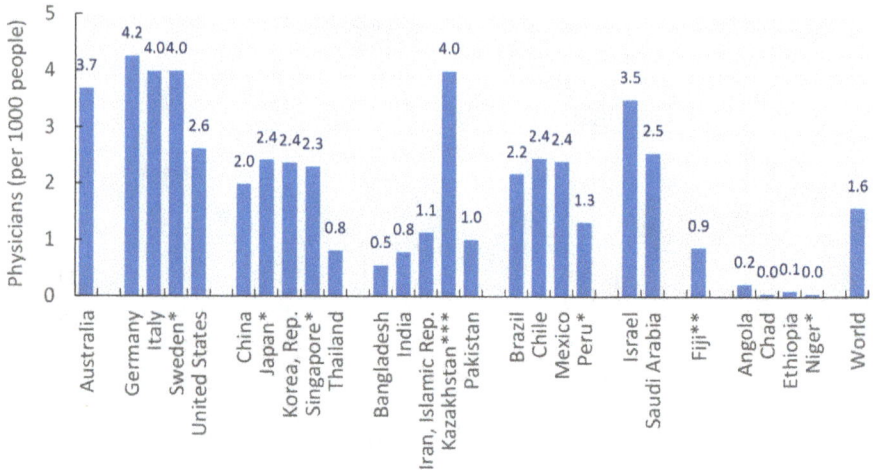

Figure 3.10   *Number of physicians per thousand people by selected SDG
countries 2017 (or nearest). Notes: * figures for 2016, ** figures
for 2015, *** figures for 2014. Data Source: World Health
Organisation, Global Health Observatory Data Repository.
(https://data.worldbank.org/indicator/SH.MED.PHYS.ZS).*

3.3   Challenges and issues of population ageing

3.3.1   Challenges to the healthcare system

Together with population ageing, the world is facing an epidemiological transition
in which the main health concerns are shifting from 'infectious and parasitic diseases that often claimed the lives of infants and children' to non-communicable
diseases (NCDs) that commonly affect adults and older people [8, p. 3]. Although
communicable diseases, maternal, perinatal and nutritional conditions constitute
more than half of the disease burden in low-income countries, in 2008, NCDs –
most notable among others include heart disease, cancer and diabetes – accounted
for more than 65% in middle-income countries and 86% in high-income countries.
These figures are expected to grow and NCDs are expected to account for the majority of the health burden in low-income countries too by 2030. Among the population
60 years or older, NCDs already account for 87% of the burden in low-, middle and
high-income countries in 2008 [8, p. 9]. This epidemiologic transition, linked to
the changes in lifestyle in favour of high fat, sugar and salt diet, sedentariness and
smoking, is expected to be particularly evident in middle-income countries [9, p. 7].

There is a concern regarding whether the world is prepared for such a transition.
For one thing, there is a huge disparity in terms of the healthcare system. Among the
selected countries, 11 countries have lower than the world average density of physicians including Thailand, all of the Southern Asian countries, Peru in Latin America,
Fiji and particularly low in all of the sub-Saharan African countries (Figure 3.10).

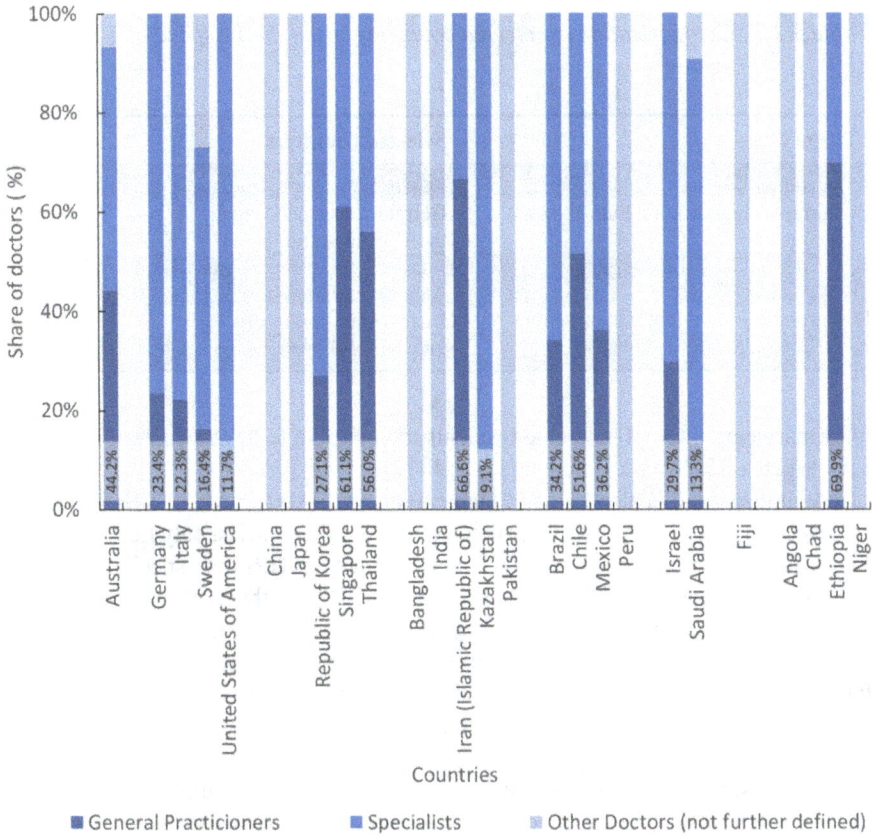

Figure 3.11   *Share of doctors by categories in 2014 (or nearest year). Data source: World health organisation, global health observatory datarepository. (https://www.who.int/data/gho).*

In addition, dealing with multiple NCDs requires a strategy focused on primary care system (PHC) which is commonly known to provide 'higher quality, better outcomes and lower costs' across major population subgroups [10] and WHO recognizes it as the key to advancing universal health coverage [11]. The primary care system often involves a network of healthcare providers – such as general practitioners (GPs), nurses, physician assistants – working together with social workers and other community partners. The actual institutional characteristics differ widely from country to country making it difficult to compare across countries. Yet, various reports point to the shortage of GPs even in developed countries [10, 12–17].

Taking the US as an example, Dall *et al.* [17] estimated a shortage of up to 31 000 adult care generalists by the year 2025 [17], and Steinwald *et al.* [16] noted that in 2016, 38% of practising physicians were primary care practitioners and the proportion should be increased to at least 40% [10]. Despite this shortage, Long *et al.* [18] report, '80 per cent of internal medicine residents, including nearly two-thirds

Table 3.2   Categorization of selected countries based on the speed of population ageing

Category	Selected countries
A: Currently high- and fast-ageing	Korea, Singapore, Thailand, China, Italy
B: Currently high but medium-to-slow ageing	Germany, Sweden, Japan, the US, Australia, Israel
C: Currently low but fast-ageing	Mexico, Chile, Brazil, Peru, Iran, Saudi Arabia, Bangladesh
D: Currently low- and medium-ageing	Kazakhstan, India, Fiji
E: Currently low- and slower-ageing	Pakistan, Ethiopia, Angola, Chad, Niger

of primary care internal medicine residents, do not plan to have a career in primary care or general internal medicine' [18, p. 1472].

A similar trend is also found in many countries outside the US. WHO statistics arranged in Figure 3.11 shows that among the selected countries, only Ethiopia, Iran, Singapore, Thailand and Chile show a clear majority in GPs over specialists, while Australia comes close at 44%. Kazakhstan and the US are the lowest with 9.1% and 11.7%, respectively. Some of the fast ageing countries, such as Italy, South Korea and Saudi Arabia, also have a low proportion of GPs. A report by the Organisation for Economic Cooperation and Development (OECD) also confirms this, as only Chile, Canada and Portugal have GPs accounting for more than 40% of all doctors among all OECD countries [7].

The reason for such a shortage can be found in the income gap between specialists and GPs. The average income gap between these two groups is assumed at approximately 104 000 USD in the US [10, p. 5]. OECD also confirms the main reason to be the existence of the income gap favourable to specialists as the incentive for doctors to specialize [7, pp. 174–7]. This naturally entices medical students towards the specialist track. Besides, the medical training in the US is also reported to be favourable to specialists in that teaching hospitals regard speciality residents and fellows as the most valuable producers of healthcare services [16], and residents in general practices often complain inadequate training and resources to successfully manage patients' social needs [18].

Another health challenge associated with population ageing is dementia, which can be caused by a variety of brain disorders including Alzheimer's disease. Alzheimer's is one of the diseases with no cure or treatment proven to be effective despite billions of dollars spent on research [7, p. 224]. According to Alzheimer's Disease International's estimate, there were 46.8 million people worldwide with dementia in 2015. In terms of regions, East Asia has the most number of people with dementia (9.8 million), followed by Western Europe (7.4 million), South Asia (5.1 million) and North America (4.8 million). In terms of country, ten countries were estimated to have more than a million people with dementia. The ten countries include China (9.5 million), the US (4.2 million), India (4.1 million), Japan (3.1 million), Brazil (1.6 million), Indonesia (1.2 million) and France (1.2 million). The total

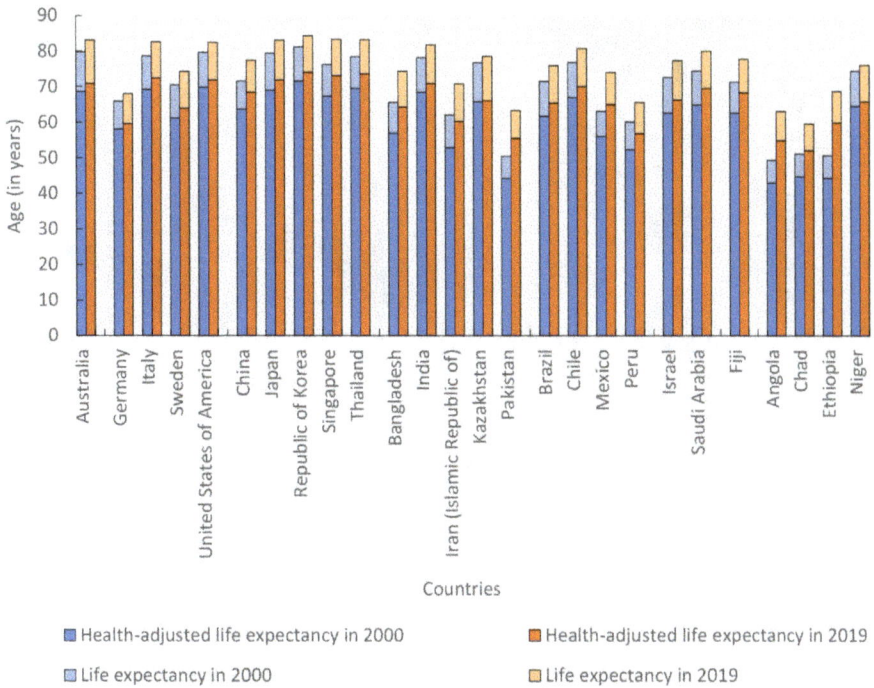

Figure 3.12 *Health-adjusted life expectancy and life expectancy for selected countries, 2000–19. Data source: World health organisation, global health observatory data repository. (https://www.who.int/ data/gho).*

number of people with dementia worldwide is expected to increase to 131.5 million by 2050, and much of the growth will be attributable to low- and middle-income countries, rising from 58% of all people with dementia in 2015 to 68% in 2050 [9, pp. 22–25].

It is also significant to note that the main costs for dementia are incurred not as medical costs but the costs of providing care either through social institutions or informally. According to Alzheimer's Disease International, direct medical costs accounted for 19.5% of the total costs while social sector costs account for 40.1% and informal care costs account for 40.4% [9, p. 56]. There were significant regional differences in terms of the cost structure, in that, the relative contribution of informal care costs to the total was the highest in Africa and lowest in North America and Western Europe, while the reverse was true for social care costs [9, p. 60].

This leads to another challenge of providing long-term care (LTC). Neurocognitive disorders such as dementia are not the only conditions that make the elderly population unable to live independently: limited mobility, frailty and other declines in cognitive function that come with old age, together with disabilities that could also be developed from NCDs, make more numbers of elderly persons seek

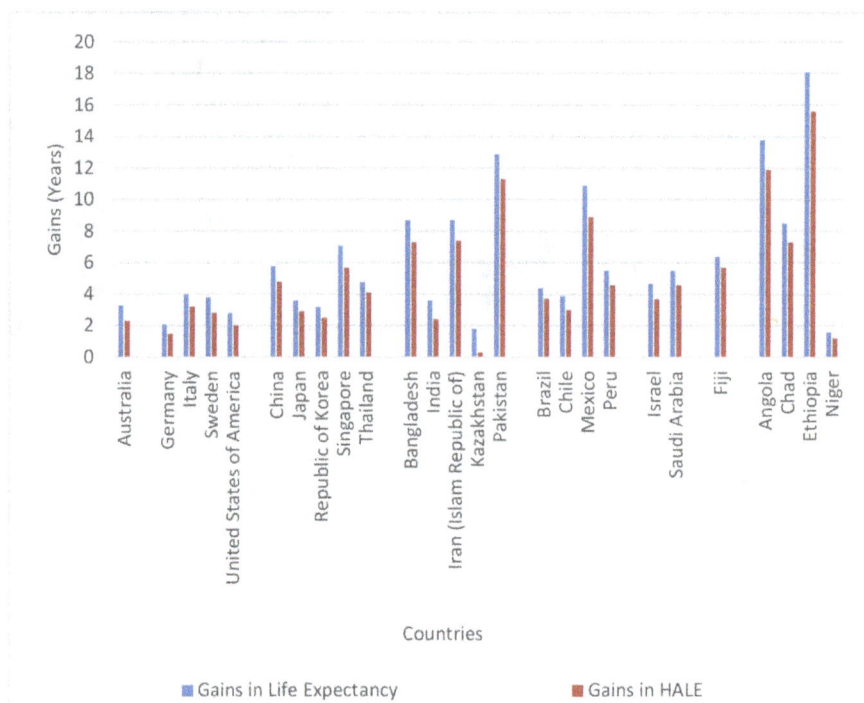

Figure 3.13   Gains in life expectancy and health-adjusted life expectancy
for selected countries, 2000–19. Data source: World health
organisation, global health observatory data repository. (https://
www.who.int/data/gho).

LTC services. The number of people seeking LTC is expected to increase with the
population ageing. OECD reports that an average of 10.8% of people aged over 65
across OECD countries received LTC services in 2017, doubling in proportion from
2007 [7, p. 234]. Even in countries that do not have well-developed LTC infrastructure, such as home nursing, community care and assisted living, residential care and
long-stay hospitals, providing LTC has economic costs because the informal caregivers might need to withdraw from employment or school to take care of the older
family members [8, p. 23]. Providing LTC is a labour-intensive service and informal
care is also often used as a complement to formal institutions even in developed
countries. Institutional LTC facilities, on the other hand, are used by especially frail
or dependent elderly and much care is needed to avoid other adverse health events
such as healthcare-associated infections and pressure ulcers.

Besides, ageing often accompanies multimorbidity and requires older patients to
take multiple medicines for long periods. Although necessary, such practice of polypharmacy increases the risk of adverse drug events, medication error and harm, creating another challenge [7, p. 238]. Together with the provision of LTC, the prospect
of long-term medical attention needed by the ageing population has raised concerns

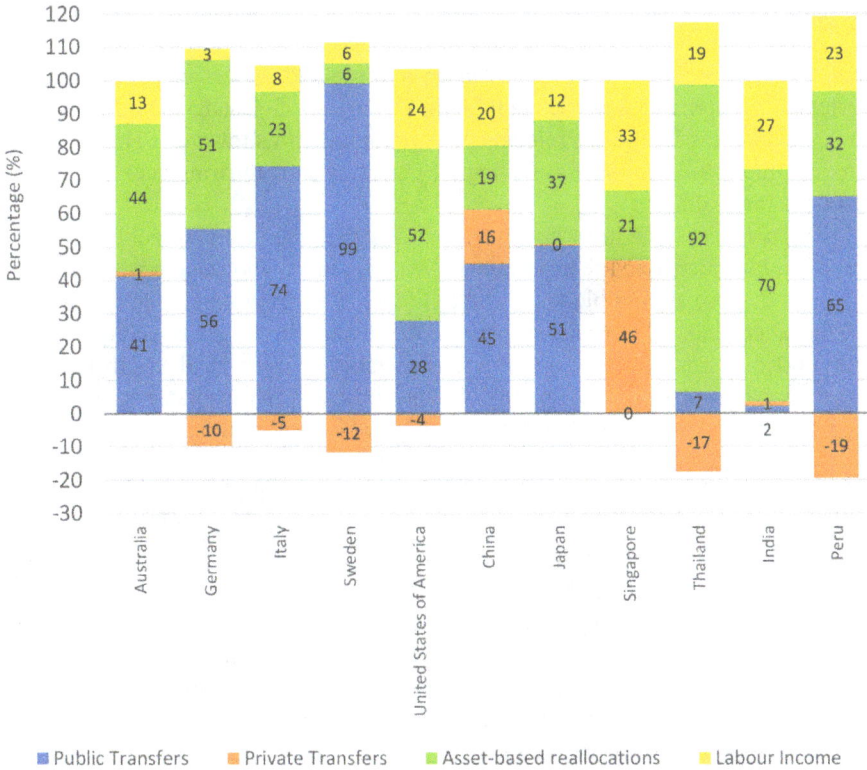

Figure 3.14   *Income sources to finance old-age consumption at ages 65 and over. Data source: National transfer accounts (https://ntaccounts. org/).*

relating to healthcare expenditure burden on household and economy [19, 20]. There are, however, debates on the relationship between population ageing and increasing medical expenditure [21–24]. Getzen [21] recognized population ageing as having a significant impact on healthcare cost [21] but Zweifel *et al.* [22] call it a red herring and suggest that per capita healthcare expenditure is independent of population ageing [22]. Smith *et al.* [23] further argue that the largest contributor to the increasing healthcare expenditure in the US is technological advances, not ageing population [23]. Colombier [24] agrees that advances in medical technology are a crucial cost driver in healthcare but cautions not to brush aside the role of population ageing [24]. Outreville [25] and Geueet *et al.* [26], on the other hand, found that per capita healthcare expenditure is independent of population ageing but is increased by high healthcare expenditure closer to the time of death – which is more likely to happen among the older population than younger individuals [25, 26].

More research results in a different context need to be compiled to resolve the question. Yet, two messages are clear. First, whether the healthcare costs are increasing because of technological advances or because people spend more on healthcare close to the time of death, the implication for the ageing population is that people will need to prepare to pay higher medical expenses in their old ages after retirement. This will either create a burden on a household budget or public pension system, if not prepared well. Second, for the countries with fast ageing but relatively low preparedness for ageing-related epidemiological shifts towards PHC and LTC services, there will be costs for making the transition and preparing necessary infrastructure for healthcare.

The practical issue here, however, is to lengthen the years in health. The scenario in which increased life expectancy is lived mostly in good health while disability is put as close as possible to the end of life is called 'compression of morbidity'. On the other hand, the opposite scenario in which disability in old age comes sooner and most of the increased years of life expectancy is lived in ill health is called 'expansion of morbidity' [27, p. 13]. Which of these scenarios pan out in a country will have a considerable impact on healthcare expenditure for government and household. Under the compression of morbidity, the overall impact of population ageing on individual and national health expenditure would be mild, whereas the expansion of morbidity will exponentially increase healthcare and LTC costs.

WHO tracks health-adjusted life expectancy (HALE) for this purpose. Although the method with which the health of the elderly population of a country is measured is subjective, making it difficult to compare across countries, it still gives us a rough idea about reality. Figure 3.12 compares HALE and life expectancy in selected countries for the years 2000 and 2019. During the two decades, all the selected countries increased healthy years in life as well as overall life expectancy. Yet, the gains in healthy years are lower than the gains in life expectancy in all countries as shown in Figure 3.13, which compares gains in life expectancy against gains in HALE. On average, 78% of gains in life expectancy were healthy for the selected countries, with Fiji recording the highest (89.1%). The lowest was recorded in Kazakhstan, with only 16.7%, or 0.3 years in HALE increase against 1.8 years in life expectancy gain. Kazakhstan is a country that has a high density of physicians per 1 000 population matching that of European countries but with a very low focus on GPs. Although it is not expected to face a serious ageing population yet, if the current trend continues, Kazakhstan might be heading into an expansion of morbidity scenario. Other countries that have lower than average in terms of HALE gains as a percentage of life expectancy gains include India (66.7%), Australia (69.7%), Germany (71.4%), the US (71.4%), Sweden (73.7%), Niger (75.0%) and Chile (76.9%) but not far below the world average of 78%.

3.3.2   Challenges to economy

The last discussion on healthcare expenditure has already brought the discussion into economic consideration. If the ageing population increases the healthcare burden, who will shoulder the burden is very much dependent on the financing structure of the elderly in different countries. National Transfer Accounts project provides useful statistics by identifying sources of income for different age groups dividing into four categories: public transfer, private transfer, asset reallocation and labour income.(Figure 3.14) Payments from public pension and healthcare benefits count towards 'public transfer'; cash and other financial supports received from family and friends constitute 'private transfer'; savings, private capital/property income, including private pension funds, are considered 'asset-based reallocations' and the payments and earnings from employment (including self-employment) contribute to the last category of 'labour income' [28, pp. 3–9].

The future challenges to the financial sustainability of the elderly population depend on the different mix of financial sources available for them and how this will change in the future. For example, countries that rely heavily on public transfers, such as Sweden, Italy and Peru will face challenges in fiscal sustainability, especially when faced with slow economic growth and declining tax-base or other sources of government income. In countries with a high proportion of private transfers, such as Singapore, population ageing will cause challenges to household budget issues. Where asset reallocation is large, maintaining the stability of the prices of such assets – financial health – will be an important issue. Developing countries with a currently low share of public transfers will need to improve pension to prepare for the elderly population – especially when accompanied by increasing independence of the elderly.

The public pension system, especially the pay-as-you-go types have been the cause of concern for population ageing. In 1994 World Bank published a landmark report titled 'Averting the Old Age Crisis', which focused on this very issue and warned the world of the fiscal burden it will cause in the future [29]. Indeed, according to OECD, pension expenditures in G20 countries increased by 1.7% reaching 9% of GDP in 2017. Public health expenditure, on the other hand, reaching 7% of GDP in 2017 up by 5.5% from 2000 [30, p. 21]. This creates much concern especially in the context of low economic growth and declining workforce [31, 32]. World Economic Forum also published a white paper in 2017 which estimated the shortfall in pensions by examining eight countries with the largest established pension systems including Australia, Canada, China, India, Japan, Netherlands, the UK and the US. The 'retirement savings gap' or the shortfall in pension saving, for these eight countries, was estimated at 70 trillion USD in 2015, and if the gap grows at the current rate without major government intervention, WEF predicts, it will grow to 400 trillion USD by 2050 [33, p. 8].

Yet there are only a few countries, according to Mercer Global Pension Index, which have a resilient and sufficient pension system. Out of 39 countries, when it traces to benchmark adequacy and sustainability of their pension system, only two countries, Denmark and Netherlands, received A. Twelve countries including Chile, Germany, Israel, Sweden and Singapore are placed in B meaning these countries have a sound structure but with some areas of improvement. A total of 17 countries including the UK, the US, Saudi Arabia, Italy and South Korea received C+ and C, which means they have good features but also major risks with questionable long-term sustainability. Then come 8 countries with D, including China, India, Japan, Mexico and Thailand, whose pension systems are reviewed as containing some desirable features but doubtful efficacy and sustainability without addressing major weaknesses or omissions [34, p. 13].

The problem with the pension system is exacerbated by the prospect of low economic growth. According to OECD predictions, the G20 countries will have to increase the tax revenue between 4.5 and 11.5 percentage points of GDP by 2060, to keep up with the increases in pension, healthcare and other expenditure associated with population ageing [30]. Yet, an ageing population might also usher in a prolonged period of low economic growth through slower investment and productivity growth. Some empirical evidence from Japan [35, 36] and other advanced economies [37–39] seem to suggest a positive correlation between population ageing and low interest rates or deflation. There are speculations as to why this is likely. Ageing could drive down aggregate employment rates because employment rates tend to decline with age. This will induce the price of labour to rise relative to the price of capital, forcing firms to increase capital per worker. This will be especially so if savings increase: with more proportion of the population preparing for their retirement with savings, interest rates will remain low. Yet, low interest rates may not result in expanding the economy if the investment moves away into relatively younger economies experiencing expansion [29, 30].

In contrast to the aged economies, countries with a young population are expected to enter a period of economic growth with the coming of the global demographic change. Such speculations are often based on the demographic dividend theory, which stipulates that a certain change in population structure creates conditions that are conducive to economic growth. For example, when the fertility of a country starts to fall rapidly, it soon leads to fewer young dependents to the working-age population, hence freeing more resources available to be invested in economic development and welfare for the future. This in turn starts a phase of economic expansion for the country which is termed the 'first demographic dividend'. A second demographic dividend is also possible when the enlarged working-age population is facing a longer period of retirement due to longer life expectancy. This gives the upper section of the working-aged population a strong incentive to accumulate assets which will push up national income [40]. East Asian countries economic growth in the second half of the twentieth century are attributed to this [41, 42], while Southern Asian countries are said to have entered this period to be followed by African countries [31]. Whether this theory truly explains the past is up for debate and whether this will pan out in the future for the countries also remains to be seen. For a country to benefit from a demographic dividend, it must also have the appropriate infrastructure, educated labour and other policies that creates conditions for channelling the growing working-age population towards productive activities [43].

3.4   Analysis and policy implications

Five categories of countries among the selected countries can be identified based on the current extent of the aged population and the expected rates of population ageing in the next thirty years as discussed in Section 3.2. These are arranged in Table 3.2. There are some countries with a relatively high proportion of population above 65 of age currently but are expected to experience slow growth including, especially,

Germany, and, to a lesser extent, Sweden, Japan, the US and Australia among the selected countries. Israel is a marginal case as the country had the same level of the aged population as Japan in 1985 but also has high fertility rate and the growth of the aged population is the slowest and expected to converge to the world average by 2050. Some Eastern and South-Eastern Asian countries such as Korea, Singapore, Thailand and China, together with Italy, on the other hand, are expected to experience relatively high population ageing while already having above the world average in terms of the proportion of people above 65. In other regions, Chile, Brazil, Iran, Peru, Saudi Arabia and Bangladesh are ageing fast and will have an older population above the world average by 2050. Kazakhstan currently stays slightly lower than the world average and will experience relatively slow growth and could be grouped with India and Fiji. Although the latter two countries will experience slightly faster growth than Kazakhstan these countries will remain close to the world average. Other countries, Pakistan, Ethiopia, Angola and Chad are expected to have a relatively young population although ageing is also increasing in those countries.

Those countries that experience fast ageing (categories A and C) will face the most serious challenges as they will also face a fast increase in OADR (see Figure 3.5). This could become a burden to the household if old age accompanies more years in ill health and most of the responsibility of looking after the elderly population falls on the household. It will become a source of a fiscal burden if following urbanization, more elderly people live on their own with a government pension. Countries that are regarded as having adequate and resilient pension system according to Mercer Global Pension Index [33] are mostly concentrated in category B with Germany, Sweden and Israel with the addition of Singapore in category A and Chile in category C. Most of the other selected countries, however, received the lowest rating including all the countries in group C, except for Saudi Arabia. Thailand and China in group A, as well as Japan in Group B, received the lowest ranking and coupled with the high level of population ageing in these countries, it will be an important issue going forward. OECD and World Economic Forum both advise countries to increase savings rate to 10–15% of an average annual salary to ensure financial sustainability after retirement as well as increasing financial literacy while making accurate information on various pensions plans and savings products to prevent a major crisis in old age [30, 33, 34].

All in all, sustainable economic growth will be key for all these countries to prevent increasing poverty among the elderly. Developing countries in groups D and E will have to make efforts to harness the benefits of demographic dividend and generate sustainable economic growth through which they can invest in the healthcare system and other social protection systems while promoting access to healthy financial institutions to prepare for the future changes and improve the welfare of the elderly population. For the countries facing high population ageing as those in group A and B, maintaining economic growth in the context of high ratio of the older population to working-age population will be an important issue to ensure the continuing provision of welfare for the elderly and prevent increasing inequality among the older individuals [44]. This is also going to become important for other countries but especially for those in group C facing relatively fast population ageing. Proposed solutions for this include prolonging the economic participation of older people. Indeed, OECD estimates that giving older employees greater opportunities could raise GDP per capita by 19% over the next three decades [45, p. 31]. There are some positive signs as employment rates among 55–64 grew in most of the G20 countries between 2000 and 2018 – which was most obvious among elderly people with higher education [30, p. 13]. There are also some concerns regarding raising the retirement age that it might affect youth employment negatively, but the evidence from developed countries suggests that during the 1990s and 2000s, there was about 8% increase in employment among the age group 55–64 and 5 percentage points increase for youth, and youth unemployment fell by 2.6 percentage points, showing that both older employment and youth employment can increase together [32].

Increasing economic participation of the elderly, however, does not have to take the form of raising the retirement age. Increasing flexibility and formally recognizing informal labour are also required to address the interrelated challenges of reducing labour force, potential productivity loss and low growth. It will be necessary to increase skills development and life-long learning for older individuals so that they can adapt to the changing world and also to their changing physical and mental capacities to remain active in flexible arrangements. Expanding the use of technology in the workplace, such as automation and artificial intelligence (AI), is also regarded as a way that helps create the age-inclusive workplace. At the same time, the UN has been urging governments to take steps to formally recognize the contribution old people, especially female, make to the economy through informal ways as carers for the young and providing financial and emotional support for the younger generation that goes through hardship, not to mention those involved in the informal sector in developing countries and rural areas [46]. These measures also prolong the social participation of the elderly for win-win outcomes for both the elderly and the society and should be accompanied by other measures such as encouraging regular and orderly migration and promoting higher fertility [30].

Yet another way will be promoting senior entrepreneurship. According to the findings of Global Entrepreneurship Monitor in 2017, older individuals have the lowest confidence in their own ability to start and run a business, lacking in personal contacts with a start-up entrepreneur who can work as a role model, but they have the higher risk-willingness compared to the younger generation, are more likely to hire others to form larger teams and are more likely to engage in social entrepreneurship [47]. Engaging old individuals in the economy also brings their human capital (experience, knowledge, management skills) and social capital (wider and more developed networks) as well as financial resources into business and economy. Fried calls this the '3rd Demographic Dividend', which will bring 'additional and sustainable benefits' by activating the 'large unrealized social capital of older adults', conferring benefits both economically and in other measures of societal well-being [48]. Older people can bring 'experience and accrued knowledge and expertise, greater creative problem-solving, and ability to make even-handed decisions – particularly in emotionally charged situations' [49]. OECD stipulates that senior entrepreneurship might be the best way to tackle economic challenges of population ageing and benefit from the 'silver economy' [30], targeting people over 60, who are 'on track to generate more than half of urban consumption growth in developed economies, fueled by spending on healthcare, transport, housing and entertainment' [50].

As Fried eloquently puts it, increasing social engagement will benefit the older people through ...

> staying engaged in activities that are meaningful to the individual, feeling productive and that one has 'given back'; engaging in meaningful activities on flexible schedules; having a structure to one's life and a reason to get up in the morning; not feeling lonely; and feeling positive about one's older age. [49, p. 79]

For all the above, however, building an age-inclusive society and removing outdated stereotypes and ageism must be one of the priorities. Age-based discrimination is what the UN Secretary-General pointed out as one of the main barriers faced by older persons in the labour market. It could be individual, institutional, systemic or structural practices, could be both explicit and implicit, and gets exacerbated by other coexisting variables such as gender and disability [51].

Another condition for increasing social engagement of the elderly is, of course, that old people remain healthy and active. Improving healthcare system is going to be important for many countries, especially for those fast ageing countries with inadequate healthcare infrastructure. As shown in Figure 3.6, some of the countries in group A and C characterized by fast ageing have a particularly low ratio of physicians per 1 000 people including Bangladesh (0.5), Thailand (0.8), Iran (1.1) and Peru (1.3). The situation is more serious for other countries in group D and E. All the countries, however, face the needs for building affordable, flexible and patient-centred primary and preventive healthcare systems. Doing so will involve increasing healthcare professionals serving in this capacity as well as strengthening coordination among relevant medical and nonmedical practitioners in different sectors [32, 44, 52]. Apart from this general direction, WHO/UNICEF provides a list of policy guidelines that countries can mix and adopt as is warranted by the country-specific evidence. One thing to note in the list is the relevance of mobile technology to all the major components of PHC systems [52, p. 37]. In fact, WHO, together with International Telecommunication Union, has launched Integrated Care for Older People and mAgeing Initiative to scale up mHealth services reaching millions of people in cooperation with governments around the globe [53].

OECD also summarises the importance of technology for maintaining health and autonomy for the elderly as below:

> telemedicine and mobile clinics can help improve healthcare in underserved areas, while home-based health monitoring through smart devices and wearable technologies communicating with health professionals can enable more personalised care. Data-driven innovation could provide practical solutions to enhance elderly people's quality of life and facilitate independent living while reducing financial costs and freeing up time for family caregivers to continue participating in the labour market. Advances in robotics (e.g. development of 'carebots'

in Japan), intelligent sensors (e.g. fall detection) and neuroscience are particularly likely to meet rising demand, as well as voice-activated technologies and
autonomous vehicles [7].

It is not just in healthcare that technology can help us address the challenges of
population ageing. As noted by the UN Secretary-General, information and computer technologies (ICTs) can help us to fight age-based discrimination, build smart
cities, ensure financial inclusion and support caregivers [51]. Technologies can also
encourage social engagements of the elderly by assisting with the mobility and
making flexible arrangements of gatherings possible. Providing flexibility in labour
arrangements and facilitating flexible, customised life-long learning and training are
crucial elements in helping old people engaged in society. These are, of course, beneficial not only to the elderly but to the society in general, and all these innovations
will move the world towards a more inclusive and sustainable future.

3.5   Concluding remarks

This chapter identified the areas of reform necessary in preparation for population
ageing: Healthcare reforms oriented towards primary care system, preventive measures and flexible LTC service arrangements; increasing flexible arrangements in job
markets while expanding recognition and remuneration for informal works; building
diverse and resilient financial options for post-retirement life; removing age-based
biases and encouraging participation of elderly in society. These are not only the
measures aimed at benefitting the elderly in an already-aged world of the future but
the pathways towards a broader concept of the sustainable future. In other words,
pursuing a resilient society in the context of the ageing population is not a separate
challenge from pursuing a sustainable world. Neither are these tasks to be put in
governments' to-do lists only: there are works cut out for entrepreneurs and companies – large and small, NGOs, healthcare providers, educators, community leaders,
artists and all works of life. Hence, these are a list of burdens, failure to accomplish
which will lead to an apocalypse: they are a list of opportunities towards which there
are already people leading us with examples.

Averting the Old Age Crisis was the title of the 1994 World Bank Report [27],
and there is no dearth of sensational headlines that chime with the word 'crisis' concerning the ageing population. The 2019 UN report on 'World Population Ageing',
by contrast, ends with a positive proclamation that 'population ageing can spur economic growth while maintaining fiscal sustainability' and continue to list 10 policy
directions that population ageing has brought to our attention which will also bring
us closer to SDGs [6, pp. 35–36]. Indeed, the future is not set in stone, and our efforts
to bring a better future – whether stored in the visions of sustainable development,
universal healthcare, inclusive growth, green jobs, or healthy ageing – will bring
new opportunities for us along the way. In turn, these will shape what our future will
be like in 30 years. Enough alarms have been raised regarding the potential problems
of population ageing. It is now time to focus our energy on making the best out of the

future, of which the ageing population is an integral part, and make preparations, so that we can celebrate longevity, not just for individuals but for society as a whole.

References

[1] United Nations. *Political* declaration and madrid international plan of action on ageing [online]. 2002. Available from https://www.un.org/en/events/pastevents/pdfs/Madrid_plan.pdf [Accessed Jan 2021].

[2] World Health Organisation. *Global strategy and action plan on ageing and health [online]*. 2017. Available from https://www.who.int/ageing/WHO-GSAP-2017.pdf?ua=1.

[3] UN General Assembly. *United Nations decade of healthy agDecade of Healthy Ageing (2021–2030).* Resolution adopted by the general assembly on 14th December 2020. A/RES/75/131. 2020. Available from https://undocs.org/en/A/RES/75/131.

[4] United Nations. *The sustainable development goals report 2019 [online].* 2019. Available from 10.18356/55eb9109-en.

[5] United Nations General Assembly. *Transforming our world: the 2030 Agenda for Sustainable Development.* Resolution adopted by the general assembly on 25 September 2015. (A/RES/70/1). 2015. Available from 10.1002/9781119541851.app1.

[6] United Nations Department of Economic and Social Affairs. *World population ageing 2019 [online].* 2020. Available from 10.18356/6a8968ef-en.

[7] OECD. *Health at a glance 2019: OECD indicators [online].* 2019. Available from 10.1787/4dd50c09-en.

[8] World Health Organization. *Global health and ageing [online].* 2011. Available from https://www.who.int/ageing/publications/global_health.pdf.

[9] Alzheimer's Disease International. *World Alzheimer report 2015: the global impact of dementia, an analysis of prevalence, incidence, cost and trends [online].* 2015. Available from https://www.alzint.org/resource/world-alzheimer-report-2015/.

[10] Steinwald B., Ginsburg P., Brandt C., Lee S., Patel K. *We need more primary care physicians: Here's why and how. USC-Brookings Schaeffer Initiative for Health Policy [online].* 2019. Available from https://www.brookings.edu/blog/usc-brookings-schaeffer-on-health-policy/2019/07/08/we-need-more-primary-care-physicians-heres-why-and-how/.

[11] World Health Organization. *Quality primary care key to advancing universal health coverage [online].* 2019. Available from https://www.who.int/southeastasia/news/detail/05-04-2019-quality-primary-care-key-to-advancing-universal-health-coverage-who.

[12] Groenewegen P.P., Jurgutis A. 'A future for primary care for the Greek population'. *Quality in Primary Care.* 2013, vol. 21(6), pp. 369–78.

[13] Groenewegen P., Heinemann S., Greß S., Schäfer W. 'Primary care practice composition in 34 countries'. *Health Policy.* 2015, vol. 119(12), pp. 1576–83.

[14]   Teljeur C., Thomas S., O'Kelly F.D., O'Dowd T. 'General practitioner work-force planning: assessment of four policy directions'. *BMC health services research.* 2010, vol. 10(148).

[15]   Storey C., Ford J., Cheater F., Hurst K., Leese B. 'Nurses working in primary and community care settings in England: problems and challenges in identifying numbers'. *Journal of Nursing Management.* 2007, vol. 15(8), pp. 847–52.

[16]   Steinwald B., Ginsburg P., Brandt C., Lee S., Patel K. *Medicare graduate medical education funding is not addressing the primary care shortage: we need a radically different approach [online].* 2018. Available from https://www.brookings.edu/research/medicare-graduate-medical-education-funding-is-not-addressing-the-primary-care-shortage-we-need-a-radically-different-approach.

[17]   Dall T., West T., Chakrabarti R., Iacobucci W., Brunec P. *The Complexities of Physician Supply and Demand: Projections from 2013 to 2025 Final Report.* Washington, DC: Association of American Medical Colleges; 2015.

[18]   Long T., Chaiyachati K., Bosu O. 'Why aren't more primary care residents going into primary care? A qualitative study'. *Journal of General Internal Medicine.* 2016, vol. 12, pp. 1452–9.

[19]   Westerhout W. 'Does ageing call for a reform of the health care sector?' *CESifo Economic Studies.* 2016, vol. 52:1, pp. 1–31.

[20]   Hsiao W., Heller P. 'What should macroeconomists know about health care policy'? [online]. IMF Working Paper 07/13. Washington, DC: IMF. 2007. Available from https://www.imf.org/external/pubs/ft/wp/2007/wp0713.pdf.

[21]   Getzen T.E. 'Population aging and the growth of health expenditures'. *Journal of Gerontology.* 1992, vol. 47(3), pp. S98–104.

[22]   Zweifel P., Felder S., Meiers M. 'Ageing of population and health care expenditure: a red herring?' *Health Economics.* 1999, vol. 8(6), pp. 485–96.

[23]   Smith S., Newhouse J.P., Freeland M.S. 'Income, insurance, and technology: why does health spending outpace economic growth?' *Health Affairs.* 2009, vol. 28(5), pp. 1276–84.

[24]   Colombier C. 'Population ageing in healthcare – a minor issue? Evidence from Switzerland'. *Applied Economics.* 2018, vol. 50(15), pp. 1746–60.

[25]   Outreville J.F. 'The ageing population and the future of healthcare plans'. *Geneva Papers on Risk and Insurance – Issues and Practice.* 2001, vol. 26(1), pp. 126–31.

[26]   Geue C., Briggs A., Lewsey J., Lorgelly P. 'Population ageing and healthcare expenditure projections: new evidence from a time to death approach'. *The European Journal of Health Economics.* 2014, vol. 15(8), pp. 885–96.

[27]   National Institute on Aging. *Why population aging matters: a global perspective [online].* 2007. Available from https://2001-2009.state.gov/documents/organization/81775.pdf.

[28]   United Nations Department of Economic and Social Affairs. *National transfer accounts manual: measuring and analysing the generational economy [online].* 2013. Available from https://www.un.org/en/development/desa/population/publications/pdf/development/Final_March2014.pdf.

[29] World Bank. *Averting the old age crisis: policies to protect the old and promote growth [online]*. 1994. Available from https://documents.worldbank.org/en/publication/documents-reports/documentdetail/973571468174557899/averting-the-old-age-crisis-policies-to-protect-the-old-and-promote-growth.

[30] OECD. 'Fiscal challenges and inclusive growth in ageing societies'. *OECD Economic Policy Paper*. 2019, vol. 27, pp. 1–69.

[31] Mejido M. *Harnessing the second demographic dividend: population ageing and social protection in Asia and the Pacific [online]*. Social Development Working Papers. 2019. Available from https://www.unescap.org/sites/default/files/SDWP%202019-03_Demographic%20Dividend.pdf.

[32] United Nations Economic and Social Commission for Asia and the Pacific. *Ageing and its economic implications [online]*. Social Development Policy Papers. 2020. Available from https://www.unescap.org/sites/default/d8files/knowledge-products/Ageing%20and%20its%20economic%20implications.pdf.

[33] World Economic Forum. *We'll live to 100 – How can we afford it? [online]*. WEF White Paper. 2017. Available from http://www3.weforum.org/docs/WEF_White_Paper_We_Will_Live_to_100.pdf.

[34] Mercer CFA Institute. *Melbourne mercer global pension index 2020 [online]*. 2020. Available from https://www.mercer.com.au/content/dam/mercer/attachments/private/asia-pacific/australia/campaigns/mcgpi-2020/MCGPI-2020-full-report-1.pdf.

[35] Ikeda D., Saito M. 'The effects of demographic changes on the real interest rate in Japan'. *Japan and the World Economy*. 2014, vol. 32(2), pp. 37–48.

[36] Anderson D., Botman D., Hunt B. *Is Japan's population ageing deflationary?. [online]* IMF Working Paper WP/14/139. 2014. Available from https://www.imf.org/external/pubs/ft/wp/2014/wp14139.pdf.

[37] Gagnon E., Johannsen B.K., Lopez-Salido D. 'Understanding the new normal: the role of demographics'. *Finance and Economics Discussion Series*. 2016, vol. 2016(080).

[38] Lisack N., Sajedi R., Thwaites G. *Demographic trends and the real interest rate. [online]* Bank of England Staff Working Paper 701. 2017. Available from https://www.frbsf.org/economic-research/files/4-Thwaites-demographic-trends-and-the-real-interest-rate.pdf.

[39] Carvalho C., Ferrero A., Nechio F. 'Demographics and real interest rates: inspecting the mechanism'. *European Economic Review*. 2016, vol. 88, pp. 208–26.

[40] Lee R., Mason A. 'What is the demographic dividend?' *Finance & Development*. 2006, vol. 43, pp. 16–17.

[41] Mason A., Kinugasa T. 'East Asian economic development: two demographic dividends'. *Journal of Asian Economics*. 2008, vol. 19(5-6), pp. 389–99.

[42] Gonand F., Jouvet P.-A. 'The "second dividend" and the demographic structure'. *Journal of Environmental Economics and Management*. 2015, vol. 72(2), pp. 71–97.

[43]   United Nations Department of Economic and Social Affairs. *World popula-tion prospects: the 2015 revision [online]*. 2015. Available from https://popu-lation.un.org/wpp/Publications/Files/Key_Findings_WPP_2015.pdf.

[44]   OECD. *Preventing ageing unequally [online]*. 2017. Available from 10.1787/9789264279087-en.

[45]   OECD. *Promoting an Age-Inclusive workforce: living learning and earning longer [online]*. 2020. Available from 10.1787/59752153-en.

[46]   United Nations Department of Economic and Social Affairs. *World popula-tion ageing 2020 highlights. [online]* ST/ESA/SER.A/451. 2020. Available from https://www.un.org/development/desa/pd/sites/www.un.org.develop-ment.desa.pd/files/undesa_pd-2020_world_population_ageing_highlights.pdf.

[47]   Global Entrepreneurship Monitor. *Report on senior entrepreneurship [online]*. 2017. Available from https://gemconsortium.org/report/gem-2016-2017-report-on-senior-entrepreneurship.

[48]   Fried L.P. 'Investing in health to create a third demographic dividend'. *The Gerontologist*. 2016a, vol. 56 Suppl 2,S2,pp. 167–77.

[49]   Fried L.P. 'Building a third demographic dividend: strengthening intergenera-tional well-being in ways that deeply matter'. *Public Policy & Aging Report*. 2016, vol. 26(3), pp. 78–82.

[50]   Irving P., Beamish R., Burstein A. *Silver to gold: the business of aging. Milken Institute Research Report [online]*. 2018. Available from https://as-sets1c.milkeninstitute.org/assets/Publication/ResearchReport/PDF/FINAL-Silver-to-Gold-0226.pdf.

[51]   U.N. General Assembly. *Follow-up to international year of older persons: Second world assembly on ageing: Report of the Secretary-General. A/75/218. UN [online]*. 2020a. Available from https://undocs.org/A/75/218.

[52]   World Health Organization & United Nations Children's Fund. A vision for primary health care in the 21st century: towards universal health coverage and the sustainable development goals. *Technical Series on Primary Health Care [online]*. 2018. Available from https://apps.who.int/iris/handle/10665/328065.

[53]   World Health Organization and ITU. *Be He@lthy be mobile: a handbook on how to implement m-Ageing [online]*. 2020. Available from http://handle.itu.int/11.1002/pub/814a72ca-en.

Chapter 4

Digital health and elderly care in low- and middle-income countries: opportunities and challenges

Fatema Khatun[1], Sabrina Rasheed[1], Sifat Parveen Sheikh[1], Kazi Nazmus Saqeeb[1], and Daniel D. Reidpath[1]

4.1 Introduction

The trends in population growth among the elderly have changed within the last 40 years due to declining birth and death rates and rising life expectancy [1]. From 1980 to 2019, the global population aged 65 years increased more than twofold, the current number being about 703 million [2]. Currently, more than two-thirds of the elderly population reside in low- and middle-income countries (LMICs) [3] while the numbers are projected to expand to 1.5 billion by 2050, with about 79% of the elderly population predicted to live in LMICs [2]. This increase in the number of older adults has important implications for health systems in developing countries, as elderlies present a wide range of morbidities, particularly attributable to non-communicable diseases (NCDs) [4]. Diabetes, cardiovascular diseases, cancer and respiratory diseases are the "big four NCDs," contributing to majority of deaths (87%) and disability-adjusted life years (54%) attributable to NCDs [4]. Elderly individuals with pre-existing chronic conditions are also more likely to develop severe manifestations of certain communicable diseases as revealed during the recent COVID-19 outbreak [5]. In 2012, the World Health Assembly set the target of a relative reduction in NCD-related deaths by 25% by 2025, known as the "25×25 target" [6]. The lack of resources and scarcity of healthcare providers in LMICs make it extremely difficult to meet this target [7]. The inequities in healthcare, particularly among elderlies in LMICs, can potentially be addressed through digital health technology [8].

The use of digital technology is now ubiquitous, even in low-resource settings [9]. In developed countries, digital health has been used in geriatric care for providing disease-related information and appointment reminders [10], delivering consultation services through telemedicine [11], remote monitoring of vital signs and patient self-management [12], clinical and pharmacy decision-support systems [13],

[1]Health Systems and Population Studies Division, International Centre for Diarrhoeal Disease Research, Dhaka, Bangladesh

prevention of fall [14] and improving the continuum of care [15]. The effectiveness of the use of mobile health (mHealth) technology in supporting geriatric care has been tested in several LMICs, although in a limited scale [16]. Several challenges exist including relatively poor penetration of technology among the elderly population, inadequate financial resources, lower technical competence and skills among users and healthcare providers and lack of knowledge and trust in digital health among the patients and their caregivers [17]. Despite the bottlenecks, digital health presents an opportunity for improving the access, efficiency and affordability of elderly healthcare in LMICs [18]. This chapter discusses the context of using digital technology for geriatric care in LMICs, e.g., the use of such tools in elderly care in low-resource settings, the associated challenges, ethical issues and policy implications. We also propose a conceptual framework with relevant case studies for integrating the technology in geriatric care in the developing world.

4.2   Context of elderly care in LMIC

In LMICs, elderly people mostly live with family members or within the support network of family and friends [19]. Institutional living for the elderly is still underdeveloped in such countries [20]. This creates opportunities to think about involving family and social networks to support elderly care [21]. However, the efficiency of professional management of the care that is more likely to be available through an institutional setting will not be achievable. Another important challenge in the context of LMICs is the lack of focus and readiness of the health systems to provide elderly care at the primary level. In many LMICs, primary care is designed to provide maternal and child health services along with limited curative care and often these services are being provided by paraprofessionals rather than trained doctors or nurses. In addition, many of these countries suffer from a shortage of trained workforce both in numbers [22] and in distribution (concentrated in urban areas) [23]. In this context, digital health can be potentially employed to strengthen the gaps in the service provision for the elderly. Till now most of the eHealth or mHealth projects tested in LMICs have focused on reproductive maternal and child health and selected NCDs, and a very few have focused on the elderly population. However, the experience of providing health service solution shows promise. Major elderly care includes chronic diseases care (respiratory diseases, heart disease, cancer and diabetes), fall prevention, psychological supports for depression, neurocognitive disorder and medication adherence. Self-management skills and the use of newer technology can find out innovative ways for their appropriate care.

4.3   The digital divide

Despite the promise of using digital technology to provide health information and services to the elderly, it is important to consider the existing digital divide that has been shown to affect the uptake of technology in LMICs. The term digital divide is used to describe the gaps in access, usage and uptake of technology among individuals or groups, which may be attributable to both voluntary and involuntary factors [24]. Involuntary factors include the lack of opportunities, such as financial constraints that limit the purchasing power for electronic gadgets and voluntary factors consider the lack of interest or motivation, from the user's side [25].

For example, women are 8% less likely to own a mobile phone and 20% less likely to possess a smartphone, when compared to men [26]. Also, females are 20% less likely to use the internet to access health-related information [26]. Older individuals' usage of technology is significantly lower compared to the young [27]. Richer individuals are more likely to be able to afford electronic devices and have the knowledge and skills to use them adequately. In urban settings, the penetration of technology is usually higher compared to rural areas in LMICs [18]. However, higher penetration or access to technology does not necessarily imply optimum utilization. For example, an elderly person may use an android phone for voice calls only but may not be oriented to other available functions such as video calling, internet browsing, etc. [28]. A person's ability to optimally use existing digital technology has been categorized by Van Dijk *et al.* [29] into five criteria: (1) Material (financial ability, possession), (2) Mental (technical skills, motivation), (3) Social (a social support system to assist the use), (4) Temporal (adequate time to use electronic device) and (5) Cultural (status and liking of use) [29]. The first three factors largely determine the use of technology among the elderly in LMICs. For elderly individuals, the inadequacy of time may not be an issue. Also, little is known about the perceived cultural barriers for the use of technology in an LMIC among the elderly.

Eynon *et al.* [25] have described the digital divide among the elderly at two levels. The first level of the digital divide is "uptake," which stems from an involuntary exclusion from electronic devices and the internet [25]. In low-resource settings, elderly individuals usually have financial limitations and are less likely to invest in technology that is expensive [30]. Moreover, in some rural and remote areas, internet access is still inadequate. The second-level digital divide is related to the "use" of digital devices and deals with differences in willingness or skills of using technology [31]. Majority of older individuals lack the skills to adopt new and complex technologies compared to younger people [32]. Older adults may not feel comfortable in integrating technology within their daily lives and reduced cognitive function may not allow the usage of complex electronic devices. Low English proficiency can also be a barrier to the use of digital devices as mobile phones often need additional input to allow local languages [29]. Moreover, older people have various physical and functional limitations such as poor visual acuity, limited manual dexterity and, in many cases, impaired cognitive function, which may limit their ability to use technology [33]. Studies have shown that age-related frailty significantly reduces the uptake of technology [34]. Another important barrier reported that impedes the use of digital technology is the issue of trust [35]. However, positive experiences of using digital technology for elderly health in LMICs have also been documented [17].

4.4   Use of digital tools for elderly care

In developing countries, digital initiatives for elderly care are few due to resource constraints and higher priority given to reproductive, maternal, newborn and child health and infectious diseases to achieve sustainable development goals [16]. In this section, we will discuss existing studies that utilized digital tools in low-resource settings for elderly care to identify some common elements that must be incorporated for the future.

In LMICs, mHealth has been employed for appointment reminders, health education, data collection, surveillance, supervision and monitoring [17]. However, there is limited data available on the impact of such interventions [36]. A handful of experimental studies involving the elderly population and digital health in LMICs focused on specific NCDs such as diabetes and cardiovascular diseases [37]. Beyond the pilot phase, however, evidence for scalability and integration of such projects into existing healthcare systems remains inadequate [38]. Studies discussed in Table 4.1 have been categorized according to WHO classification of digital health intervention. All studies discussed in Table 4.1 do not necessarily include the elderly patient population but apply to disease and disability associated with ageing (Table 4.1).

4.5   Framework for caregiver-mediated digital health support for elderlies in LMICs

We propose a conceptual framework based on the socio-ecological model (SEM) that involves the use of digital health targeted at different levels (individual, family, community and health system) in caring for the elderly (Figure 4.1) [46].

The framework will consider case studies that employed digital health tools for elderly care at different levels (individual, interpersonal, community and organizational) and in various healthcare settings.

Based on the case studies, we have identified some commonalities between the levels that are impacted by digital health interventions (Table 4.2). All of the interventions included individual and the health systems/organisation levels, as touchpoints. The case study involving the psychosocial support intervention in India was able to create a bridge between the individual, family (informal caregiver), community and the organisation. Based on Table 4.2 and case studies, we recommend an integrated design for elderly care in LMICs, where the informal caregiver can support the use of digital tools for the elderly individual's healthcare needs and communication with the formal health system. Well-designed digital health intervention follows the "human-centred design" an approach to interactive systems development that aims to make systems usable and useful by focusing on user requirements, which enhances effectiveness, accessibility, sustainability, improves user well-being and satisfaction [51]. However, for elderly care, the digital health intervention program needs to include the elderly and their caregivers (community healthcare providers, peer networks, formal healthcare providers) during the design phase [52].

Table 4.1 *Studies that dealt with elderly care in LMICs*

WHO classification of digital health intervention [39]	Disease/disability addressed	Location	Target population	Digital intervention	Healthcare domain	Outcome
1.1 Targeted client communication	Type 2 diabetes	India [40]	Patients with HbA1c >7%, insulin therapy ≥3 months	Cell phone-based text messaging	Adherence to a dietary regimen, physical activity and drug schedules)	Lower HbA1c in comparison to control group
1.1 Targeted client communication	Cervical cancer (Ca Cervix)	Kenya [41]	25–69 years who did not perform Ca Cervix screening before	Cell phone-based reminders for screening	Clinical compliance for screening of cancer	Intervention group: 8 times more likely to adhere to scheduled rescreening
1.1 Targeted client communication 2.3 Healthcare provider decision support	Cardiovascular disease (CVD)	India [42]	Patients aged 40–84 years with or at high risk of CVD	Multifaceted intervention with decision support, SMS reminders, etc.	• Treatment adherence • Healthcare quality • Continuum of care	Significant improvement in the use of blood pressure medication in the intervention group
1.1 Targeted client communication 2.4 Client-to-provider telemedicine	Type-2 diabetes	Pakistan [43]	Older adults, HbA1c≥8.0% and having functional mobile phone	Mobile phone voice calls	Clinical compliance	Lowered HbA1c levels in the intervention group
1.1 Targeted client communication	Cardiovascular risk factors	Iran [44]	Post-menopausal women. Age: 40–60 years; BMI >25	Cell phone-based text messaging	Lifestyle modification (physical activity and healthy food choices)	Increased consumption of vitamin A-rich fruits and vegetables and increased fish intake

(Continues)

Table 4.1   Continued

WHO classification of digital health intervention [39]	Disease/disability addressed	Location	Target population	Digital intervention	Healthcare domain	Outcome
1.1 Targeted client communication 2.4 Client-to-provider telemedicine	Psychiatric illness	Iran [45]	Male, war veterans with post-traumatic stress disorder (PTSD)	Mobile phone calls and SMS/ telenursing	Reduction of recurrence, treatment adherence	• Reduced severity of symptoms • Lower recurrence of PTSD • Improved quality of life

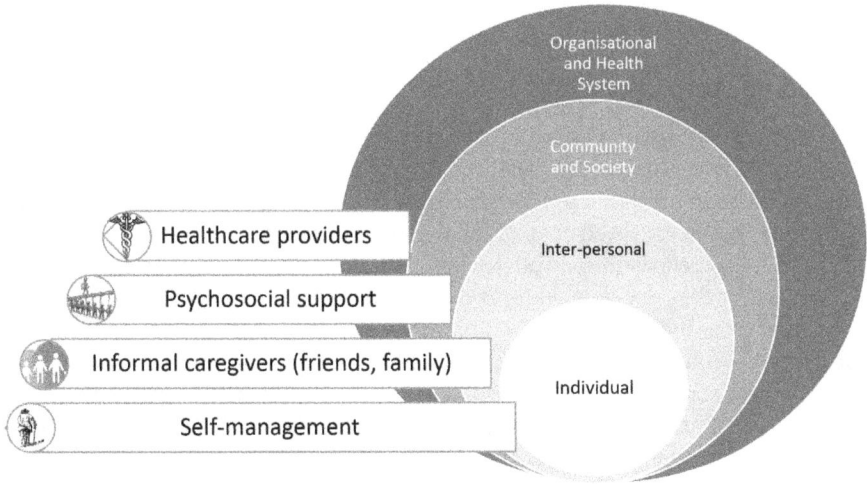

Figure 4.1   Socio-ecological framework applied to digital health in geriatric care

The "human-centred design" follows the sensitive issues that meet users' cultural, historical and societal requirements. Moreover, the ethics and policy implication of the intervention need to be taken into account [53].

4.6   Ethics and policy implications

The use of digital tools in elderly healthcare in LMICs has the potential to address critical gaps in health systems. However, the widespread use of such technologies in healthcare may give rise to ethical issues related to data privacy and governance [54]. The issues around privacy are related to the collection of passive health data through wearable devices, health-related apps, internet of things and android phones [55]. Moreover, data related to a patient's home environment can also yield sensitive information that patients or caregivers may not be comfortable sharing [56]. Researchers have argued that most patients and their caregivers, especially in low-resource setting, do not know about the extent and implications of the health data collected [57]. This problem is compounded by the lower literacy rates and lack of technical competency among users in developing countries. The personal identifier must be deleted from the data set according to the General Data Protection Regulation [58], which is not often followed in LMICs. Health-related data contains personal information, which may be easily used to reveal a person's identity in cases of caregiver-mediated digital health program [59]. Individuals intending to hack such data sources can obtain sensitive information about a patient, breaching security and confidentiality [60].

Individual

Case study 1: Role of digital health in self-management by elderly patients

An experimental study conducted in Iran compared the effectiveness of a tele-monitoring intervention with usual care for patients with heart failure [47]. Each patient in the intervention group received telemonitoring tailored to their needs. The intervention consisted of an evaluation of the patient's self-care status related to heart failure, education and advice on self-management, follow-up and revaluation. Self-management includes monitoring of symptoms such as dry cough and measuring body weight daily, recording and managing any new symptoms, restricting diet and fluid and performing exercise daily to prevent complications. Following discharge from the hospital, patients were contacted for telemonitoring by trained nurses throughout a period of 8 weeks, at weekly intervals. All study participants underwent post-test evaluation twice via phone calls, at 4 and 8 weeks after intervention. During this time, any history of readmission due to heart failure was asked and recorded. Self-care behaviours among heart failure patients significantly improved due to telemonitoring. Hospital readmission rates for the intervention group was about half of that of the control group, though insignificant.

Interpersonal (family and friends, informal caregivers)

Case study 2: Role of digital health in supporting the informal caregiver and elderly patients

In rural Thailand, experimental research was conducted upon one hundred patient-caregiver dyads attending a cardiac clinic for heart failure [48]. The intervention group received face-to-face counselling, a manual, a DVD and telephone support for heart failure. The control group received the usual care. Patients in the intervention group had higher scores for knowledge, better self-management, and quality of life scores at three and six months than those who received usual care. At six months, subjects who received digital education had better self-care management scores and at three months, informal caregivers had higher perceived control scores. Therefore, this digital intervention involving the informal caregiver helped to improve patient knowledge, behaviours around self-care, quality of life and caregiver knowledge and perceived control over care related to heart failure.

Community and society

Case study 3: Role of digital health in providing psychosocial support for elderly patients

The MINDS Foundation, India offers a spectrum of services related to mental health in rural India [49]. The project has three major components: (1) education

(Continues)

and awareness on mental illnesses and how it can be addressed through this service; (2) free conveyance for patients to the hospital to reduce cost-related barriers; and (3) a cell phone-based data collection app for community health workers to enable them to check up on the mental health status of the people in the community. The aim of the project is to empower patients so that they can gain control over their mental health with the help of family support and community resources. Moreover, through this project, individuals and their families received training for additional technical skills, assistance with job searching to help them find a place within their communities.

Organizational and health systems

Case study 4: Role of digital health in supporting communication between the healthcare provider and elderly patients

An intervention trial was conducted in Japan, to assess the effectiveness of telenursing in reducing or preventing postoperative complications in patients with prostate cancer (CA prostate) [50]. The intervention was designed to address postsurgical symptoms, thereby improving the quality of life (QOL) among patients who underwent surgery for CA prostate. First, the participants received face-to-face education from doctors and nurses about recommended postsurgical lifestyles and behaviours. After discharge from hospital, the participants were asked to log in through a tablet into a designated website and enter information regarding postoperative symptoms, from the comfort of their homes. They were asked to report symptoms such as urinary incontinence, bowel movement changes, symptoms of erectile dysfunction, sleep patterns, etc. Symptoms entered were automatically charted as virtual progress reports that was visible to both patients and providers. E-mail and chat functions were available that provided individualized nursing support in real time. The results of this study showed that QOL improved 3 months later. Telenursing helped patients improve their disease condition by sharing their goals, through constant communication with a healthcare provider.

4.6.1   Policy implications

To ensure the implementation of data governance, a formal structure for enforcement is necessary. Tiffin and colleagues recommend a framework of data governance for LMICs that incorporate the main pillars – ethics and consent, data access, sustainability and a legal framework (Figure 4.2) [61]. The components are discussed below.

4.6.1.1   Ethics and consent

First and foremost, it is essential to ensure that health-related data remains confidential. The standard practices include de-identification and maintaining the anonymity

Table 4.2   Commonalities of caregiver-mediated digital health support in the case studies

	Individual	Interpersonal	Community/ society	Organizational and health systems
Self-management	√			√
Informal caregiver	√	√		√
Psychosocial support	√	√	√	√
Healthcare provider	√			√

of data, though this may not be adequate to ensure the security and privacy of the patient information [62]. More robust approaches such as IT system administration and firewall restrictions should ensure limited access by designated individuals only [63]. Vulnerable populations such as the elderly, marginalized populations and those in humanitarian and conflict situations must be identified [64]. An additional layer of protection is necessary to prevent the higher potential of harm associated with breach of privacy of health data of such vulnerable individuals.

The informed consent process should include detailed information on (a) intended data use, (b) anonymity, (c) data protection, (d) risks, benefits and remuneration and (e) contact information for possible concerns/questions [61]. Any secondary use of data by third parties should also be clearly mentioned [65]. Moreover, the consenting procedure should be adapted to meet the ability of the user (literacy, tech-savviness, etc.) to ensure that the patient and their caregivers fully understand the implications of sharing such information [66].

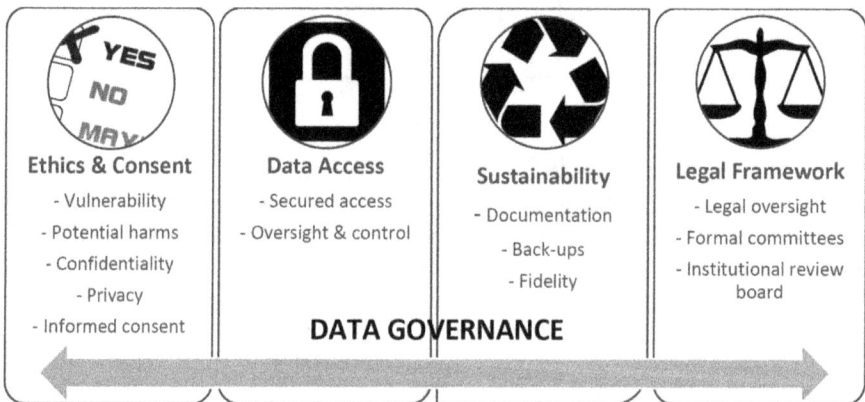

Ethics & Consent
- Vulnerability
- Potential harms
- Confidentiality
- Privacy
- Informed consent

Data Access
- Secured access
- Oversight & control

Sustainability
- Documentation
- Back-ups
- Fidelity

Legal Framework
- Legal oversight
- Formal committees
- Institutional review board

DATA GOVERNANCE

Figure 4.2   Pillars of governance of digital health data, adapted from Tiffin et al. [61]

4.6.1.2 Data access

Data protection and data access restrictions should include firewalls, encryptions, password protections in addition to system administration [67]. Tiered access to data as suited to the need of specific users is also another way of ensuring data privacy [68]. In addition to the storage of data, apps that are used for communication must also ensure controlled assess. A recent study shows that the WhatsApp chat app has been widely used in telemedicine in LMIC settings, with minimum emphasis on health data privacy or security [69]. This highlights the need for a low-cost, user-friendly, yet secure platform for patient-provider communication.

4.6.1.3 Sustainability

In LMICs, the lack of sustainability planning has led to experimentation of short-lived mobile and other digital health tools without adequate integration within the existing health system [36]. Ensuring sustainability requires formal data steward-ship with clear, consistent error-free data availability and storage. There should be adequate documentation and backup, along with adherence to the FAIR (F = Findable, A = Accessible, I = Interoperable and R = Reusable) principles of data management and stewardship [70].

4.6.1.4 Legal framework

Though not as formal as developed countries, many LMICs have implemented regulations to protect the privacy of patient information. For example, the Protection of Personal Information Act of South Africa provides guiding principles for safeguarding healthcare data [71]. In countries where formal legislative structures are not in place, Institutional Review Boards should act as gatekeepers for the protection of participants in digital health-related studies [61]. While ensuring robust digital data governance structure may be defined as the government's responsibility, researchers and relevant institutions have an important role to play in ensuring the consent and privacy of users.

4.7 Conclusion

This chapter focused on the use of digital tools in healthcare for elderly population in LMICs. Digital health presents a window of opportunities to provide health-related education, consultation, treatment, prevention services with the potential of improving the quality of life for elderlies. In this chapter, we provided a concise review of studies that employed digital tools for the management of diseases and disabilities of the elderly in developing countries. We also highlighted the role of family members or informal caregivers within the support system for elderlies. Furthermore, we adopted the SEM to introduce a conceptual framework through case studies that employed digital tools for elderly care in LMICs. Through this conceptual framework, our objective was to highlight the potential role of digital tools in connecting the informal support system with formal health services to minimize the gaps in elderly care in LMICs. Despite the rationale of employing digital tools in the field of elderly care, there are some unique barriers among the elderlies in a low-resource setting, such as the scarcity of resources, the digital divide and lack of policies to ensure data governance (and/or stewardship) giving rise to healthcare data-related ethical issues for vulnerable populations. Thus, the last section of this chapter meets our objectives of discussing possible ethical and policy implications, which are important considerations for both researchers and policymakers to ensure data security and foster the elderly patient's trust in digital health.

References

[1]   Bongaarts J. 'Human population growth and the demographic transition'. *Philosophical Transactions of the Royal Society B: Biological Sciences*. 2009, vol. 364(1532), pp. 2985–90.

[2]   United Nations Department of Economic and Social Affairs. 'Population division'. *World Population Ageing 2017 – Highlights (ST/ESA/SER.A/397)*. 2017.

[3]   Phillips D.R., Gyasi R.M. 'Global aging in a comparative context'. *The Gerontologist*. 2021, vol. 61(3), pp. 476–7.

[4]   Islam S.M.S., Purnat T.D., Phuong N.T.A., Mwingira U., Schacht K., Fröschl G. 'Non-communicable diseases (NCDS) in developing countries: a symposium report'. *Globalization and Health*. 2014, vol. 10(1), pp. 1–8.

[5]   Daoust J.-F. 'Elderly people and responses to COVID-19 in 27 countries'. *Plos One*. 2020, vol. 15(7),e0235590.

[6]   Kontis V., Mathers C.D., Bonita R., *et al.* 'Regional contributions of six preventable risk factors to achieving the 25×25 non-communicable disease mortality reduction target: a modelling study'. *The Lancet Global Health*. 2015, vol. 3(12), pp. e746–57.

[7]   Sharma A., Ladd E., Unnikrishnan M. 'Healthcare inequity and physician scarcity: empowering non-physician healthcare'. *Economic and Political Weekly*. 2013, pp. 112–17.

[8]   Griffiths F., Watkins J.A., Huxley C., *et al.* 'Mobile consulting (mConsulting) and its potential for providing access to quality healthcare for populations living in low-resource settings of low- and middle-income countries'. *Digital health*. 2020, vol. 6, pp. 1–17.

[9]   Ahmed T., Rizvi S.J.R., Rasheed S., *et al.* 'Digital health and inequalities in access to health services in Bangladesh: mixed methods study'. *JMIR mHealth and uHealth*. 2020, vol. 8(7),e16473.

[10] Meessen B. 'The role of digital strategies in financing health care for universal health coverage in low- and middle-income countries'. *Global Health: Science and Practice*. 2018, vol. 6(Supplement 1), pp. S29–40.

[11] Lupton D. 'Critical perspectives on digital health technologies'. *Sociology Compass*. 2014, vol. 8(12), pp. 1344–59.

[12] Lupton D. 'The digitally engaged patient: self-monitoring and self-care in the digital health era'. *Social Theory & Health*. 2013, vol. 11(3), pp. 256–70.

[13] O'Connor P.J., Sperl-Hillen J.M., Rush W.A., *et al*. 'Impact of electronic health record clinical decision support on diabetes care: a randomized trial'. *The Annals of Family Medicine*. 2011, vol. 9(1), pp. 12–21.

[14] Kannan M., Hildebrand A., Hugos C.L., Chahine R., Cutter G., Cameron M.H. 'Evaluation of a web-based fall prevention program among people with multiple sclerosis'. *Multiple Sclerosis and Related Disorders*. 2019, vol. 31, pp. 151–6.

[15] Mathews S.C., McShea M.J., Hanley C.L., Ravitz A., Labrique A.B., Cohen A.B. 'Digital health: a path to validation'. *NPJ Digital Medicine*. 2019, vol. 2(1), pp. 1–9.

[16] Mechael P.N. 'The case for mHealth in developing countries'. *Innovations: Technology, Governance, Globalization*. 2009, vol. 4(1), pp. 103–18.

[17] Latif S., Rana R., Qadir J., Ali A., Imran M.A., Younis M.S. 'Mobile health in the developing world: review of literature and lessons from a case study'. *IEEE Access*. 2017, vol. 5, pp. 11540–56.

[18] Wallis L., Blessing P., Dalwai M., Shin S.D. 'Integrating mHealth at point of care in low- and middle-income settings: the system perspective'. *Global health action*. 2017, vol. 10(sup3), pp. 29–36.

[19] Perkins J.M., Subramanian S.V., Christakis N.A. 'Social networks and health: a systematic review of sociocentric network studies in low- and middle-income countries'. *Social Science & Medicine*. 2015, vol. 125, pp. 60–78.

[20] Shetty P. 'Grey matter: ageing in developing countries'. *The Lancet*. 2012, vol. 379(9823), pp. 1285–7.

[21] Garay Villegas S., Montes de Oca Zavala V., Guillén J, Villegas S.G, de Oca Zavala V.M. 'Social support and social networks among the elderly in Mexico'. *Journal of Population Ageing*. 2014, vol. 7(2), pp. 143–59.

[22] Anyangwe S.C.E., Mtonga C. 'Inequities in the global health workforce: the greatest impediment to health in sub-Saharan Africa'. *International Journal of Environmental Research and Public Health*. 2007, vol. 4(2), pp. 93–100.

[23] Zurn P., Dal Poz M.R., Stilwell B., Adams O., *et al*. 'Imbalance in the health workforce'. *Human Resources for Health*. 2004, vol. 2(1), pp. 1–12.

[24] Mossberger K., Tolbert C.J., Stansbury M. *Virtual Inequality: Beyond The Digital Divide*. Georgetown University Press; 2003.

[25] Eynon R., Helsper E. 'Adults learning online: digital choice and/or digital exclusion?' *New Media & Society*. 2011, vol. 13(4), pp. 534–51.

[26] Rowntree O., Shanahan M. Connected women: the mobile gender gap report 2020. London, UK: GSMA; 2020. pp. 4–5. Available from www.gsma.com/mobilefordevelopment/wp-content/uploads/2020/05/GSMA-The-Mobile-Gender-Gap-Report-2020.pdf.

[27] Cosco T.D., Firth J., Vahia I., Sixsmith A., Torous J. 'Mobilizing mHealth data collection in older adults: challenges and opportunities'. *JMIR Aging*. 2019, vol. 2(1),e10019.

[28]   Campbell R.J., Nolfi D.A. 'Teaching elderly adults to use the Internet to access health care information: before-after study'. *Journal of Medical Internet Research*. 2005, vol. 7(2),e19.

[29]   Van Dijk J.A. 'A theory of the digital divide'. *The Digital Divide*. 29; 2013. pp. 29–51.

[30]   Friemel T.N. 'The digital divide has grown old: determinants of a digital divide among seniors'. *New Media & Society*. 2016, vol. 18(2), pp. 313–31.

[31]   Van Deursen A., Van Dijk J. 'Internet skills and the digital divide'. *New Media & Society*. 2011, vol. 13(6), pp. 893–911.

[32]   Henriquez-Camacho C., Losa J., Miranda J.J., Cheyne N.E., *et al.* 'Addressing healthy aging populations in developing countries: unlocking the opportunity of eHealth and mHealth'. *Emerging Themes in Epidemiology*. 2014, vol. 11(1), pp. 1–8.

[33]   Gell N.M., Rosenberg D.E., Demiris G., LaCroix A.Z., Patel K.V. 'Patterns of technology use among older adults with and without disabilities'. *The Gerontologist*. 2015, vol. 55(3), pp. 412–21.

[34]   Keränen N.S., Kangas M., Immonen M., *et al.* 'Use of information and communication technologies among older people with and without frailty: a population-based survey'. *Journal of Medical Internet Research*. 2017, vol. 19(2),e29.

[35]   Adjekum A., Blasimme A., Vayena E. 'Elements of trust in digital health systems: Scoping review'. *Journal of Medical Internet Research*. 2018, vol. 20(12),e11254.

[36]   Huang F., Blaschke S., Lucas H. 'Beyond pilotitis: taking digital health interventions to the National level in China and Uganda'. *Globalization and Health*. 2017, vol. 13(1), pp. 1–11.

[37]   Devi R., Kanitkar K., Narendhar R., Sehmi K., Subramaniam K. 'A narrative review of the patient journey through the lens of non-communicable diseases in low- and middle-income countries'. *Advances in Therapy*. 2020, vol. 37(12), pp. 4808–30.

[38]   Shuvo T.A., Islam R., Hossain S., *et al.* 'eHealth innovations in LMICs of Africa and Asia: a literature review exploring factors affecting implementation, scale-up, and sustainability'. *Healthcare*. 2015, vol. 2, pp. 95–106.

[39]   World Health Organization. WHO guideline: recommendations on digital interventions for health system strengthening. Geneva: World Health Organization; 2019. pp. 1–175. Available from WHO-RHR-19.7-eng.pdf.

[40]   Boels A.M., Rutten G., Zuithoff N., de Wit A., Vos R. 'Effectiveness of diabetes self-management education via a smartphone application in insulin treated type 2 diabetes patients – design of a randomised controlled trial ("TRIGGER study")'. *BMC endocrine disorders*. 2018, vol. 18(1),74.

[41]   Wanyoro A., Kaburi E. 'Use of mobile phone short text message service to enhance cervical cancer screening at Thika level 5 Hospital, Kiambu County, Kenya: a randomised controlled trial'. *Research in Obstetrics and Gynecology*. 2017, vol. 5(1), pp. 10–20.

[42] Praveen D., Patel A., Raghu A., *et al.* 'SMARTHealth India: development and field evaluation of a mobile clinical decision support system for cardiovascular diseases in rural India'. *JMIR mHealth and uHealth*. 2014, vol. 2(4),e54.

[43] Shahid M., Mahar S.A., Shaikh S., Shaikh Z. 'Mobile phone intervention to improve diabetes care in rural areas of Pakistan: a randomized controlled trial'. *Journal of the College of Physicians and Surgeons—Pakistan : JCPSP*. 2015, vol. 25(3), pp. 166–71.

[44] Vakili M., Abedi P., Afshari P., Kaboli N.E. 'The effect of mobile phone short messaging system on healthy food choices among Iranian postmenopausal women'. *Journal of Mid-Life Health*. 2015, vol. 6(4),154.

[45] Haghnia Y., Samad-Soltani T., Yousefi M., Sadr H., Rezaei-Hachesu P. 'Telepsychiatry-based care for the treatment follow-up of Iranian war veterans with post-traumatic stress disorder: a randomized controlled trial'. *Iranian Journal of Medical Sciences*. 2019, vol. 44(4),291.

[46] Bronfenbrenner U. *The Ecology of Human Development*. Harvard University Press; 1979.

[47] Negarandeh R., Zolfaghari M., Bashi N., Kiarsi M. 'Evaluating the effect of monitoring through telephone (tele-monitoring) on self-care behaviors and readmission of patients with heart failure after discharge'. *Applied Clinical Informatics*. 2019, vol. 10(2), pp. 261–8.

[48] Srisuk N., Cameron J., Ski C.F., Thompson D.R. 'Randomized controlled trial of family-based education for patients with heart failure and their carers'. *Journal of Advanced Nursing*. 2017, vol. 73(4), pp. 857–70.

[49] Shah S.H., Byer L.E., Appasani R.K., Aggarwal N.K. 'Impact of a community-based mental health awareness program on changing attitudes of the general population toward mental health in Gujarat, India—a study of 711 respondents'. *Industrial Psychiatry Journal*. 2020, vol. 29(1),97.

[50] Sato D. 'Effectiveness of telenursing for postoperative complications in patients with prostate cancer'. *Asia-Pacific Journal of Oncology Nursing*. 2020, vol. 7(4), p. 396.

[51] Holeman I., Kane D. 'Human-centered design for global health equity'. *Information Technology for Development*. 2020, vol. 26(3), pp. 477–505.

[52] Portz J.D., Ford K.L., Doyon K., *et al.* 'Using grounded theory to inform the human-centered design of digital health in geriatric palliative care'. *Journal of Pain and Symptom Management*. 2020, vol. 60(6), pp. 1181–92.

[53] Jokinen A., Stolt M., Suhonen R. 'Ethical issues related to eHealth: an integrative review'. *Nursing Ethics*. 2021, vol. 28(2), pp. 253–71.

[54] Ho C.W.L., Soon D., Caals K., Kapur J., Ho C. 'Governance of automated image analysis and artificial intelligence analytics in healthcare'. *Clinical Radiology*. 2019, vol. 74(5), pp. 329–37.

[55] Cornet V.P., Holden R.J. 'Systematic review of smartphone-based passive sensing for health and wellbeing'. *Journal of Biomedical Informatics*. 2018, vol. 77, pp. 120–32.

[56] Segura Anaya L.H., Alsadoon A., Costadopoulos N., Prasad P.W.C., Anaya L.S. 'Ethical implications of user perceptions of wearable devices'. *Science and Engineering Ethics*. 2018, vol. 24(1), pp. 1–28.

[57] Hossain N., Yokota F., Sultana N., Ahmed A. 'Factors influencing rural end-users' acceptance of e-health in developing countries: A study on portable health clinic in bangladesh'. *Telemedicine and e-Health*. 2019, vol. 25(3), pp. 221–9.

[58] Kelman C.W., Bass A.J., Holman C.D.J. 'Research use of linked health data—a best practice protocol'. *Australian and New Zealand Journal of Public Health*. 2002, vol. 26(3), pp. 251–5.

[59] Pharow P., Blobel B. 'Mobile health requires mobile security: challenges, solutions, and standardization'. *Studies in Health Technology and Informatics*. 2008, vol. 136,697.

[60] Maher N.A., Senders J.T., Hulsbergen A.F.C., *et al.* 'Passive data collection and use in healthcare: a systematic review of ethical issues'. *International Journal of Medical Informatics*. 2019, vol. 129, pp. 242–7.

[61] Tiffin N., George A., LeFevre A.E. 'How to use relevant data for maximal benefit with minimal risk: digital health data governance to protect vulnerable populations in low-income and middle-income countries'. *BMJ Global Health*. 2019, vol. 4(2),e001395.

[62] Nelson G.S. 'Practical implications of sharing data: a primer on data privacy, anonymization, and de-identification'. SAS Global Forum Proceedings; Dallas, Texas, March, 2015; 2015. pp. 1–23.

[63] Mackenzie I.S., Mantay B.J., McDonnell P.G., Wei L., MacDonald T.M. 'Managing security and privacy concerns over data storage in healthcare research'. *Pharmacoepidemiology and Drug Safety*. 2011, vol. 20(8), pp. 885–93.

[64] Perakslis E.D. 'Using digital health to enable ethical health research in conflict and other humanitarian settings'. *Conflict and Health*. 2018, vol. 12(1),p. 23.

[65] Caine K., Hanania R. 'Patients want granular privacy control over health information in electronic medical records'. *Journal of the American Medical Informatics Association*. 2013, vol. 20(1), pp. 7–15.

[66] William C. '22 Privacy and security: privacy of personal ehealth data in low-and middle-income countries'. *Global Health Informatics: Principles of eHealth and mHealth to Improve Quality of Care*. 2017, vol. 14, pp. 269–76.

[67] Cucoranu I.C., Parwani A.V., West A.J., *et al.* 'Privacy and security of patient data in the pathology laboratory'. *Journal of Pathology Informatics*. 2013, vol. 4,4.

[68] Broes S., Lacombe D., Verlinden M., Huys I. 'Toward a tiered model to share clinical trial data and samples in precision oncology'. *Frontiers in Medicine*. 2018, vol. 5,6.

[69] Mars M., Scott R.E. 'WhatsApp in clinical practice: a literature review'. *Studies in Health Technology and Informatics*. 2016, vol. 231, pp. 82–90.

[70] Boeckhout M., Zielhuis G.A., Bredenoord A.L. 'The fair guiding principles for data stewardship: fair enough?' *European Journal of Human Genetics.* 2018, vol. 26(7), pp. 931–6.

[71] Buys M. 'Protecting personal information: implications of the protection of personal information (POPI) act for healthcare professionals'. *South African Medical Journal.* 2017, vol. 107(11), pp. 954–6.

Chapter 5

Health co-benefits in climate action policies for healthy ageing

Sardar Masud Karim[1], Siaw-Teng Liaw[2], and Pradeep Ray[2,3]

5.1 Introduction

"Ageing is like climbing a mountain, you get out of breath but you have a magnificent view" (Ingmar Bergman). The world has seen a rapid rise in life expectancy and a reduction of morbidity, thanks to the advances in medical science. However, healthy life cannot be achieved only by taking medications and it depends on various factors in a person's life including economic condition, social and environmental factors, education, upbringing, etc. The WHO Report on Global Age-friendly Cities provides a holistic view involving six key determinants of Active Ageing (personal, physical environment, economic, social, behavioural and social+health services) [1].

"Healthy ageing is the process of optimising opportunities for physical, social and mental health to enable older people to take an active part in society without discrimination and to enjoy an independent, good quality of life." The determinants of Healthy Ageing include access to health care in rural/urban areas, physical environment, transport and infrastructure, employment and working conditions, housing, education, social issues, pensions, justice, violence and abuse. The European Union (EU) Project called 'Healthy Ageing' looked into various aspects of healthy ageing (including physical environment) from a global policy perspective. The project concluded that it is important to address the impact of climate change, a major threat to the survival in the long run and poses many potential risks to the health of the vulnerable sections of the global population [2]. As health benefits of low-carbon measures and technologies can contribute to healthy ageing both directly (e.g. reducing lung diseases) and indirectly (e.g. reducing co-morbidities due to

[1]CRC for Low Carbon Living, UNSW, Sydney, New South Wales, Australia
[2]WHO Collaborating Centre on eHealth (AUS-135), School of Population Health, UNSW, Sydney, New South Wales, Australia
[3]Centre For Entrepreneurship, University of Michigan-Shanghai Jiao Tong University Joint Institute, Shanghai, China

ageing) policymakers should purposefully consider the health benefits of climate action policies in planning for healthy ageing. Over the past decade, there has been substantial development in terms of developing frameworks, methodologies and assessment tools that can support policymakers to identify, assess and incorporate health benefits of climate action policies in planning for healthy ageing.

There have been many studies and worldwide efforts (e.g. the Paris Climate Agreement) to tackle the problem by the reduction of carbon emission and energy consumption. These global policies are important given the ubiquitous impact of climate change on all areas of business and society, such as agriculture, oceanology, economy and health. At the same time, there is a need for actions at the government and business levels for a tangible impact.

In this chapter, we focus on the development and implementation of government planning policies on climate action, which are found to have wide-ranging non-climate-related benefits including significant health benefits that contribute to healthy ageing. This focus is defined by terming these additional benefits of climate action policies as 'co-benefits'. These co-benefits motivate governments to frame climate change mitigation in a positive light to operationalise broader economic, social, health and environmental benefits of low-carbon policies within the concept of sustainable development. This holistic approach has been globally formalised through the UN Sustainable Development Goals (UN SDGs).

The objectives of this chapter are to highlight the awareness of the importance of climate action in healthy ageing and how that can be implemented in a holistic manner through low-carbon planning of sustainable development. The chapter starts with Section 5.2 on the basics of climate action and relevance of co-benefits in accelerating climate action. Section 5.3 introduces the concept of co-benefits and its various applications in climate change-related policy studies. Section 5.4 discusses the frameworks, various methods and assessment tools which are used to integrate co-benefits into policy-decision-making process. Section 5.5 discusses how *Health Impact Assessment* (HIA) can be used to formally integrate health impacts of all planning policies. This is followed by a discussion in Section 5.6 of health co-benefits in the holistic context of healthy living as per UN SDGs. Section 5.7 discusses the current situation on the practical usage of health co-benefits in climate policy development in local councils in Australia. Section 5.8 concludes the chapter with some pointers to future work.

5.2   Co-benefits of climate action

Climate change is a major challenge to sustainable development [3]. Following the signing of the 2015 Paris Climate Agreement, countries who signed the agreement have been trying to develop national climate policies to cut their greenhouse gas (GHG) emissions. So far, the United Nations Framework Convention on Climate Change has received 165 pledges from these countries to lower their GHG emissions, which is known as Intended Nationally Determined Contributions (INDCs) [4]. Nevertheless, these INDCs are widely considered as insufficient to limit global temperature rise by 2°C, as targeted in the Paris Agreement [5, 6]. The review of global politics around climate change and international efforts to reach an agreement on climate change suggests that there are many reasons why countries are unable to consider climate change as a priority on their national agenda. These reasons include domestic politics around climate change, concerns about the costs of climate action on the economy and fairness of sharing the burden of the costs across various sectors of the economy [7]. The realisation that the goal of mitigating climate change alone may not be enough to draw public support for implementing GHG emissions-reduction measures in part has led to a growing awareness in and research on other non-climate-related benefits resulting from emissions-reduction measures. Over the years, research in the assessment of climate policies has found that these policies also have impacts on areas other than climate. A wide range of positive macro-economic, environmental, human health, social and equity effects are associated with most of the GHG emissions reduction measures. In many cases these non-climate-related benefits are greater than the value of benefits obtained from mitigating climate change per se. These additional benefits from climate change mitigation are often referred to as 'co-benefits'. Sections 5.3 and 5.4 provide an understanding of co-benefits in terms of what they are, how the concept is applied in climate action and how they can be incorporated into policy-decision-making process.

5.3 Defining co-benefits

A basic understanding of what does 'co-benefits' mean is necessary to navigate a wide spectrum of concepts found in the literature that are related to co-benefits. Generally, in public policy discourse, the positive effects of a policy that happen apart from the planned primary goal of that policy are commonly considered as 'co-benefits' [8]. However, in climate change-related policy discourse, the co-benefits concept is applied as a 'win-win strategy' aimed at capturing both 'development and climate benefits' in one or a specific set of policies or measures [9].

The use of the term 'co-benefits' was first observed in the literature during the 1990s. At that time, it focused mostly on reconciling environmental and developmental goals. Later, co-benefits generated wider interest when the Intergovernmental Panel on Climate Change (IPCC) in the Third Assessment Report differentiated co-benefits as 'the intended positive side-effects of a climate policy from its unintended positive side-effects' [10].

More recently, the use of the co-benefits terminology in literature can be distinguished in four distinct streams of climate policy-related studies:

- 'Development co-benefits' denote the non-climate benefits that occur from climate policies at a local level. These include a wide variety of benefits such as health benefits from reduced air pollution to economic benefits from reduced energy usage to the creation of more jobs through use of cleaner and energy-efficient technologies.

- 'Climate co-benefits' refer to the climate benefits of GHG emissions reduction resulting from policies and measures planned for the purpose of development. This view of co-benefits originated given the need of developing countries to give priority to development over climate when considering climate change [11].
- 'Climate and air co-impacts' relate to the multiple effects of policies designed to reduce air pollution at local and regional levels. This view is held by researchers in air-pollution research when focusing on the impacts of short-lived climate pollutants, such as hydrofluorocarbons, black carbon and ozone or short-term climate coolers, such as sulphur dioxide [12].
- 'Climate and health impacts' relate to the effects of climate change on human health. Climate change is causing enormous adverse impact on the livelihood of common people due to the rising sea levels. For example, researchers of International Centre for Diarrhoeal Disease Research, Bangladesh, have identified that the health of the villagers in coastal areas of Bangladesh, is adversely affected by drinking underground water that has become saline due to rising sea levels [13].

The above observations suggest that the application of the co-benefits concept is not rigid. The concept has no clearly identifiable boundaries, and there is a notable absence of a unanimous definition of the term in the literature. Depending on the way the term is used in targeted areas or sectors of policy studies, the definition may vary. Several notable definitions of co-benefits used by major organisations in co-benefits studies related to climate change policies are presented here:

> 'The benefits of policies that are implemented for various reasons at the same time including climate change mitigation — acknowledging that most policies designed to address greenhouse gas mitigation also have other, often at least equally important rationales (e.g. related objectives of development, sustainability, and equity). The term *co-impact* is used in a more generic sense to cover both positive and negative side of benefits.' [10]
> 'Co-benefits approach refers to the development and implementation of policies and strategies that simultaneously contribute to tackling climate change whilst addressing local environmental and developmental problems.' [14]
> 'For GHG mitigation policies, co-benefits can best be defined as effects that are additional to direct reductions of GHG and impacts of climate change and have estimated to be large, relative to the costs of mitigation (e.g. anywhere from 30% to over 100% of abatement costs).' [15]

A critical review of these definitions suggests that they are based on a common understanding that policies explicitly formulated to address climate or development objectives can generate other benefits. Therefore, in the discourse on climate change-related policy, co-benefits are widely understood as the set of benefits occurring due

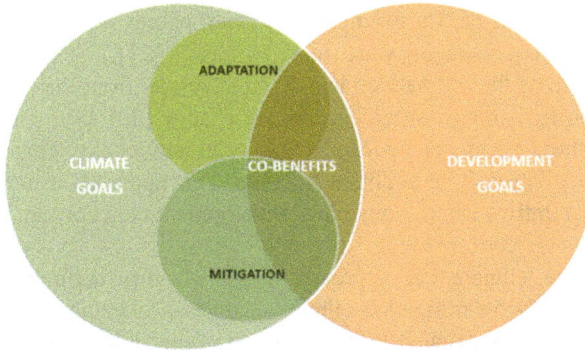

Figure 5.1   Co-benefits – conceptual diagram

to actions that connect the climate-change goals (both mitigation and adaptation) with other development goals (see Figure 5.1).

The IPCC in its Fifth Assessment Report (AR5) has used the terms 'co-benefits' and 'adverse side-effects' with respect to 'the positive and negative side-effects', respectively, of climate change 'mitigation policies and measures' [16]. The IPCC also used the term 'co-impacts' to include both positive and negative side-effects [17, 18]. This chapter will be consistent with this and considers all positive side-effects of policies and programmes related to climate change mitigation as co-benefits.

5.4   Co-benefits: applications, frameworks, methods and assessment tools

This section discusses various application of co-benefits concept, frameworks, methods and assessment tools that are commonly used in co-benefits studies to identify, quantify and incorporate co-benefits in existing policy-decision-making frameworks.

5.4.1   Applications of co-benefits concept

Policy-makers prioritise and value policy goals differently when addressing climate change in their policies. They rarely devise policies with the aim to mitigate climate change alone, but most policies that are intended to address climate change typically serves other purposes as well. What policy-makers consider as the primary aim of a policy determines what benefit(s) of that policy would be co-benefit(s) to the primary (or direct) benefit of that policy. Depending on the valuation policy-makers place on climate-change mitigation compared with other goals, three different applications of the co-benefits concept can be distinguished in the empirical research, resulting in notable difference in the approach and valuation of climate-policy goals.

First, is the 'development first' approach. In this category, policies are not specifically planned to address climate change but may nonetheless contribute towards mitigating climate change as a side-benefit (i.e. co-benefit). The main objective of these policies could be, for example, achieving energy security [19], obtaining health benefits [20] or managing waste more efficiently [21]. Climate change mitigation is referred to as the 'climate co-benefit' that results from the positive impacts of the development policies on global climate change [22]. The idea behind such application of the 'co-benefits' concept is that it can facilitate creating a pathway for development that is sensitive to climate change. This approach is mainly observed in developing countries where immediate development concerns are given priority over climate change concerns [23].

Second, is the 'climate first' approach. In this category, the policies studied are formulated primarily for mitigating climate change or adapting to climate change. Local positive impacts of such policies, for example, low-carbon energy policy might have positive effects on economic policy goals such as job creation [24] as well as health policy goal of improved public health [25], one example given in Section 5.3 [13]. These are considered as 'development co-benefits'. This is usually referred to as the 'climate first' approach.

Third, is the 'climate and other goal' approach. In this category the policies studied are characterised by the non-prioritisation of either goal (i.e. development or climate change mitigation) and are planned to attain both goals concurrently. A common example of such application of the co-benefits concept is 'climate and pollution co-benefits' [26] where policy measures to reduce GHGs simultaneously reduce other air-polluting gases (such as N_2O, NOx, NH_3), thereby automatically resulting in air-pollution control as a 'co-benefit'. The fundamental principle is to 'co-control of atmospheric emissions to yield simultaneous benefits for climate change and air quality' [27], with the benefits considered together as co-impacts or co-benefits.

5.4.2   *Identifying, quantifying and incorporating co-benefits into policy-decision-making*

Irrespective of various definitions of co-benefits and different applications of the co-benefits concept found in the literature, all co-benefits studies are essentially based on an overarching methodological framework that consists of three distinct phases: (i) identification, (ii) quantification and (iii) incorporation of co-benefits (see Figure 5.2).

Each phase relies on a specific set of assumptions, has certain limitations and faces specific methodological challenges in performing its respective tasks. This section provides a detailed guide for understanding these three phases of the co-benefits framework. It includes discussion of (a) some general challenges faced by each phase, (b) the assumptions and limitations of the methods utilised in respective phases and (c) a discussion of how to address these limitations of the existing framework in the context of future co-benefits studies.

5.4.2.1   Identifying and considering co-benefits

In general, most co-benefits studies focus on studying climate change mitigation as the main benefit instead of considering it as one of the multiple benefits of a policy. This is because the majority of co-benefits studies are focused on the benefits within

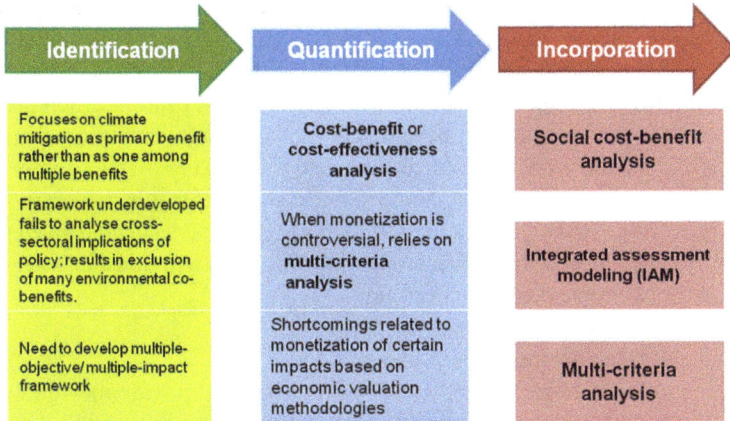

Figure 5.2   Three phases of co-benefits framework. Source: Collated and developed from Pearce, Japanese Ministry of Environment, UNEP, Williams et al., Ürge-Vorsatz et al. and Floater et al. [28–33].

a single sector rather than on the benefits across multiple sectors. This limitation is due to the absence of a multi-objective policy-perspective and integrated framework necessary for a proper assessment of co-benefits across multiple sectors [32].

The UNEP's climate policy evaluation framework addressed this limitation to some extent by promoting the adoption of a multi-objective policy perspective when evaluating various policy options. While UNEP's framework acted as a major catalyst in developing other similar frameworks [34] based on multi-criteria analysis (MCA), these efforts are still at the development stage and yet to be employed and assessed carefully.

To understand the net benefits of a policy, including all effects resulting from its interactions with other policies, a rigorous and comprehensive analysis of co-benefits is required. Considering the time and resources required for conducting such an analysis it is often not feasible in practice. Particularly, for developing countries where policy operates within a resource-constrained environment, this type of analysis may be considered superfluous. In such circumstances, even if the magnitude of the effects cannot be assessed, efforts to explicitly consider possible co-benefits of a policy and to measure them can nonetheless be considered sufficient for decision-making.

In theory, net welfare impacts of a given climate policy should be measured considering all direct and indirect effects, including cross-sectoral interactions of that policy with other policies. In practice, however, welfare impacts are assessed using 'general equilibrium models' (general equilibrium models try to represent the functioning of 'the economy as a whole'), which 'typically do not include externalities and thus exclude a large range of environmental co-benefits' [32].

In some cases, it is difficult to undertake a correct evaluation of co-benefits of certain climate policies due to lack of information about relevant contextual factors.

For example, when considering the social impacts of a particular mitigation policy, it would be misleading if the assessment is based only on the net welfare effects as the same intervention may have different effects on different stakeholder groups. For example, improved air quality resulting from the adoption of low-carbon measures (i.e. low-carbon public transport) benefit people from lower-income brackets more as they often live and work in polluted areas and more likely to have poorer health than the average. To ensure proper assessment of co-benefits it is necessary to consider all relevant groups of stakeholders who might be impacted by the given policy.

All these challenges involving proper identification and consideration of co-benefits in the literature point to a need for

    i.   a detailed taxonomy of co-benefits and
   ii.   a multiple-objective and multiple-impact assessment framework.

An ideal taxonomy that would cover distinct, independent co-benefits for individual sector of the economy – or particular sector-based classification of co-benefits that are identified in the literature – has not been developed [32, 33]. In any event, it may not be possible because of the complexity of the task such a taxonomy would demand. In the absence of such an ideal taxonomy of co-benefits, the key is twofold:

    i.   to detect the cause-and-effect relations and interactions between the effects, and
   ii.   to differentiate between co-benefits based on their points of origin, end points and intermediate phases that affect other outcomes.

This approach is used in the 'Impact Pathway Methodology' devised by the 'ExternE Project' for assessing the economic effect of atmospheric pollution in the EU [32].

Figure 5.3 illustrates a conceptual diagram of such a process for mapping pathways of different co-benefits. Using common mitigation measures (e.g. energy efficiency, renewable energy, active transport and lifestyle/behaviour change) as examples, the diagram tracks the impact chains and identify possible intermediate impact points and their interactions with each other that may occur . Notably, the diagram highlights the wide variety of multiple impacts of each measure and how their interactions with each other may affect the final impact.

5.4.2.2   Quantifying and valuing co-benefits

Perhaps the most challenging part of the co-benefits framework is the valuation of the identified co-benefits in some form of quantifiable units that would enable their integration into existing decision-making processes. Since existing decision-making frameworks rely heavily on cost-benefit or cost-effectiveness analysis, which is mainly based on the monetary valuation of units, a monetary value of the co-benefit needs to be estimated first before it can be incorporated into such a valuation process. This results in a number of challenges.

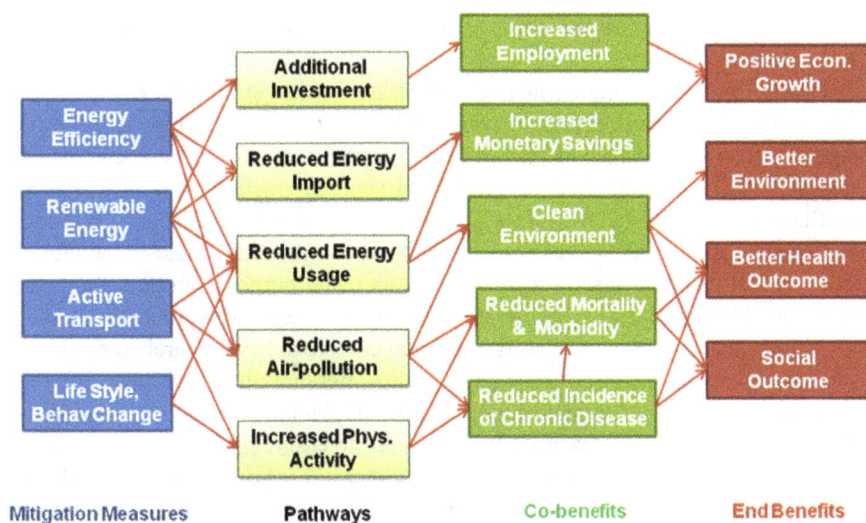

Figure 5.3   Conceptual framework for mapping pathways of co-benefits

First, theoretically, it is possible to estimate monetary value for some of the co-benefits of policies related to climate change mitigation (e.g. amount of energy saved, reduced amount of air pollutants, reduced amount of waste, number of additional jobs created, etc.) based on certain economic valuation methodologies [35]. However, monetisation of certain 'non-climate' and 'non-energy'-related co-benefits (such as environmental- and health-related co-benefits) is questionable, as methodologies used to monetise such co-benefits are criticised for commodifying ecosystem services for which no market value exist [36] or to the ethical impli-cations of differential valuation of human life in countries and regions based on income levels [37].

Second, another major challenge is co-benefits are always dependent on the policy context. While direct costs and benefits of a given policy can be assessed with some degree of certainty, the size of its welfare effects largely depends on the local situation. This includes how policies are applied and under what conditions. This makes it difficult to judge the size of the impact of different co-benefits and provide simplified methodologies for precise assessment of co-benefits.

Third, there is the possibility of 'double counting' for some co-benefits as they are closely related and often overlap. For example, parks designed as part of building a healthy physical environment result in better environments which in turn result in better health outcome through improving some of the dimensions of 'aged-friendly environments' – these benefits partly overlap (see Figure 5.3). There is a risk of 'double counting' these co-benefits when their monetary values are incorporated into the cost-benefit analysis of the present decision-making frameworks. Therefore, to avoid double counting, careful analysis is necessary. However, if it is not pos-sible to completely eliminate this risk, it is worth considering whether such risk is significant to compromise the effort of integrating them into the decision-making frameworks.

Fourth, to avoid complex analysis most studies target specific categories of co-benefits. Such selection fails to consider the specific relationships and the full range of interactions and feedback loops that exist between different co-benefits. For example, studies of sustainable energy policies generally focus on assessing only the benefits resulting from reduced air pollution and related health benefits. While such policies may also result in decreases in healthcare costs and associated savings of resources that can be utilised for other developmental purposes, these benefits are not included in the analysis [38]. As a result, in the majority of co-benefits studies, the total positive and negative effects of a given climate policy are rarely considered.

Fifth, in certain cases, when climate policy/measures likely to have different effects on different stakeholder groups, it is not sufficient to consider the net positive effect of the given policy/measures. In such cases, to ensure proper evaluation of co-benefits, the distributional effects of the policy/measures should also be considered. This is critical particularly when measures undertaken to mitigate climate change also contribute to reducing inequality across socioeconomic groups. For example, a policy measure such as promoting public transport which has climate change mitigation benefit as well as net non-climate benefits (through reduced air pollution, reduced congestion, savings in energy cost, etc.) can also facilitate access to economic opportunities for the disadvantaged section of the society by lowering their travel cost [39].

The above discussion has identified some limitations of the existing co-benefits framework and the challenges it faces in quantifying and valuing certain co-benefits. The most important shortcoming is the absence of valuation techniques for certain categories of co-benefits (e.g. health benefits, social benefits, ecosystem services, etc.) appropriate for incorporation into the cost-benefit analysis of the existing decision-making framework. In those cases, when monetary valuation of a co-benefit is considered questionable, valuation in physical units is often advisable. Such valuation needs to be combined with alternative assessment techniques (instead of cost-benefit analysis), such as Multi-criteria analysis (MCA) (which is discussed in Section 5.4.2.3).

5.4.2.3 Incorporating co-benefits into policy-decision-making process

Generally, co-benefits studies on policies to mitigate climate change is framed within a cost-benefit analysis approach. Such approach generally evaluates co-benefits in financial terms. It means it only considers the benefits of a given policy which have or can be quantified in monetary units and benefits that do not have any monetary value are generally excluded from the analysis. To address this limitation, there is a growing trend of using welfare analysis in co-benefits studies where different methods are used. Most of these methods are capable of assessing most of the co-benefits including non-monetary valuation of those co-benefits that often occur as a nonmarket benefit. Three main methods are commonly used to incorporate the identified co-benefits into climate change-related policy-decision-making process:

    i.   social cost-benefit analysis,
    ii.   integrated assessment modelling (IAM) and
    iii. multi-criteria analysis (MCA).

Social cost-benefit analysis

Social cost-benefit analysis is considered a more appropriate tool than financial cost-benefit analysis in co-benefits studies on climate policies. This is because it considers costs and benefits of a particular policy as variations in human well-being. Such approach permits the evaluation of benefits of defined climate policy options in terms of their contribution to the net welfare of society. This approach to cost-benefit analysis distinguishes social cost-benefit from financial cost-benefit [35, 40]. The method is particularly relevant when quantifying and valuing certain climate co-benefits, which frequently arise as non-market costs and benefits. For this, the method uses various economic valuation tools (such as computable general equilibrium models, contingent valuation, energy pricing, hedonic pricing, input-output analysis, etc.) [41].

Integrated assessment modelling

IAM is developed specifically for climate change mitigation policy analysis, which evaluates the costs of different mitigation policies. As IAM operates within a cost-effectiveness system, the model does not consider the primary benefit or the welfare implications of climate change mitigation. The IPCC relied on IAM in analysing different mitigation policy options in its Fourth Assessment Report and AR5 [42]. IAM estimates direct costs of mitigation based on partial or general equilibrium analysis where macroeconomic feedback typically remains limited [43]. In such analysis, 'the employment effects of climate policies, implications for investment flows and trade balances, or interactions between climate policy and the fiscal setting are not captured' [32]. The strength of IAM lies in its ability to include assessments in monetary as well as physical units. This permits the evaluation of environmental, social and health-related impacts of mitigation policies in non-monetary way. The process requires complex modelling and a large amount of data that make IAM unsuitable, particularly for policy context where resources are limited.

Multi-criteria analysis

MCA is perhaps the most suitable method available for incorporating all categories of co-benefits into existing policy-decision-making framework. It has three important strengths that distinguish it from social cost-benefit analysis in considering most climate co-benefits:

•   First, it provides an appropriate framework that can bring quantitative and qualitative information together. This allows consideration of the co-benefits for which quantitative or monetary information is not obtainable or cannot be estimated through available valuation techniques [44].

- Second, there is provision for the incorporation of stakeholders' diverse perspectives and preferences into the decision-making based on a process of weighting objectives [45].
- Third, 'it frames decision-making in procedural terms by embedding it within a structured process of deliberation and discussion' [32]. Utlising a deliberative process, the method ensures relevant stakeholders' perspectives are duly considered for productive use of qualitative information in the analysis. This ultimately helps to achieve better decision over time [46].

Collectively, these aspects make the MCA capable of productively processing qualitative and quantitative information together and achieving better policy outcomes. Its methodological specificity of arriving at decisions through stakeholder deliberation distinguishes MCA from the other two methods – social cost-benefit analysis and IAM.

As discussed earlier in this chapter, the most comprehensive effort to develop a climate policy evaluation framework adopting MCA was initiated by the UNEP [30]. There is a growing body of literature where MCA is used in environmental decision-making [30, 47] – for example, using MCA studies were conducted to understand the wider development implications of introducing carbon markets for conservation of forests [48].

However, when applying MCA its limitations need to be carefully considered alongside its strengths. As the method relies on subjective values and weights for some benefits, all implicit values and weights are required to be explicit for ensuring transparency and credibility of the process. Therefore, to be reliable, MCA requires a supportive social process where these subjective values and weights are given 'explicit' consideration in discussion and decision-making [32]. This means the MCA requires extensive background work to (i) clearly explain all assumptions, source details and opinions; (ii) clearly transmit the outcomes and (iii) record all streams of argumentation and analysis leading to the results, among all the stakeholders.

5.4.3   Impact assessment tools of climate action policies

The co-benefits framework (see Section 5.4.2) relies on various impact assessment tools to assess the impacts of climate change mitigation policies, projects and programmes in different sectors. The use of appropriate impact assessment tools is considered critical as they assist policymakers to verify the impacts of their policies and their actual co-benefits. In this section, we focus our discussion on four key impact assessment tools: environmental impact assessment (EIA), strategic environmental assessment (SEA), sustainability assessment (SA) and Health Impact Assessment (HIA). These impact assessment tools are used in case studies focusing on GHG emissions reduction policies, projects and programmes in urban planning at the city level [49].

Based on the various ways these impact assessment tools are used in the studies, EIA can be defined as 'a planning instrument for predicting the effects on the environment from altering or building a new establishment' [50]. SEA can be defined as 'a decision-making support instrument for the formulation of sustainable spatial and sector policies, plans and programmes, aiming to ensure an appropriate consideration of the environment' [51]. SA can be defined as 'a method of assessment and optimisation, that examines the social, economic, and environmental effects of policies, programs, and projects' [52]. HIA can be defined as 'a combination of procedures, methods and tools by which a policy, program or project may be judged as to its potential effects on the health of a population, and the distribution of those effects within the population' [53].

Among these, EIA is regarded as the most developed, recognised and institutionalised impact assessment tool [54] which is adopted by over 100 countries in their institutional processes [55]. Both EIA and SEA focus on ensuring that environmental issues are clearly addressed and incorporated into the decision-making process. While EIA's concerns are limited to environmental impacts of infrastructural projects, SEA addresses environmental issues at a higher planning level (policy, plan, programme) [55]. As for SA and HIA, while both focus on diverse policies, programmes and projects beyond urban planning [52, 54], HIA exclusively focuses on assessing the health impacts of policies, programmes and projects [53].

It has been observed that there are some shortcomings in the consideration of health impacts in the use of SEA, EIA and SA. A case study on GHG emission reduction policies of the city of Geneva focusing on three projects in urban planning, heating and transportation found a narrow vision of health in the application of these impact assessment tools on all three projects [49]. As the relevant legislation relating to these tools required to review only the effects of the projects on the determinants of the physical environment, broader health effects of these projects that cannot be assessed based on these determinants were not considered. Furthermore, the EIA does not require the integration of the health dimension in its impact assessment process. As for SA, consideration of health is superficial as it is conducted primarily through the analysis of 'health and safety' criteria [49]. These observations suggest that compared to SA, SEA or EIA; HIA is the appropriate tool which provides the most elaborate assessment of the consequences for the health of the GHG reduction policies, projects and programmes.

5.5   HIA as a framework to integrate health dimension in all policies

HIA emerged as a prospective decision-making aid tool in the context of development projects in the early 1990s [56, 57] which aims to improve the qualities of policies, programmes or projects through recommendation that promote health [58]. The *Gothenburg Consensus* defines HIA as 'a combination of procedures, methods and tools by which a policy, programme or project may be judged as to its potential effects on the health of a population, and the distribution of those effects within the population' [53].

HIA is developed based on the methodology of EIA which uses

'a similar screening stage to decide whether an assessment should take place, followed by scoping which defines the perimeter, methodology, management and participants of the process. The assessment itself then produces its results and recommendations. After the decision is taken and implemented, the effects of the decision are monitored to examine whether predicted impacts have materialised. This approach has much in common with the policy appraisal process. HIA strengthens this process by allowing a systematic review of the health consequences' [58].

HIA is an important component of four prospective impact assessment tools currently used in Europe: EIA, SEA, SA and HIA [49].

5.5.1   Case study: HIA in phases IV and V of the WHO European Healthy Cities Network

HIA was introduced into the WHO European Healthy Cities Network (EHCN) during Phase IV (2003–08) as one of four core themes. The objectives were to raise awareness and create a common understanding of HIA, provide leadership and strengthen capacity, share results and evidence from HIA practice with other European cities and provide evidence of HIA's contribution to areas such as healthy urban planning and healthy ageing. Another objective was to work towards mainstreaming HIA as a framework for integrating health and well-being concerns into all urban policies and projects [58].

Despite changes in the core themes of the WHO EHCN between 2008 and 2013, HIA remained linked with the overarching theme of health and health equity in all local policies and a requirement regarding capacity building. This viewpoint is founded on the Adelaide Statement on *Health in All Policies* (HiAP), which promotes HIA as one of the most effective tools for HiAP operationalisation [58]. The main objective of the EHCN Phase V evaluation was to investigate the effects of the implementation of HIA methodology at a local level across Europe in over 30 countries with widely differing economies and administrative and socio-political backgrounds.

5.5.2   Methods

The methodology used in the EHCN Phase V evaluation was driven by a Realist Evaluation framework which was used to collect and aggregate data obtained through three methods: an HIA factors analysis, a case-study template analysis using Nvivo software and a detailed General Evaluation Questionnaire. The use of such a multi-method approach in the study allows for triangulation of data and information [58].

5.5.3   Results

The results of the impact appraisal (based on submitted case studies on the implementation of HIA in nine cities) show that HIA clearly makes the link between impacts of policies (projects) and positive health outcomes (progress in most health issues) for all the cities.

5.5.3.1 HIA implementation process

Based on the different ways the HIA and/or its different components were used in the case studies, the HIA implementation processes were broadly categorised into three main groups:

    i.   Impact assessment of individual projects
    ii. Impact assessment within planning policy
    iii. Policy and strategy development.

5.5.3.2 Securing city's (council's) mandate for HIA implementation

For all cases, securing the city's (city council's) mandate to implement HIA was identified as an essential prerequisite step of the HIA implementation process. Depending on the city's intention of how it wanted to use the HIA, the scope of the mandate for the HIA work among the cities varied. For cities that wanted to incorporate HIA (or health and equity issues) into their existing processes and procedures, the mandate was a statutory requirement that allowed them to undertake other forms of impact assessments such as EIA or equality impact assessment. For cities seeking to incorporate health and equity issues into the policymaking process, the mandate was in the form of a formal commitment to the objectives of Healthy Cities Phase V, including health and health equity in all local policies. For example, in one case the mandate was for introducing HIA into the municipality in the form of assessing a strategic infrastructure project. In another case, the mandate was in the form of City Council passing a resolution requiring all strategic documents for the city discussed by the City Council to be sent to the Healthy City Foundation for assessment based on Healthy Cities principles and the method of HIA. For a city concerned to develop a systemic approach to HIA in planning policy decisions, the mandate was a commitment in the local Core Spatial Strategy to improving the health of the local population.

It appears from this research that HIA is the tool that provides the most elaborate assessment, compared to SA, SEA or EIA, of the potential effects on the health of the GHG reduction policies undertaken by local decision-makers at the city level. This study also highlights the complementarity between EIA and HIA for assessing the potential impacts of a proposal. Indeed, HIA can add information regarding the health outcomes of changes in the environment [49]. Table 5.1 illustrates an example of a HIA analysis based on a study by Diallo *et al.*, pp. 9–10 [49].

Table 5.1   A generic case-study template for HIA analysis based on a study by Diallo et al., pp. 9–10.

Policy/Project/ Programme (examples)	Output (physical manifestation of action, such as infrastructure, improved/new facility, legislation)	Outcome (change caused by output)	HIA process of planning for active transport at the local level	
			Issues analysed	Summary of results (medium- or long-term effect of outcome)
Planning for active transport modes – public transport, cycling and walking, etc.	Installation of public transport/bicycle or pedestrian networks and facilities.	Increased use of active modes of travel and decreased use of private vehicles by local population.	Air quality and climate	Reduced air pollution and cleaner environment with associated health co-benefits resulting from reduced health hazards (accidents), disease and death with the project compared to no action.
			Noise	Reduced traffic congestion resulting in less noise pollution and associated health co-benefits (reduced stress, discomfort to aged population) with the project compared to no action.
			Physical activity	Significant increase in the use of sustainable modes of transport (walking, cycling and public transport) during morning peak and evening peak with the project compared to no action.
			Energy	Reduced fuel consumption with reduction in carbon emissions resulting in reduced energy cost and positive health impacts and maximising co-benefits with the project compared to no action.

Adapted from table 3, summary of the results of the impact appraisal, from Diallo *et al.* [49], pp. 9–10.

5.6   Health co-benefits in the context of UN SDG

Health-related co-benefits of climate policies are amongst the largest group of co-benefits and often dominate the literature in terms of importance compared with other categories of co-benefits [59]. This has also been confirmed by IPCC's findings in the human health chapter (Chapter 11) of its AR5: Chapter 3, 92

> … the short-term and relatively localised health co-benefits from reducing greenhouse gas emissions could be very large. Opportunities to capture health co-benefits include reducing health-damaging, climate-altering air pollutants (CAPs) through energy-efficiency measures; shifting to cleaner energy sources; shifting consumption away from animal products toward less CAP-intensive healthy diets; and designing transport systems that promote active transport. In economic terms, these health co-benefits from reducing emissions would be extremely cost-beneficial. [60]

Health co-benefits studies of climate policies can be categorised into six groups [61]:

i.   Reduce emissions of health-damaging pollutants, either primary or precursors to other pollutants in association with changes in energy production, energy efficiency or control of landfills
ii.   Increase access to reproductive health services
iii. Decrease meat consumption (especially from ruminants) and substitute low-carbon healthy alternatives
iv.   Increase active transport particularly in urban areas
v.   Increase urban green space [60]

A large body of health-related co-benefits studies focuses on reduced air pollution impacts on human health resulting from reduced GHG emissions [12, 60]. Improvements in human health are estimated based on either decrease in mortality, morbidity and disease prevalence, or reduced healthcare costs. The methods to do such estimation are developed through establishing a link between people's exposure to concentration of air pollutants and public-health outcomes. Such research found that reduced exposure to air pollution has beneficial effects on human health in the form of reductions in cardiovascular, respiratory and other non-communicable diseases on a large scale [62]. Such 'reductions in health damages are by far the largest category of co-benefits arising from abating GHG emissions and account for 70–90 per cent of the total value of quantified co-benefits in energy-related co-benefits analyses' [31]. Section 5.7 discusses the issue from the perspective of HIA.

Measures to increase active travel (such as walking, cycling and use of public transport) that increase physical activity are identified for their zero-carbon emissions, less air pollution and a wide range of health benefits such as reduced obesity; reduced non-communicable diseases, improved mental health and associated

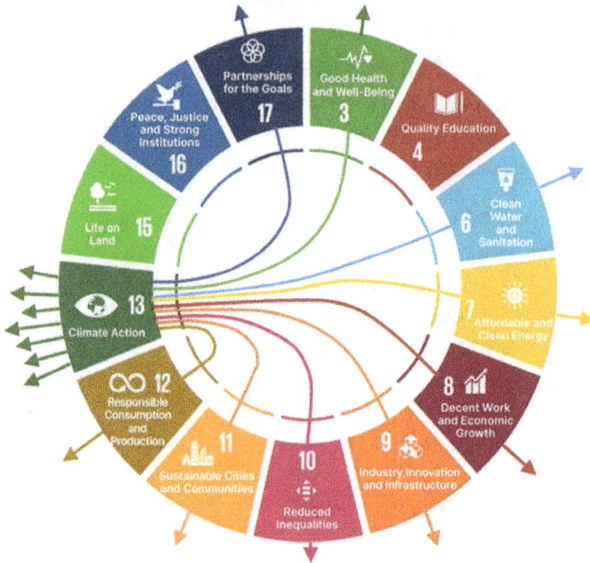

Figure 5.4   Potential co-benefits linking climate policy goal with other SDGs.
Source: Adapted from UN SDGs 2015.

savings in health care costs [63]. The expansion of public transport is found to save human lives because it involves less deadly and non-fatal injuries [64].

Observing the above large body of health-related co-benefits as well as a wide range of environmental and social co-benefits that result from various GHG emissions reduction measures, Article 6.4 of the Paris Climate Agreement provides for a new mechanism by which governments and non-government stakeholders can support developing policies and projects that can simultaneously deliver GHG emission reductions and UN's sustaibale development goals (see Figure 5.4). The UNEP's climate policy evaluation framework (see Figure 5.5) support policy makers in linking climate policy goals with other SDGs.

5.6.1   *Co-benefits as potent motivator for local climate action*

It has been observed that if the wider benefits of climate actions can be demonstrated to the communities, the communities are more likely to support councils in taking actions on climate change [65]. This is because while the primary benefits of GHG mitigation occur at the global level which cannot be experienced locally, most co-benefits of climate actions occur at the local level. Since these co-benefits have some immediate welfare effects on the communities who bear the costs of climate actions (typically as the taxpayers and/or the consumers), highlighting these co-benefits councils can convince them of the justification of acting on climate change [66]. Hence, these co-benefits provide incentives for local government policy-makers to engage in stricter climate action and are considered more politically feasible. On the

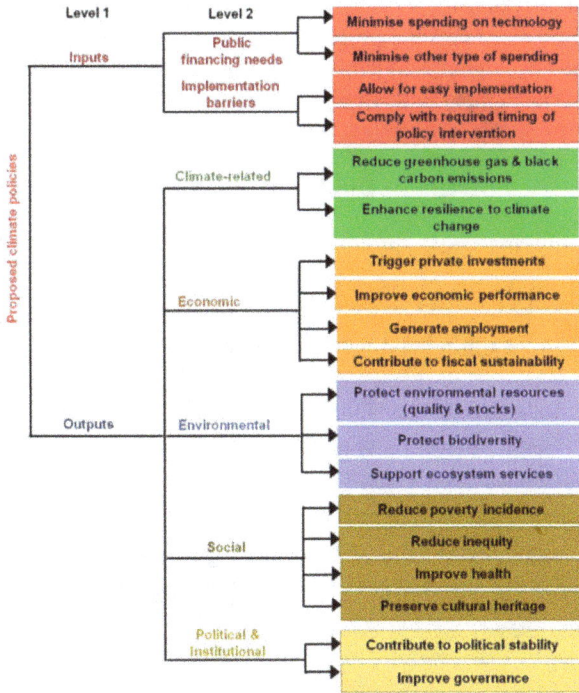

Figure 5.5   Multi-objective climate policy evaluation framework. Source: Adapted from UNEP [30], p. 49.

other hand, it has also been observed that local government policies which are designed based on innovation and aimed to deliver wider economic, environmental and social benefits to their communities could potentially lead to key climate co-benefits (e.g. substantial reduction of GHG emissions).

5.6.2   The Australian perspective

In Australia, local climate action mainly started when some 238 local councils joined the International Council for Local Environmental Initiatives (ICLEI)'s 'Cities for Climate Protection' (CCP) programme to lower GHG emissions from their operations and communities [67]. While there is a difference of opinion about individual council motivation in joining the CCP program, it has been widely acknowledged that the programme's 'win-win' potential to reduce the energy usage, and resulting reduction of GHG emissions, as well as securing significant monetary savings, predominantly motivated these councils in joining the programme [68]. Other common motivations were: the responsibility in planning for the future, demonstrate leadership to their community through adopting measures that reduce emissions from councils' operations and concern about the possibility of facing litigations from the communities, businesses and other stakeholders [69, 70]. The CCP programme successfully demonstrated that local climate action can be constructed as a local issue which can be resolved with local issues and priorities that can lead to cutting of GHG emissions. This means the program managed to synthesise the climate policy goal with local development objectives in taking up climate change actions that resulted in GHG abatement with significant co-benefits.

5.7 Health co-benefits in policy process: Australian case study

In Australia, while the 'co-benefits approach' is adopted by local governments in pursuing low-carbon policies, the approach is limited in targeting certain 'energy-related' monetary benefits. 'Non-climatic and non-energy-related' benefits, which include significant health-related gains, rarely enter climate change-related policy discourse [71]. This section presents the main findings of a broader investigation [7] focusing on local governments' understandings of the 'co-benefits approach' in considering the health dimension in planning for climate change.

5.7.1 Background

Part of Karim's study [7] focused on investigating whether, how and to what extent local government's climate change-related policies consider the public health needs of their communities. The specific objective has been to understand the extent to which local councils target health-related co-benefits in planning for climate change.

5.7.2 Methods

The research methods comprised a comprehensive online survey and review of New South Wales (NSW) councils' climate change-related policies, as well as interviews of selected council officers. The geographic area of investigation for this study was the *Sydney Greater Metropolitan Region* and surrounding local government jurisdictions. The investigation focused primarily upon policy processes at the local government level, but the research also investigated the links of local to state and broader national processes.

5.7.3 Results

The findings show that local government policymakers rarely consider whether their GHG reduction policies also yield health co-benefits. In many instances, the health co-benefits of their climate policies, projects and programmes are not identified, let alone measured by local governments. In most councils, climate planning activities and work on public health are happening separately and in parallel, rather than through an integrated approach. The primary focus on cost minimisation has largely limited climate policies' targets to reducing GHG emission costs, together with the attainment of energy-related monetary savings. This focus on monetary considerations, together with constrained authority, absence of stable policy, legislative support and clear direction from higher levels of government, and lack of data and technical knowledge to assess health benefits collectively have influenced limited consideration of health dimension in NSW local government's climate planning [7].

5.7.4   Discussion

The results of this study suggest the need for a clear policy direction from the state to local government to link climate change planning with health; inter-agency coordination and training to conduct health impact analyses of all policies; development of tools, methods for identifying, quantifying and incorporating health-related co-benefits; and regulatory or statutory changes to support actions in certain areas that are currently beyond local governments' sphere of control.

5.8   Conclusion

This chapter has discussed the role of climate action in promoting healthy ageing and age-friendly environments in the context of sustainable development and planning, using a concept called 'co-benefits'. The definition and meaning of co-benefits have been discussed in the context of *Climate Action*, SDGs and HIA. The Australian case study demonstrated the application of 'co-benefit' in local government climate change-related policy-decision-making. However, more work is required to ascertain their adoption and impact in policymaking to promote sustainable development and climate change mitigation.

References

[1] World Health Organisation (WHO). *Global age-friendly cities: a guide [online]*. 2007. Available from https://www.who.int/ageing/publications/age_friendly_cities_guide/en/ [Accessed Feb 2021].

[2] Costongs C. *Healthy ageing, presentation of EuroHealthNet, European network of national public health and health promotion institutes [online]*. 2007. Available from https://ec.europa.eu/employment_social/social_situation/docs/costongs_slides_en.pdf [Accessed 03 Feb 2021].

[3] IPCC [Intergovernmental Panel on Climate Change]. 'Summary for policymakers' in Edenhofer O., Pichs-Madruga R., Sokona Y., Brunner S. (eds.). *Climate Change 2014: Mitigation of Climate Change. Contribution of Working Group III to the Fifth Assessment Report of the Intergovernmental Panel on Climate Change*. Cambridge, United Kingdom and New York, NY, USA: Cambridge University Press; 2014.

[4] UNFCCC [UN Framework Convention on Climate Change Secretariat]. *Paris Agreement. United Nations [online]*. 2015. Available from https://unfccc.int/files/essential_background/convention/application/pdf/english_paris_agreement.pdf [Accessed 2 Jan 2017].

[5] UNFCCC [UN Framework Convention on Climate Change Secretariat]. *Synthesis report on the aggregate effect of the intended nationally determined contributions. COP21. UNFCCC [online]*. 2015a. Available from http://unfccc.int/resource/docs/2015/cop21/eng/07.pdf [Accessed 02 Jan 2017].

[6]   Falkner R. 'The Paris agreement and the new logic of international climate politics'. *International Affairs.* 2016, vol. 92(5), pp. 1107–25.

[7]   Karim S.M. *Co-benefits of low-carbon policies in the built environment: an Australian investigation into local government co-benefits policies* [online] A thesis in fulfilment of the requirements for the degree of Doctor of Philosophy, UNSW-Australia. 2020. Available from http://handle.unsw.edu.au/1959.4/62960 [Accessed 01 Mar 2021].

[8]   Mayrhofer J.P., Gupta J. 'The science and politics of co-benefits in climate policy'. *Environmental Science & Policy.* 2016, vol. 57(4), pp. 22–30.

[9]   Puppim de Oliveira J.A., Doll C.N.H., Kurniawan T.A., Geng Y., Kapshe M., Huisingh D. 'Promoting win–win situations in climate change mitigation, local environmental quality and development in Asian cities through co-benefits'. *Journal of Cleaner Production.* 2013, vol. 58(1), pp. 1–6.

[10]   IPCC [Intergovernmental Panel on Climate Change]. *Climate Change 2001: Mitigation [online]. (2001a).* Contribution of Working Group III to the Third Assessment Report (TAR) of the Intergovernmental Panel on Climate Change. (Editor: R. Pachauri). Available from https://www.ipcc.ch/site/assets/uploads/2018/03/WGIII_TAR_full_report.pdf [Accessed 27 Feb 2021].

[11]   Schipper L. *'Automobile fuel economy and CO_2 emissions in industrializing countries: troubling trends through 2005/6'. Earlier Faculty Research Series, University of California Transportation Center.* Berkeley, CA: University of California; 2008.

[12]   Nemet G.F., Holloway T., Meier P. 'Implications of incorporating air-quality co-benefits into climate change policymaking'. *Environmental Research Letters.* 2010, vol. 5(1), p. 014007.

[13]   Teh K.Y., S.-C R., Ray P. Student-led engineering designs to meet the challenges of climate change and public health, ieee leader *[online].* 2020. Available from https://www.ieee-tems.org/student-led-engineering-designs-to-meet-the-challenges-of-climate-change-and-public-health/ [Accessed 03 March 2021].

[14]   UNU-IAS [United Nations University Institute of Advanced Studies]. *Urban Development with Climate Co-benefits: Aligning Climate, Environmental and Other Development Goals in Cities.* Yokohama, Japan: UNU-IAS Policy Report; 2013.

[15]   OECD [Organisation for Economic Co-operation and Development]. *Benefits of Climate Change Policies.* Paris: OECD; 2018.

[16]   IPCC [Intergovernmental Panel on Climate Change], (2014a). *'Climate change 2014: mitigation of climate change'* in Edenhofer O., Pichs-Madruga R., Sokona Y., Minx J.C. (eds.). *Contribution of Working Group III to the Fifth Assessment Report of the Intergovernmental Panel on Climate Change.* Cambridge, UK/NY: Cambridge University Press; 2014b.

[17]   Edenhofer O., Kadner S., von Stechow C., Schwerhoff G., Luderer G. 'Linking climate change mitigation research to sustainable development' in Atkinson G., Dietz S., Neumayer E., Agarwala M. (eds.). *Handbook of*

Sustainable Development. 2nd edn. Cheltenham, UK: Edward Elgar; 2014. pp. 476–99.

[18] Pachauri R.K., Allen M.R., Barros V.R., 'IPCC [Intergovernmental Panel on Climate Change]'. in Pachauri R.K., Meyer L.A. (eds.) *Climate Change 2014: Synthesis Report. Contribution of Working Groups I, II and III to the Fifth Assessment Report of the Intergovernmental Panel on Climate Change*. Geneva, Switzerland: IPCC; 2014b. p. 151.

[19] Alam Hossain Mondal M., Kamp L.M., Pachova N.I. 'Drivers, barriers, and strategies for implementation of renewable energy technologies in rural areas in Bangladesh—an innovation system analysis'. *Energy Policy*. 2010, vol. 38(8), pp. 4626–34.

[20] de Nazelle A., Nieuwenhuijsen M.J., Antó J.M., *et al.* 'Improving health through policies that promote active travel: a review of evidence to support integrated health impact assessment'. *Environment International*. 2011, vol. 37(4), pp. 766–77.

[21] Kurniawan T.A., Puppim de Oliveira J., Premakumara D.G.J., Nagaishi M. 'City-to-city level cooperation for generating urban co-benefits: the case of technological cooperation in the waste sector between Surabaya (Indonesia) and Kitakyushu (Japan)'. *Journal of Cleaner Production*. 2013, vol. 58(3), pp. 43–50.

[22] Bradley B.A., Houghton R.A., Mustard J.F., Hamburg S.P. 'Invasive grass reduces aboveground carbon stocks in shrublands of the Western US'. *Global Change Biology*. 2006, vol. 12(10), pp. 1815–22.

[23] Spencer B., Lawler J., Lowe C., *et al.* 'Case studies in co-benefits approaches to climate change mitigation and adaptation'. *Journal of Environmental Planning and Management*. 2017, vol. 60(4), pp. 647–67.

[24] Cai Q., Lee J., Eluru N., Abdel-Aty M. 'Macro-level pedestrian and bicycle crash analysis: incorporating spatial spillover effects in dual state count models'. *Accident Analysis & Prevention*. 2016, vol. 93(2), pp. 14–22.

[25] Haines A., McMichael A.J., Smith K.R., *et al.* 'Public health benefits of strategies to reduce greenhouse-gas emissions: overview and implications for policy makers'. *The Lancet*. 2009, vol. 374(9707), pp. 2104–14.

[26] Bollen J., van der Zwaan B., Brink C., Eerens H. 'Local air pollution and global climate change: a combined cost-benefit analysis'. *Resource and Energy Economics*. 2009, vol. 31(3), pp. 161–81.

[27] Thambiran T., Diab R.D. 'Air pollution and climate change co-benefit opportunities in the road transportation sector in Durban, South Africa'. *Atmospheric Environment*. 2011, vol. 45(16), pp. 2683–9.

[28] Pearce D.W. *Policy Frameworks for the Ancillary Benefits of Climate Change Policies*. London: Centre for Social and Economic Research on the Global Environment; 2000.

[29] Japanese Ministry of the Environment. *Manual for Quantitative Evaluation of the Co-Benefits Approach to Climate Change Projects: Version 1.0*. Tokyo: Author; 2009.

[30] UNEP [United Nations Environmental Programme]. *A Practical Framework for Planning Pro-Development Climate Policy*. Paris: Author; 2011.

[31] Williams C.A., Hasanbeigi, Price L., Wu G. *International Experiences with Quantifying the Co-Benefits of Energy-Efficiency and Greenhouse-Gas Mitigation Programs and Policies*. Berkeley: Ernest Orlando Lawrence Berkeley National Laboratory, University of California; 2012.

[32] Ürge-Vorsatz D., Herrero S.T., Dubash N.K., Lecocq F. 'Measuring the co-benefits of climate change mitigation'. *Annual Review of Environment and Resources*. 2014, vol. 39(1), pp. 549–82.

[33] Floater G., Heeckt C., Ulterino M., *et al.* 'Co-benefits of urban climate action: A framework for cities'. *A Working Paper by the Economics of Green Cities Programme, LSE Cities*. London School of Economics and Political Science; 2016.

[34] Dubash N.K., Hagemann M., Höhne N., Upadhyaya P. 'Developments in national climate change mitigation legislation and strategy'. *Climate Policy*. 2013, vol. 13(6), pp. 649–64.

[35] Azqueta D. *Introducci´on a la econom´ıa ambiental*. 2nd Ed. Madrid, Spain: McGraw-Hill; 2007.

[36] Luck G.W., Chan K.M.A., Eser U., *et al.* 'Ethical considerations in on-ground applications of the ecosystem services concept'. *BioScience*. 2012, vol. 62(12), pp. 1020–9.

[37] Miller T.E. 'Variation between countries in the values of statistical life'. *Journal of Transport Economic Policy*. 2000, vol. 34, pp. 169–88.

[38] Shih Y.-H., Tseng C.-H. 'Cost-benefit analysis of sustainable energy development using life-cycle co-benefits assessment and the system dynamics approach'. *Applied Energy*. 2014, vol. 119(1), pp. 57–66.

[39] Hosking J., Mudu P., Dora C. *Health Co-Benefits of Climate Change Mitigation—transport Sector: Health in the Green Economy*. Geneva: World Health Organization; 2011.

[40] Eur. Comm. [European Commission]. 'Guide to cost-benefit analysis of investment projects: structural funds, cohesion fund and instrument for pre-accession. brussels: European commission directorate general regional policy'; 2008.

[41] Tirado Herrero S., Ürge-Vorsatz D., Petrichenko K. 'Fuel poverty alleviation as a co-benefit of climate investments: evidence from Hungary'. Proceedings European Council for an Energy Efficient Economy; Summer Study, Belambra/Presqu'ıle de Giens, France, June 3–8; 2013.

[42] IPCC [Intergovernmental Panel on Climate Change]. 'Climate change 2007: The physical science basis' in Solomon S., Qin D., Manning M. (eds.). *Contribution of Working Group I to the Fourth Assessment Report of the Intergovernmental Panel on Climate Change*. Cambridge University Press; 2007.

[43] Shukla P.R. *Review of Linked Modelling of Low-Carbon Development, Mitigation and Its Full Costs and Benefits*. Cape Town, S. Africa: Mitigation Action Plans Scenario (MAPS); 2013.

[44] Munasinghe M. *Making Development More Sustainable: Sustainomics Framework and Practical Applications*. Colombo, Sri Lanka: Munasinghe Institute for Development; 2007.

[45] Böhringer C., Keller A., van der Werf E. 'Are green hopes too rosy? employment and welfare impacts of renewable energy promotion'. *Energy Economics*. 2013, vol. 36(1), pp. 277–85.

[46] Munda G. 'Social multi-criteria evaluation: methodological foundations and operational consequences'. *European Journal of Operational Research*. 2004, vol. 158(3), pp. 662–77.

[47] Ramanathan R. 'Abc inventory classification with multiple-criteria using weighted linear optimization'. *Computers & Operations Research*. 2006, vol. 33(3), pp. 695–700.

[48] Brown K., Corbera E. 'A multi-criteria assessment framework for carbon-mitigation projects: putting 'development'in the centre of decision-making'. *Tyndall Centre for Climate Change Research Working Paper*; 2003. p. 29.

[49] Diallo T., Cantoreggi N., Simos J., Christie D.P.T.H. 'Is HIA the most effective tool to assess the impact on health of climate change mitigation policies at the local level? A case study in Geneva, Switzerland'. *Global Health Promotion*. 2017, vol. 24(2), pp. 5–15.

[50] Lenzen M., Murray S.A., Korte B., Dey C.J. 'Environmental impact assessment including indirect effects—a case study using input–output analysis'. *Environmental Impact Assessment Review*. 2003, vol. 23(3), pp. 263–82.

[51] Fischer T.B. 'Strategic environmental assessment in post-modern times'. *Environmental Impact Assessment Review*. 2003, vol. 23(2), pp. 155–70.

[52] Conseil fédéral Suisse. *Stratégie pour le développement durable 2012–2015 (2012). Office fédéral du développement territorial, section développement durable, section développement durable, 3003*. Berne: Conseil fédéral Suisse; 2012.

[53] World Health Organisation (WHO). *Health Impact Assessment: Main Concepts and Suggested Approach. The Gothenburg Consensus Paper*. Copenhagen: WHO Regional Office for Europe; 1999.

[54] Fehr R., Viliani F., Nowacki J., Martuzzi M. (eds.). *Health in Impact Assessments: Opportunities Not to Be Missed*. Copenhagen: WHO Regional Office for Europe; 2014.

[55] Simos J. 'Introducing health impact assessment (HIA) in Switzerland'. *Sozial- und Präventivmedizin SPM*. 2006, vol. 51(3), pp. 130–2.

[56] Birley M., Peralta G. *Guidelines for the Health Impact Assessment of Development Projects, Environment Paper*. Manila: Asian Development Bank; 1992.

[57] Birley M. *Health Impact Assessment. Principles and Practice*. Earthscan, London; 2011.

[58] Simos J., Spanswick L., Palmer N., Christie D. 'The role of health impact assessment in phase V of the healthy cities European network'. *Health Promotion International*. 2015, vol. 30 Suppl 1, pp. i71–85.

[59]   Arrow K.J., Dasgupta P., Goulder L.H., Mumford K.J., Oleson K. 'Sustainability and the measurement of wealth'. *Environment and Development Economics.* 2012, vol. 17(03), pp. 317–53.

[60]   Cambridge University Press. 'Human health: impacts, adaptation, and co-benefits' in Smith K.R., Woodward A., Campbell-Lendrum D., Sauerborn R (eds.). *Climate Change 2014: Impacts, Adaptation, and Vulnerability.* Cambridge, United Kingdom and New York, NY, USA: Cambridge University Press; 2014. pp. 709–54.

[61]   Smith K.R., Jerrett M., Anderson H.R., *et al.* 'Public health benefits of strategies to reduce greenhouse-gas emissions: health implications of short-lived greenhouse pollutants'. *Lancet.* 2009, vol. 374(9707), pp. 2091–103.

[62]   Jack D.W., Kinney P.L. 'Health co-benefits of climate mitigation in urban areas'. *Current Opinion in Environmental Sustainability.* 2010, vol. 2(3), pp. 172–7.

[63]   Woodcock J., Givoni M., Morgan A.S. 'Health impact modelling of active travel visions for England and Wales using an integrated transport and health impact modelling tool (ITHIM'. *PLoS ONE.* 2013, vol. 8(1),p. e51462.

[64]   Creutzig F., He D. 'Climate change mitigation and co-benefits of feasible transport demand policies in Beijing'. *Transportation Research Part D: Transport and Environment.* 2009, vol. 14(2), pp. 120–31.

[65]   Bain P. G., Milfont T. L., Kashima Y., *et al.* 'Co-benefits of addressing climate change can motivate action around the world'. *Nature Climate Change.* 2016, vol. 6(2), pp. 154–7.

[66]   Markandya A., Rübbelke D.T.G. 'Ancillary benefits of climate policy'. *Journal of Economics and Statistics.* 2003, vol. 224(4), pp. 488–503.

[67]   Hoff J. 'Local climate protection programs in Australia and New Zealand: Results, dilemmas and relevance for future actions'. *CIDEA Project Report No. 1, Department of Political Science.* Denmark: University of Copenhagen; 2010.

[68]   Bulkeley H. 'Down to earth: local government and greenhouse policy in Australia'. *Australian Geographer.* 2000, vol. 31(3), pp. 289–308.

[69]   LGNSW [Local Government New South Wales]. *Local government needs in responding to climate change in NSW, Australia [online].* 2010. Available from http://www.lgsa-plus.net.au/ClimateChangeActionPack [Accessed 18 Aug 2017].

[70]   Zeppel H. 'Climate change governance by local councils: Carbon mitigation by Greater Adelaide councils'. ACELG Local Government Researchers Forum: Local Governance in Transition'. UTS Sydney; 2011.

[71]   Karim S.M., Thompson S., Williams P. 'Co-benefits of low carbon policies in the built environment: an investigation into the adoption of co-benefits by Australian local government'. *Procedia Engineering.* 2017, vol. 180(1), pp. 890–900.

Chapter 6

Health data privacy for aged population in Australia

Koel Ghorai[1], Guneet Randhawa[2], and Jan M. Smits[3]

Abstract: More than 15.9% of Australia's population is aged 65 years or above as of 2019 and this group is projected to increase more rapidly over the next decade. Over the last few years, there has been an active push by healthcare providers to have patient health data and records uploaded online for better and faster healthcare services. Due to Covid-19, many health service providers are taking their patients' records to online platforms. Even though accessing these online health records has become much easier and more cost-effective than working with physical documents, there has been increased awareness and concerns regarding health data privacy. In this chapter, we will look at the Australian health data privacy and how it is applicable to online health data of the aged population.

Keywords: health data privacy, healthcare service, health records, aged population

6.1 Introduction

There has been an increased use of electronic technology in the past two decades for the delivery of healthcare. This has led to a growth in the use of Electronic Health Records (EHRs) and Personal Health Records (PHRs) in various healthcare sectors [1]. EHR are patient-centred medical records that are stored on a central database in digital format and can be shared with different healthcare providers linked to that database [2]. EHRs originate from and are controlled by doctors. PHR is also a health record but it differs from an EHR in the sense that it can be generated by anyone including doctors, patients, pharmacies, hospitals and other sources but it is controlled by the patient. There is various literature that document the advantages of EHRs and PHRs over paper-based health records including benefits like improved

[1]School of Population Health, University of New South Wales, Australia
[2]NetsetSoftware, Australia
[3]Law and Technology, Industrial Engineering & Innovation Sciences, University of Technology, The Netherlands

quality, reduced medical errors and cost-effectiveness, among others [3]. Another benefit is accurate and timely information exchange between healthcare providers [4]. However, with the healthcare data being shared by multiple providers for various uses, it has become crucial to keep control of the privacy aspects of the data once it is collected from patients with legal consent. In case of any issues with the data, the legislation needs to be thoroughly checked and implemented to ensure the security and privacy of the owner of the data, such as the patient, is strictly maintained. In this chapter, we will look at what legislation is applicable in various scenarios that deal with EHRs as well as PHRs.

With the growing use of EHR, it is now possible to allow individuals to have electronic copies of their records so that they can create an electronic or a web-based PHR. A PHR is defined as an electronic application that can be used by an individual or their authorised representative to manage and share their own health information in a private, confidential and secure environment [5]. This, in turn, will allow for improved patient-centred care and health outcomes with less cost to the already-burdened healthcare system [6].

There has been considerable planning and implementation of PHR in countries such as the UK, the USA, Canada, New Zealand and Australia [7]. In the UK, for example, there is the Summary Care Record for every citizen registered under the National Health Service. It contains health-related information such as medical conditions, allergies and medications. The Summary Care Record is created for every citizen except for those who say otherwise, based around an opt-out model [8]. In the USA, there is no national provision of PHR but rather they have provider-initiated PHR where hospitals and other healthcare providers make some of their health-related information available to patients via electronic means [9]. Canada [10] and New Zealand [11] appear to be in the initial stages of planning for a national PHR. In Australia, My Health Record is the national digital health record system, sponsored by Australian Government, that allows every citizen and permanent resident to share their health information with doctors, hospitals and other healthcare providers if they want to.

While there is some research surrounding the security and privacy of PHRs from a technical perspective [12], there is limited research on the legislation surrounding the privacy and security of EHRs in Australia and especially concerning the aged population [13]. In Australia the elderly were one of the targeted groups for the initial roll-out of the My Health Record [14]. The aim of this chapter is to provide a legal analysis of health data privacy of the aged population in Australia and provide insights through two different case studies including one of My Health Record and the other for an aged care facility that houses dementia patients.

The objectives of this chapter are as follows:

i.   Mapping the regulatory environment (primarily from a privacy perspective) of an aged person entering the healthcare system
ii.   Due to the large number of potential partners involved in most cases dealing with healthcare system, the chapter aims at clarifying at a high-abstraction level the roles that all the different involved

parties have, such as data subject, data controller,data processor and third parties

iii. Suggest potential solutions that might help overcome issues in the current regulatory framework for healthcare systems.

6.2   Regulations dealing with Australian online health data

The privacy and security of Australian online health data of Australian citizens, including senior citizens, is governed by various legislation and laws and these regulations would generally be executed through the National Health Record Service provider (such as Federal Government departments and their partners) or service providers including aged care facilities, home care providers, hospitals, primary health centres and doctors. Federal Government and the service providers would be the custodians of patient data and they would be governed by legislation and laws. In this section, we will discuss the different legislation that is applicable to parties or organisations that deal directly or indirectly with Australian EHR.

6.2.1   General regulations

6.2.1.1   Tort

In Australia, Torts are common law actions that are applicable for civil wrongs. Individuals are entitled to sue other people or the state unless barred by statute for the purpose of obtaining a legal remedy for the wrongs committed. Torts include battery, deceit, trespass to land or goods, assault, false imprisonment, conversion of goods, private and public nuisance, intimidation and negligence (the very expansive tort). Torts might be applicable to some entities in relation to Australian EHRs and their potential misuse.

The groundwork for the Australian Tort law has been established [15]. However, it is lagging behind EU General Data Protection Regulation (GDPR) [16] and other countries as far as misuse of personal information is concerned [15].

In the current legal environment, claims to be tested in courts using established traditional tort cases for data breaches[17]. An entity could test the physical harm inflicted under the intentional tort (*Wilkinson tort*) [18] or the tort of negligence (*Tame v New South Wales*) [19].

6.2.1.2   Corporations Act 2001

A data breach in an organisation could lead to reputation loss, operational disruptions, legal impact and/or financial loss. The data breach can be due to a breach of directors' duty for a listed company [20]. An example for illustration purposes was the reputation loss suffered by Yahoo through a cyberattack. Yahoo had to reduce the sale price to Verizon by almost USD 350 million.

A data breach would be classified as a cyberattack and thus would entail the engagement of the Privacy Act 1988 (APP 11) and the Corporations Act among others.

For an organisation, its reputation is the most important asset. A Director has four main duties in the Corporations Act, of which care and diligence and to act in good faith would be the most relevant duties for data protection.

Australian Securities and Investments Commission (ASIC), the company's regulator for the Corporations Act, can take an organisation to court for data breach. Though most examples in existing literature are given through the lens of a financial organisation, these are relevant to health data when a breach occurs.

6.2.1.3   Consumer Data Rights

Consumer Data Rights (CDR) datasets are data designated by the treasurer which extend the Australian consumer-based regulatory framework [21]. This data can include value-added analysed data. Entities need to be registered to be consumers of CDR data [22]. This regulatory regime is most likely a direct response to the Facebook Cambridge data scandal [23] and a confidence-building response to consumers' security and integrity of data [22].

The CDR was enacted by the Treasury Laws Amendment (CDR) Act 2019 (Cth[a]) which inserted a new Part IVD into the Competition and Consumer Act 2010 (Cth). These laws will follow the data (consumer) standards given by the Commonwealth Scientific and Industrial Research Organisation data [24]. The financial domain would lead the way and others would follow soon [25].

The data processors and data controllers (as defined in Section 6.3) would need to be registered with Australian Competition and Consumer Commission (ACCC) to ensure that the data standards of sharing are maintained.

Some of the highlights of this legislation are:

1. Under Section 56BS (1)

    i.   The ACCC can make rules if it has reasonable belief that it would harm the Australian economy. No consent is required from the minister and the public
    ii. The minister has the power to appeal or vary the emergency data rule
    iii. The ACCC must consider the effect of the rules on consumers, markets, privacy and confidentiality, competition, intellectual property and the public interest among others

2. Under Section 56EO

[a]Commonwealth

i. Data processors and data controllers take steps as outlined in the consumer data rules, to protect the CDR data from misuse, interference and loss, and unauthorised access, modification or disclosure

ii. If the data processor/controller no longer needs data, the Entity needs to take steps to destroy or de-identify that redundant data. The Entity also needs to confirm if the redundant data is not in any current or anticipated legal proceedings or a dispute resolution process (s. 56EO(2)(c)).

6.2.1.4 Criminal law

Main offences [26]:

Criminal law can be engaged if privacy data is used without permission. Penalties apply when used with criminal intent such as to harass or in any fraudulent way.

The relevant sections are as below:

i. s. 478.1(1) Criminal Code – unauthorised access to, or modification of, restricted data

ii. s. 477.3(1) Criminal Code – unauthorised impairment of electronic communication

iii. s. 474.17 Criminal Code – using a carriage service to menace, harass or cause offence.

Penalties

i. The maximum penalty for unauthorised access to, or modification of, restricted data is 2 years' imprisonment

ii. The maximum penalty for using a carriage service to menace, harass or cause offence is 3 years' imprisonment.

6.2.2 Specific to health records

6.2.2.1 Criminal offences from My Health Record

Unauthorised collection, use or disclosure of health information that is included in a healthcare recipient's My Health Record by a person who is not authorised (s 59(1) and (2)) – criminal offence – penalty is 120 penalty units or imprisonment for 2 years, or both. The civil penalty is 600 penalty units.

The person needs to have planned the disclosure, mere accident is not sufficient. A person who has received data from a Third Party (as defined in Section 6.3 of this chapter) could also be liable if the party intentionally disclosed information [27].

6.2.2.2   Mandatory notifications of Data Breach

Under the Notifiable Data Breach scheme, an organisation or agency must notify affected individuals and the Office of the Australian Information Commissioner (OAIC) about an eligible data breach. An eligible data breach [28] occurs when

    i.   there is unauthorised access to or unauthorised disclosure of personal information, or a loss of personal information, that an organisation or agency holds

    ii.   this is likely to result in serious harm to one or more individuals and

   iii. the organisation or agency has not been able to prevent the likely risk of serious harm with remedial action.

6.2.2.3   The Privacy Act 1988

[b]The Privacy Act 1988 (Cth2) is the single most comprehensive legislation for providing broad coverage for data protection, including cyber security[19]. It covers key categories required for cybersecurity breaches and analysis, which are confidentiality, integrity and availability. It also has key concepts of GDPR [GDPR16] such as Data Processor and Data Controller through the definition of Entities, which are applied across the 13 Australian Privacy Principles (APPs).

According to the Privacy act of 1988, an "Entity" can be defined as an agency (which largely refers to a federal government entity and/or office holder) or an organisation (which includes an individual, partnership, unincorporated association, body corporate or trust). This definition would cover all the actors in the use cases for our legal analysis (see Sections 6.4 and 6.5).

The Privacy Act of 1988 requires organisations (all relevant actors related directly or indirectly to EHRs and aged care service providers) to keep data secure and to take reasonable steps to implement required practices and procedures considering 13 APPs into account.

A breach in the privacy of a data subject can be further enhanced through other legislation and case laws, contracts, corporations' law and intentional tort. The elements of these domains are more explicit in GDPR. The English case ("Gulati") [29] and the European Courts recognise that GDPR Article 82 provides a fundamental structure of European Tort law [30].

6.2.2.4   Australian Privacy Principles

The APPs are principles-based laws that apply to any organisation or agency that the Privacy Act 1988 covers. The APPs provide an organisation or agency the flexibility

[b]Commonwealth

to tailor their information-handling practices to their business models and the diverse needs of individuals. These principles are technology-neutral.

There are 13 APPs that govern standards, rights and obligations around:

    i.   the collection, use and disclosure of personal information
    ii.   an organisation or agency's governance and accountability
    iii. integrity and correction of personal information
    iv. the rights of individuals to access their personal information.

A breach of an APP can lead to regulatory action and penalties. The 13 APPs are as provided in Appendix.

6.2.2.5   My Health Records Act 2012 (Cth)

The My Health Record system is a national public system for making health information about a healthcare recipient available for the purposes of providing healthcare to the recipient.

A healthcare recipient will have a My Health Record if the recipient registers in the My Health Record system and have a health record, unless the recipient elects to opt-out of the system. The My Health Record system is operated by the System Operator. The System Operator is Australian Digital Health Agency (ADHA) as of 1 July 2016. Regulation 2.1.1 of the My Health Records Regulation 2012 prescribes the ADHA to be the System Operator. The System Operator operates the National Repositories Service, which stores key records that form part of a healthcare recipient's My Health Record. Other records are stored by registered repository operators [31]. Together these records make up a healthcare recipient's My Health Record, as depicted in Figure 6.1.

If a healthcare recipient is registered in the My Health Record system, a healthcare provider may upload health information about the recipient to the system, unless the record is one which the healthcare recipient has advised the healthcare provider not to upload or the record is not to be uploaded under prescribed laws of a State or Territory.

Health information may be collected, used and disclosed from a healthcare recipient's My Health Record for the purpose of providing healthcare to the recipient, subject to any access controls set by the recipient. Under certain circumstances where health information may be collected, used or disclosed from a My Health Record, criminal and civil penalties apply if a person collects, uses or discloses information from a My Health Record without authorisation.

An authorisation to collect, use or disclose information under this Act is also an authorisation to do so for the purposes of the Privacy Act 1988. A contravention of this Act is also an interference with privacy for the purposes of the Privacy Act 1988 and so can be investigated under that Act.

The My Health Record system operates under the My Health Records Act 2012. The Act establishes:

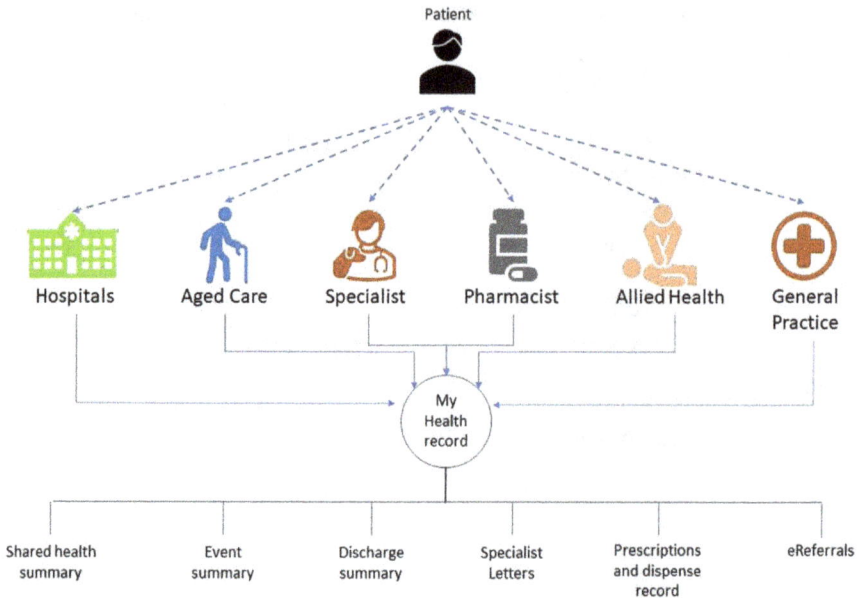

Figure 6.1   Types of records in My Health Record

    i.   the role and functions of the System Operator
   ii.   a registration framework for individuals, and entities such as healthcare provider organisations, to participate in the My Health Record system and
  iii.   a privacy framework (aligned with the Privacy Act 1988) specifying which entities can collect, use and disclose certain information in the system (such as health information contained in a healthcare recipient's My Health Record), and the penalties that can be imposed on improper collection, use and disclosure of this information.

The Commonwealth Minister for Health can make My Health Records Rules under Section 109 of the My Health Records Act, about matters required or permitted by that Act to be dealt with by My Health Records Rules, as set out in the My Health Records Act. The Rules currently in force are:

    i.   My Health Records Rule 2016 – specifying requirements for registered entities in the system
   ii.   My Health Records (National Application) Rules 2017 – providing for the national implementation of the My Health Record system opt-out model under Schedule 1 of the My Health Records Act.

A foundation of the My Health Record system is the Healthcare Identifiers Service, which is established under the Healthcare Identifiers Act 2010.

Other legislation supporting the My Health Record system are:

i.   My Health Records Regulation 2012 – this specifies additional information as identifying information and privacy laws that continue to apply to the disclosure of sensitive information

ii. Healthcare Identifiers Regulations 2010 – these provide additional detail and requirements regarding the operation of the Healthcare Identifiers Service and

iii. My Health Records (Information Commissioner Enforcement Powers) Guidelines 2016 – these set out the Information Commissioner's general approach to exercising its enforcement and investigative powers under the My Health Record system.

6.2.2.6   Contracts and blockchain

A contract is a written or spoken agreement, especially for services, that is intended to be enforceable by law. When the client or data subject pays for the services to a data controller or a data processor, there is a contract. The relationship derived from storing and managing data is part of the contract [32]. This contract would come under the aegis of consumer law among other legislation. The data subject is a defined consumer according to Australian Consumer Law. The contract would be in trade and commerce, *Concrete Construction* [33].

The current consumer legislation is broad enough to provide the data subject sufficient protection from the misuse of data. However, there is not enough case law on this subject. Legislators have provided further consumer rights through the CDR legislation.

There is another issue that could be an obstacle for the consumer, the transient nature of data would make the defaulter elusive [34].

Governing data through contractual nature would free up legislators for having to make more legislation to protect the data subject rights, the sheer volume of contacts would inherently make it complex to adjudicate. It would also be costly to the data subject.

A contractual relationship between the respective partners in the exchange between namely data subject, data processor, data controller and third parties would generate the following benefits:

i.   Question of liability is left to the contracting parties such as responsibility of the integrity of the data.

ii. Freedom to choose the jurisdiction

iii. Contract laws are being implemented to govern internet transactions and thus could easily be used to govern data protection [35].

Current data protection through different types of regulations and the path to jus-tice is complex and expensive for a litigant. Having access to justice is a well-known and well-documented issue and it will especially be true for the elderly patient. A former High Court Justice Michael Kirby describes it as a Rolls Royce legal system. The issues which could arise out of the sole use of contract law are:

i.   that the contracts may not govern all the aspects of data protec-tion issues and especially when the data subject is the vulnerable party
ii. the doctrine of privity will hinder the data subject from pursuing a claim involving Third Parties.

Contract law implemented as a smart contract through blockchain is one pos-sible response to the deficit nature of the traditional contract formations.

Electronic contracts were established initially with the receipt of parking meters (*Thornton v Shoelane*) [36]. Electronic Data Interchange (EDI) further enhanced the for-mation of electronic contracts through the exchange of structured business information such as invoices and orders. An entity receiving the structured digital information could automatically process and integrate it in its own bookkeeping. EDI was a step forward from contracts being formed through paper, faxes and emails. However, EDI has issues due to its simplicity: current data exchange has become voluminous, complex to manage and has issues with real-time processing and security.

To cater to the changing data security and real time processing needs of clients/ data subjects, blockchain platform can be an effective way. Blockchain is a contractual platform that uses digital token for various transactions and it has been proven to be very effective for real time processing and security. Using blockchain could enhance the elec-tronic contract formation. The contract details from the EDI could be integrated into the blockchain infrastructure. In the use case of the Aged Care supply chain, the child node can hold the data subject's privacy data whereas the parent node can act as a controller for activities such as validation and execution timing of the contract. Non-repudiation is also a property of blockchain. MedRec has successfully used this platform to keep the data secure and has utilised both the EDI and blockchain features in a hybrid implementation for a better and secure outcome (Lippman, 2018) [37].

The hybrid solution gives the data subject the power to how and when the private information is to be released to the data controller, data processor and/or third parties. The hybrid blockchain solution has the following advantages:

i.   the public blockchains have no concept of central authority of a state. This means the data subject has authority over their data as compared to government
ii. blockchains provide scalability which is required for content inten-sive medical records
iii. provide confidentiality and privacy to data subjects.

6.3   Identifying and mapping legal actors to corresponding roles and regulations: legal framework

With the introduction of evolving new technologies in the electronic space, online and electronic services have been integrated into all kinds of service delivery including healthcare. Electronic delivery has the potential to under-pin all other delivery channels, providing consistent services within as well as across borders. The legal framework will provide guidance to government and private agencies, sectors as well as jurisdictions in dealing with healthcare data and the legislation that are applicable to EHRs.

6.3.1   Identifying legal actors and resources (data)

A business process is a set of logically related business activities that combine to deliver something of value (e.g. products, goods, services or information) to a patient [38]. A business process can be seen as a set of activities that create a value chain for an organisation and associate the value chain with the requirements of the actors or entities involved in the process. Thus, it is important to identify the various actors to be able to successfully understand and analyse the value chain and map it to the required level of security and privacy.

Actors: An actor is a person or an organisation or a legal entity that can par-ticipate in an activity. Four types of actors can be identified in a business process.

i.   Data Subject: The Australian Privacy Act 1988 regulates the processing of personal information about individuals, defined in Section 6.6 to mean "natural persons". A data subject is a natural person that can be at least reasonably identified from the data and it must relate to that person because of the supply of goods or ser-vices to them or one of their associates.

ii.   Data Processor: As per GDPR [GDPR16], "Processing" means any operation or a set of operations which is performed upon personal data or sets of personal data, whether or not by automated means, such as collection, recording, organisation, structuring, storage, adaptation or alteration, retrieval, consultation, use, disclosure by transmission, dissemination or otherwise making available, align-ment or combination, erasure or destruction. According to appli-cable GDPR [GDPR16], a data processor can be a legal person, a public authority, an agency or an electronic platform that car-ries out the operation or set of operations. Whilst the term "pro-cessor" is not used in the Privacy Act, the APPs naturally apply to the APP entities to the extent that they hold personal informa-tion. According to OAIC, this is sufficiently broad to encompass

	Sensitivity	Assurance Level	Examples	Requirements	Risks and access
Regulated Data	High	High	Social Security Numbers, credit card numbers, bank accounts, driver's license, **health information,** donors.	Protection of data is required by law or policy	High level of harm to reputation with financial costs, access for only those individuals with explicit authorisation, or designated for approved access. Information provides access to resources, physical or virtual.
Confidential Data	Medium	Substantial	Research details, library transactions, personnel information, information covered by non-disclosure agreements, financial information, contracts, facilities, management information.	Contractual obligation to protect.	Medium level of harm to reputation with financial costs, access for employees and non-employees who have a business need to know, delegated access privileges. Smaller subset of restricted data at a school, department, or unit level.
Public Data	Low	Low	Directory information that is not suppressed, campus maps, web pages intended for public use.	At the discretion of the data custodian.	Low level risk to privacy and reputation and general public with a need to know.

Figure 6.2   *Types of data and level of sensitivity [39]. Source: "GDPR, adopted by the European Parliament", [39] [Online]. Available: http://eur-lex.europa.eu/legal-content/EN/TXT/?uri=celex%3A32016R0679.*

outsourced service providers which, in Europe for example, might be considered "processors".

iii.   Third Party: Is any natural or legal person, public authority, agency, or any other body other than the data subject, the controller, the processor and the persons who, under the direct authority of the controller or the processor, are authorised to process the data.

iv.   Resource (Data): Resource is a component of the business process that can be shared physically or electronically between the actors. Resource applies to any kind of data, most importantly, "personal data", which can be defined as any information relating to an identified or identifiable natural person ("data subject").

6.3.2   Data types and assurance levels

A business process, not only in the health sector, often involves the exchange of data which can be personal, organisational and have a national as well as an international origin. Whenever the exchange of data is concerned, there are legal issues that are involved in the process. In order to map the data exchange to legal aspects, data has been categorised into three types according to the level of sensitivity, as given in Figure 6.2. This will pave the way for mapping data to the legal framework.

6.3.3   Mapping actors to their rights and responsibilities (as per GDPR)

Table 6.1 provides an overview of the rights and responsibilities of the various actors as defined in Section 6.3.1.

6.3.4   Identification of appropriate regulations

It is crucial for any EHR-related business process to identify and apply appropriate legislation and regulations to each actor. These regulations and legislation are

Table 6.1   Overview of the rights and responsibilities of the various related actors

Actors	**Rights/Responsibilities**
Data subject	• The rights include
	• The provision of clear and easily understandable information regarding the processing of his or her personal data
	• The right of access, rectification and erasure ("right to be forgotten") of their data
	• The right to obtain data
	• The right to object to profiling
	• The right to lodge a complaint with the competent data protection authority and to bring legal proceedings
	• The right to compensation and damages resulting from an unlawful processing operation
	• The right to data portability
Data controller	• The controller shall adopt appropriate policies and implement appropriate and demonstrable technical and organisational measures to ensure and be able to demonstrate in a transparent manner that the processing of personal data is performed in compliance with this Regulation, having regard to the state of the art, the nature of personal data processing, the context, scope and purposes of the processing, the risks for the rights and freedoms of the data subjects and the type of the organisation, both at the time of the determination of the means for processing and at the time of the processing itself.
	a. The controller shall be able to demonstrate the adequacy and effectiveness of the measures
	b. The controller shall have the right to transmit personal data inside the Union within the group of undertakings the controller is part of, where such processing is necessary for legitimate internal administrative purposes between connected business areas of the group of undertakings and an adequate level of data protection as well as the interests of the data subjects are safeguarded by internal data protection provisions or equivalent codes of conduct as referred to in Article 38

(Continues)

Table 6.1 Continued

Actors	Rights/Responsibilities
Data processor	• Where processing is to be carried out on behalf of a controller, the controller shall choose a processor providing sufficient guarantees to implement appropriate technical and organisational measures and procedures in such a way that the processing will meet the requirements of this Regulation and ensure the protection of the rights of the data subject, in particular in respect of the technical security measures and organisational measures governing the processing to be carried out and shall ensure compliance with those measures • The carrying out of processing by a processor shall be governed by a contract or other legal act binding the processor to the controller. The controller and the processor shall be free to determine respective roles and tasks with respect to the requirements of this Regulation and shall provide that the processor shall: a. process personal data only on instructions from the controller, unless otherwise required by Union law or Member State law b. employ only staff who have committed themselves to confidentiality or are under a statutory obligation of confidentiality c. take all required measures pursuant to Article 30 d. determine the conditions for enlisting another processor only with the prior permission of the controller, unless otherwise determined e. insofar as this is possible given the nature of the processing, create in agreement with the controller the appropriate and relevant technical and organisational requirements for the fulfilment of the controller's obligation to respond to requests for exercising the data subject's rights laid down in Chapter II f. assist the controller in ensuring compliance with the obligations pursuant to Articles 30 to 34 g. return all results to the controller after the end of the processing, not process the personal data otherwise and delete existing copies unless Union or Member State law requires storage of the data h. make available to the controller all information necessary to demonstrate compliance with the obligations laid down in this Article and allow on-site inspections • The controller and the processor shall document in writing the controller's instructions and the processor's obligations • If a processor processes personal data other than as instructed by the controller or becomes the determining party in relation to the purposes and means of data processing, the processor shall be considered to be a controller in respect of that processing and shall be subject to the rules on joint controllers laid down in Article 24.
Third party	• Any party that does not have access to (personal) data except on the basis of either a public legal obligation or a contract between authorised parties

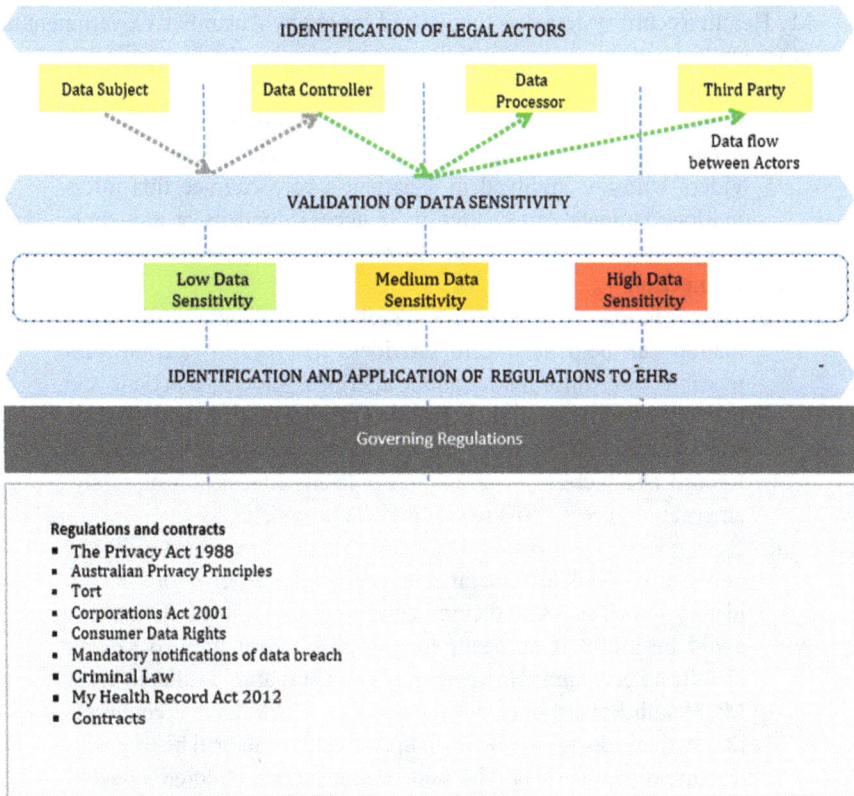

Figure 6.3   Legal framework. Source: "GDPR, adopted by the European Parliament", [39] [Online]. Available: http://eur-lex.europa.eu/ legal-content/EN/TXT/?uri=celex%3A32016R0679.

specific to each country or union. Figure 6.3 provides a snapshot of the combined legal framework as applicable for Australian EHRs. This framework can be used for identifying the various stakeholders as well as the regulations for online health data exchange and transfer.

6.4   Use case 1: My Health Record for aged care and the legal framework

6.4.1   Overview of My Health Record for aged care

My Health Record is a secure electronic healthcare data platform that hosts online summary of an individual's health information and is available to all Australians. Healthcare providers authorised by their healthcare organisation can access My Health Record to view and add to their patients' health information.

My Health Record system was funded and started by Australian Government in 2012 to provide Australians with the following benefits by 2022

    i.   Access: All documents in My Health Record are set to general access for healthcare providers by default. This means any providers who are involved in a patient's care can see this information. Patients can change their access controls at any time. They can access their health information if they have an internet connection.

    ii.   Safety: In a medical emergency, seeing the patient's health information can help healthcare providers quickly provide the best possible care. Information about allergies, adverse reactions and medical conditions helps healthcare providers give better advice and treatment. If a patient has set an access code for his Health Record and there is a serious threat to his life, health or safety, emergency access to his record may be provided.

    iii.   Convenience: If a person has a My Health Record, he will not necessarily need to remember every single detail of his health history – such as his medicines, conditions and test results – which could be useful if he needs to give this information to several healthcare providers. However, having information available in his My Health Record does not replace the need to have a conversation with his doctor to obtain an update on his medical history and/ or current medications. The same applies to his children's health, with My Health Record recording immunisations and medical tests if one wishes.

    iv.   Security: Patient can control who sees what information. There are strict regulations about who can see one's My Health Record. This protects the patient's health information from misuse or loss.

The My Health Record system has around 22.86 million (total population of Australia is 25.5 million) health records as of November 2020. From medical histories to the latest blood tests, more than 2.46 billion documents have been securely stored and uploaded on the platform.

In addition to providing healthcare providers access to their healthcare summary, users of the system can also decide which healthcare providers can view and update their record and decide what information they would like to share.

Various organisations are registered with My Health Record and are using the platform to share and upload patient details. As of November 2020, 99% of Australian pharmacies are registered and 89% are using My Health record. Of the General Practitioners (GPs), 95% are registered and 85% of them are using the My Health Record for uploading patient health documents and updates. About 96% of Australian public hospitals are registered and 94% are using My Health Record.

6.4.1.1 Benefits of My Health Record in aged care

My Health Record offers significant potential to improve care coordination and health outcomes, particularly for older Australians who generally experience a higher prevalence of chronic and complex conditions and polypharmacy and interact frequently with the health system.

My Health Record offers a range of practical uses for aged care health professionals and patients/residents, such as:

i. When meeting a patient/resident for the first time, the healthcare professional can gain an overview of the patient's/resident's health status through their shared health summary in the My Health Record system. This can include their medical conditions, medications, allergies and adverse reactions, and immunisations.

ii. When a patient/resident has been to a hospital, the healthcare professional can gain an overview of the encounter through the discharge summary in their My Health Record. This can include details of treatments, procedures and tests performed and recommendations for follow-up.

iii. The healthcare professional and the patient/resident can refer to their My Health Record for their medications information rather than relying on their memory. This can include the brand name and active ingredients, strength and dosage instructions.

iv. The patient/resident can elect a nominated representative, such as a family member or carer, to share visibility of and help to manage their My Health Record.

v. The patient/resident can upload an advance care-planning document to their My Health Record to record their wishes for end-of-life care.

6.4.2 Health record registration process and upload

Individuals need to register for a health record. This can be done through various ways including online registration via a government portal, offline methods like form submission, through healthcare providers or via government provided helplines. An individual can have only one health record in the system at any given point in time. The user needs to provide various proofs of identity to create the record. Once created, he is able to sign in to his record, view details, share and upload healthcare documents to the health record using an online portal.

All the data is stored on secured servers that are located within Australian borders and are regulated by ADHA, an Australian Govt Agency, and operated by a Federal sponsored National Operator which is an Information Technology service provider selected by ADHA through careful consideration and request for proposals.

6.4.3   Identification of legal actors

Various organisations and individuals can access the My Health Record for various purposes and they have different authorisation and access levels based on the type of service they provide. These organisations and individuals include, but not restricted to, the following

i.   Healthcare provider: Only healthcare provider organisations involved in the patient's care, who are registered with My Health Record, are allowed by law to access My Health Record. Treating healthcare providers can view documents in the patient's My Health Record as part of the default preferences. The patient can add extra privacy controls, so they can choose which healthcare organisations can access their record or individual documents in it. These can be GPs, Public hospitals or private hospitals, Nursing homes, Diagnostic imaging and pathology service providers.

ii.   Nominated representative: A nominated representative is a trusted person invited by the patient to help manage his My Health Record. They might be a family member, close friend or carer.

iii.   Authorised Representatives: An authorised representative manages the My Health Record of someone who cannot manage their own. This could be for their child under 14 years, or someone of any age who lacks the capacity to manage their own record. An authorised representative may be a parent, carer, family member or someone with an enduring power of attorney.

iv.   Access in emergency: In a medical emergency, healthcare providers can access My Health Record to see the patient's health information, so they can provide them with the best possible treatment and care.

v.   Software products: Several software products used by healthcare organisations support digital health functions, including Medical Director, Fred IT, MedTech32, Smart clinics, Genie, Best Practice and more. These software products can access, view and upload documents to the My Health Record system.

For the purpose of legal analysis using the legal framework from Section 6.3 of this chapter, the above-mentioned entities have been categorised in Table 6.2.

6.4.4   Legal analysis

Introduction of new services and technologies for data sharing and transfer entails the need to frequently re-evaluate the various risks and threats to patient's sensitive data and implement necessary measures to counter them. In this use case, the patient's personal health data is uploaded on the My Health Record system through adequate procedures, depending on the level of data sensitivity.

Table 6.2   Categorising actors and entities

Data subject	Data controller	Data processor	Third party
• Patient • Nominated representative • Authorised representative	• Federal Government • ADHA • National regulators	• National operator	• Registered public hospitals • Registered private hospitals • General practitioners (GPs) • Software products and applications • Nursing homes • Aged care facilities • Diagnostic imaging and pathology service providers

All the actors in this use case have been categorised into data subject, data con-troller, data processor and third party for ease of legal analysis. The patient, autho-rised and nominated representatives have been categorised as the data subjects who own the personal data. Service providers, private and public hospitals, GPs, software products, diagnostic imaging and pathology service providers have been categorised as third party. The national operator has been categorised as a National processor as they process all the data that is uploaded and implement required authentication and legislative technical aspects to the system. ADHA, federal government bodies have been categorised as the national operators.

6.4.4.1   Mapping actors and data to regulations

Figure 6.4 portrays the mapping of the My Health Record use-case-specific actors to their respective legislation and regulations[40]. Each actor of the use case has been mapped to the regulations they are bound by. Corresponding regulation articles have also been presented.

6.5   Use case 2: legal analysis of online health record of dementia patient in aged care

The second use case that we will delve into for this chapter is online health record of a dementia patient in an aged care facility. This scenario will look at the electronic health record creation process that is different to the My Health Record creation pro-cess as discussed in the previous use case and hence the entities and actors involved will be different as well.

6.5.1   Overview of online health record of Australian dementia patient in aged care

Dementia is the second leading cause of death of Australians (BAEvans, 2018)[41]. Dementia is described as a collection of symptoms that are caused by disorders

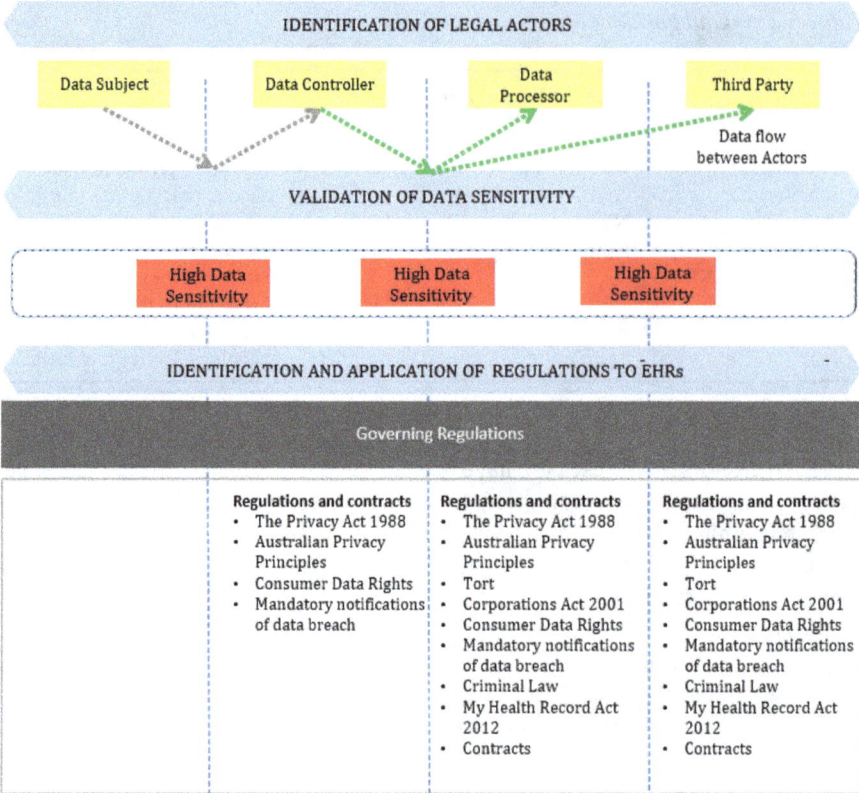

Figure 6.4   Mapping of My Health Record actors to legislation and regulations [39]

affecting the brain. It is not one specific disease. It affects thinking, behaviour and the ability to perform everyday tasks. Brain function is affected enough to interfere with the person's normal social or working life. It can happen to anybody, but it is more common after the age of 65 years.

In 2020, there is an estimated 459 000 Australians living with dementia [42] and this number is expected to increase to 590 000 by 2028. People with dementia account for 52% of all residents in residential aged care facilities.

Generally, a dementia patient is registered at an aged care facility by an authorised or a nominated representative. Once the registration is completed, most aged care facilities that provide 24 hr-care and support will create an electronic health record of the patient with all personal and health-related information. This health record would be created on third-party software or application and the record will be accessible by the staff and doctors of the aged care facility. If the facility is registered with My Health Record system, then the main aged care software or application will have the means to connect, view and upload information to My Health Record system if access is granted by the patient or their legal representative.

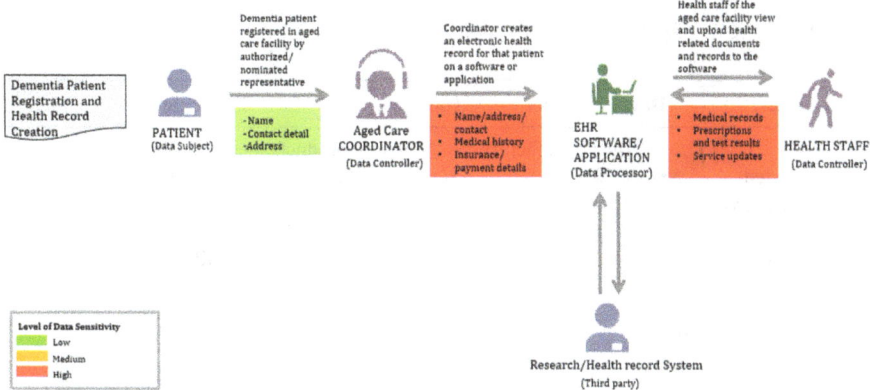

Figure 6.5   Dementia patient registration and electronic health record creation

Various government research bodies might access the patient record on My Health Record for various research purposes or statistical analysis. Figure 6.5 depicts the dementia patient registration and electronic health record creation process.

6.5.2   Identification of legal actors

In this use case, there are various legal actors that can be identified, as also depicted in Figure 6.4. The dementia patient and their authorised/nominated representative in this case would be considered as the data subject who own the patient data. The aged care facility including its coordinators, staff and healthcare providers will be data controllers. They are responsible for registering the patient and provide necessary healthcare services. The data controllers are also responsible for creating an electronic health record in their software or application that is owned or licensed by the aged care facility. In most cases the software/application is developed by an external software vendor. Hence the software or application is considered as the data processor that processes the electronic patient record. Health staff have access to the patient record as per the access levels granted by the patient and his representatives. They can view and update the record as required. The software application might need to be able to integrate with the government My Health Record for various reasons like research, health record update for funding purpose. In this use case, the My Health Record system will be a third-party entity that can read and write to the Data Processor software. Various government and research organisations can have access to the patient record through the My Health Record. Even these research organisations would be considered as third-party entities.

For the purpose of legal analysis using the legal framework from Section 6.3 of this chapter, the above-mentioned entities have been categorised in Table 6.3.

6.5.3   Legal analysis

In this use case, the patient's personal health data is uploaded to an online platform for patient management by the aged care staff and healthcare providers. All

Table 6.3   Categorising actors and entities

Data subject	Data controller	Data processor	Third party
• Patient • Nominated representative • Authorised representative	• Aged care facility • Staff • Health workers • Contracted medical providers	• Software products and platforms like Medical Director, Fred IT, MedTech32	• Registered public hospitals • Registered private hospitals • GPs • Software products and applications • Nursing homes • Aged care facilities • Diagnostic imaging and pathology service providers

the actors in this use case have been categorised into Data Subject, Data Controller, Data Processor and Third Party for ease of legal analysis. The patient and his authorised and nominated representatives have been categorised as the data subject who own the personal data. Aged care facility staff and healthcare service providers have been categorised as data controllers. The software for electronic health record creation and maintenance is categorised as the Data processor. My Health Record system and other research platforms that integrate with the software are categorised as third-party entities.

6.5.3.1   Mapping actors and data to regulations

Figure 6.6 portrays the mapping of the Aged Care Dementia Patient use-case-specific actors to their respective legislation and regulations. Each actor of the use case has been mapped to the regulations they are bound by.

6.6   Conclusion

Even though the online health data sharing systems have many advantages over paper-based processes, there are still issues that exist like

    i.   Data confidentiality is being maintained by an Australian Federal Agency (in Australia that is the ADHA who are also the National Operator for My Health Record), private health practitioners, hospitals, laboratories among others. The National operator for My Health Record can aggregate data from other data controllers even when consent is not provided by the data subject for each health record. Blanket consent is collected from the Data Subject in most cases.

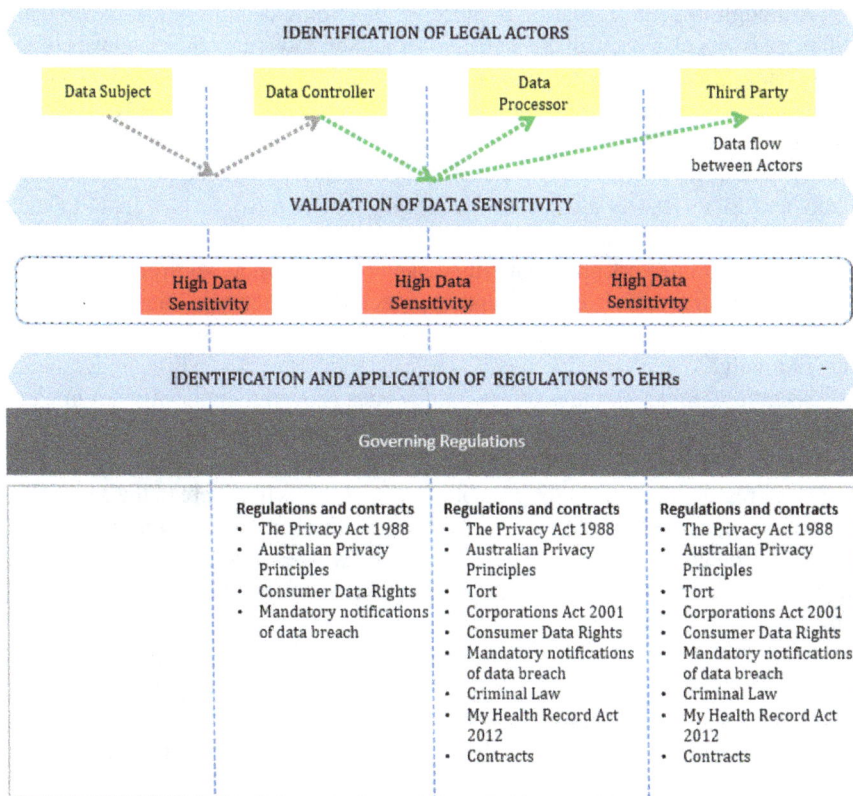

IDENTIFICATION OF LEGAL ACTORS

Data Subject   Data Controller   Data Processor   Third Party

Data flow
between Actors

VALIDATION OF DATA SENSITIVITY

High Data Sensitivity   High Data Sensitivity   High Data Sensitivity

IDENTIFICATION AND APPLICATION OF REGULATIONS TO EHRs

Governing Regulations

Regulations and contracts	Regulations and contracts	Regulations and contracts
• The Privacy Act 1988 • Australian Privacy Principles • Consumer Data Rights • Mandatory notifications of data breach	• The Privacy Act 1988 • Australian Privacy Principles • Tort • Corporations Act 2001 • Consumer Data Rights • Mandatory notifications of data breach • Criminal Law • My Health Record Act 2012 • Contracts	• The Privacy Act 1988 • Australian Privacy Principles • Tort • Corporations Act 2001 • Consumer Data Rights • Mandatory notifications of data breach • Criminal Law • My Health Record Act 2012 • Contracts

Figure 6.6   Mapping of actors to legislation and regulations [39]

ii. Public health data is kept under one central database, but copies are maintained across multiple servers for risk mitigation. This could lead to potential data security issues. Also, with the health data shared across data controller, various data processors and Third-Party applications, the potential issue of cybersecurity breach increases manifold. The problem is complex as each of the data controllers also controls its own cybersecurity environment.

iii. Third-party applications can get access to public health data via the blanket consent provided by Data Subjects to the Data Controller (or National Operator). The level of access provided in some cases might be more than the legitimate requirements of access given by the data controller or consented by the Data Subject. Data Subject has very little control over his data once it has been collected by the Data Controller in the beginning of a business process when the health record is created.

Although there is legislation in place for electronic dealing of healthcare data, still there is less clarity on all the legislation together. Laws are made to make citizen rights transparent and easy to understand. The legal framework, as described in this chapter, will provide guidance to individuals as well as organisations in identifying the responsibilities and liabilities of the parties involved in an online business process that deals with uploading and sharing of sensitive health data in the form of EHRs and PHRs. It will also help in identifying the regulations that apply to each entity involved in the process.

The legal framework proposed in this chapter has some noteworthy contributions.

First, the framework ensures that approaches to electronic data privacy and security balance the underlying risk with the need for ease of use on behalf of all parties involved.

Second, it enhances the confidence of parties (government or private) in electronic dealings, by providing more insights into the roles and responsibilities and the legislation linked with each entity involved in the process.

More research is needed for possible solutions that will adhere to the applicable legislation for processes and systems that deal with electronic healthcare data and provide adequate transparency and control to the involved parties over this data. One such possible solution might be the use of blockchains. Blockchains have garnered a lot of interest over the past few years when it comes to online-secured data. This can be used in the context of health data as well. Blockchains, if implemented, can directly involve the data subject by providing him optimum transparency and control over his data at any stage of the process. The cost of implementing a blockchain solution at the scale of a public health record system and the benefits still need to be researched more.

Appendix: Australian Privacy Principles

Principle	Title	Purpose
APP 1	Open and transparent management of personal information	Ensures that APP entities manage *personal information* in an open and transparent way. This includes having a clearly expressed and up to date APP *privacy policy.*
APP 2	Anonymity and pseudonymity	Requires APP entities to give individuals the option of not identifying themselves, or of using a pseudonym. Limited exceptions apply.
APP 3	Collection of solicited personal information	Outlines when an APP entity can collect personal information that is solicited. It applies higher standards to the collection of "sensitive" information.
APP 4	Dealing with unsolicited personal information	Outlines how APP entities must deal with unsolicited personal information.

Principle	Title	Purpose
APP 5	Notification of the collection of personal information	Outlines when and in what circumstances an APP entity that collects personal information must notify an individual of certain matters.
APP 6	Use or disclosure of personal information	Outlines the circumstances in which an APP entity may use or disclose personal information that it holds.
APP 7	Direct marketing	An organisation may only use or disclose personal information for direct marketing purposes if certain conditions are met.
APP 8	Cross-border disclosure of personal information	Outlines the steps an APP entity must take to protect personal information before it is disclosed overseas.
APP 9	Adoption, use or disclosure of government-related identifiers	Outlines the limited circumstances when an organisation may adopt a government-related identifier of an individual as its own identifier, or *use or disclose* a government-related identifier of an individual.
APP 10	Quality of personal information	An APP entity must take reasonable steps to ensure the personal information it collects is accurate, up to date and complete. An entity must also take reasonable steps to ensure the personal information it uses or discloses is accurate, up to date, complete and relevant, having regard to the purpose of the use or disclosure.
APP 11	Security of personal information	An APP entity must take reasonable steps to protect the personal information it holds from misuse, interference and loss, and unauthorised access, modification or disclosure. An entity has obligations to destroy or de-identify personal information in certain circumstances.
APP 12	Access to personal information	Outlines an APP entity's obligations when an individual requests to be given *access to personal information* held about them by the entity. This includes a requirement to provide access unless a specific exception applies.
APP 13	Correction of personal information	Outlines an APP entity's obligations in relation to *correcting the personal information* it holds about individuals.

References

[1]   Kruse C.S., Stein A., Thomas H., Kaur H. 'The use of electronic health re-
      cords to support population health: a systematic review of the literature'.
      Journal of Medical Systems. 2018, vol. 42(11), p. 214.

[2]   Kierkegaard P. 'Electronic health record: Wiring Europe's healthcare'.
      Computer Law & Security Review. 2011, vol. 27(5), pp. 503–15.

[3]   Menachemi N., Collum T.H. 'Benefits and drawbacks of electronic health
      record systems'. *Risk Management and Healthcare Policy.* 2011, vol. 4(4),
      pp. 47–55.

[4]   Silow-Caroll S., Edwards J.N., Rodin D. *'Using electronic health records
      to improve quality and efficiency: the experiences of leading hospitals'.*
      Commonwealth Fund; 2012.

[5]   Tang P.C., Ash J.S., Bates D.W., Overhage J.M., Sands D.Z. 'Personal health
      records: definitions, benefits, and strategies for overcoming barriers to adop-
      tion'. *Journal of the American Medical Informatics Association.* 2006, vol.
      13(2), pp. 121–6.

[6]   Bauman A.E., Fardy H.J., Harris P.G. 'Getting it right: why bother with
      patient-centred care?' *Medical Journal of Australia.* 2003, vol. 179(5), pp.
      253–6.

[7]   Detme D., Steen E. *Learning from Abroad: Lessons and Questions on
      Personal Health Records for National Policy.* AARP Public Policy Institute;
      2006.

[8]   N. H. Service. *Summary Care Records (SCR) – information for patients [on-
      line].* 2020. Available from https://digital.nhs.uk/services/summary-care-re-
      cords-scr/summary-care-records-scr-information-for-patients [Accessed 29
      Dec 2020].

[9]   U.S. Department of Health & Human Right Services. Privacy, security, and
      electronic health records [online]. Available from https://www.hhs.gov/sites/
      default/files/ocr/privacy/hipaa/understanding/consumers/privacy-security-
      electronic-records.pdf [Accessed 29 Dec 2020].

[10] C. H. Infoway. Canada Health Infoway [online]. Available from https://www.
      infoway-inforoute.ca/en/component/edocman/3466-infographic-infoway-s-
      strategic-plan-2017-2022/view-document?Itemid=101 [Accessed 29 Dec
      2020].

[11] Singh A.S., Jebaraj S. 'Implementing electronic health records in New Zealand:
      a critical appraisal of literature'. *Health Informatics – An International
      Journal.* 2016, vol. 5(4), p. 8.

[12] Rezaeibagha F., Win K.T., Susilo W. 'A systematic literature review on secu-
      rity and privacy of electronic health record systems: technical perspectives'.
      Health Information Management Journal. 2015, vol. 44(3), pp. 23–38.

[13] O'Keefe C.M., Connolly C.J., O'Keefe C.C. 'Privacy and the use of health
      data for research'. *Medical Journal of Australia.* 2010, vol. 193(9), pp.
      537–41.

[14] Kerai P., Wood P., Martin M. 'A pilot study on the views of elderly regional Australians of personally controlled electronic health records'. *International Journal of Medical Informatics*. 2014, vol. 83(3), pp. 201–9.

[15] Trakman L., Walters R., Zeller B. 'Tort and data protection: are there any lessons to be learnt?" *EDPR Review, UNSW Law Research*'. *EDPR Review*. 2019, vol. 5(4), pp. 1–20.

[16] E. P. a. C. o. t. E. Union. General Data Protection Regulation. 2016. Available from https://eur-lex.europa.eu/legal-content/EN/TXT/PDF/?uri=CELEX:32016R0679&from=EN [Accessed 29 Dec 2020].

[17] Office of the Australian Information Commissioner. *When to report a data breach* [online]. Available from https://www.oaic.gov.au/privacy/notifiable-data-breaches/when-to-report-a-data-breach/ [Accessed 29 Dec 2020].

[18] 'Wilkinson v Downton, *EWHC 1*, 2 QB 57, 1897'.

[19] Cyber Security – Who is liable if your business is breached? Available from https://www.s5.technology/cyber-security-who-is-liable-if-your-network-or-data-is-breached/ [Accessed 29 Dec 2020].

[20] S. T. Group. *Cyber security – who is liable if your business is breached?* [online] Available from https://www.s5.technology/cyber-security-who-is-liable-if-your-network-or-data-is-breached/ [Accessed 29 Dec 2020].

[21] Collyer A. *The* consumer data right and energy – what it means and what to do about it [online]. 2019. Available from https://www.allens.com.au/insights-news/insights/2019/03/the-consumer-data-right-and-energy-what-it-means-a [Accessed 29 Dec 2020].

[22] Linklaters A. *Consumer data right [online]*. Available from https://www.allens.com.au/insights-news/insights/hubs/consumer-data-right-hub/ [Accessed 29 Dec 2020].

[23] Wong J.C. *The Cambridge Analytica – scandal changed the world but it didnt change Facebook [online]*. 2019. Available from https://www.theguardian.com/technology/2019/mar/17/the-cambridge-analytica-scandal-changed-the-world-but-it-didnt-change-facebook [Accessed 29 Dec 2020].

[24] Ishak R., Grillakis V. *Why consumer data right will change your life [online]*. 2019. Available from https://www.williamroberts.com.au/news-and-insights/insights/articles/why-consumer-data-right-will-change-your-life [Accessed 29 Dec 2020].

[25] The Office of the Australian Information Commissioner. *CDR legislation [online]*. Available from https://www.oaic.gov.au/consumer-data-right/cdr-legislation/ [Accessed 29 Dec 2020].

[26] CDPP. *Cybercrime [online]*. Available from https://www.cdpp.gov.au/crimes-we-prosecute/cybercrime [Accessed 29 Dec 2020].

[27] Wolf G., Mendelson D. 'The my health record system: potential to undermine the paradigm of patient confidentiality?' *SSRN Electronic Journal*. 2019, vol. 42(2), pp. 619–651.

[28] Notifiable Data Breaches Privacy Amendment Act 2017 [online]. Available from https://www.oaic.gov.au/privacy/notifiable-data-breaches/when-to-report-a-data-breach/ [Accessed 29 Dec 2020].

[29]   '*EWHC 1482 (Ch*'. *[2015] EWCA Civ 1291 (CA)*. 2015.

[30]   'Liability under EU Data Protection Law - From Directive 95/46 to the General Data Protection Regulation'. *Journal of Intellectual Property, Information Technology and E-Commerce Law*. 2016, vol. 7(217).

[31]   My Health Records Act 2012 [online]. Available from https://www.legislation.gov.au/Details/C2018C00509 [Accessed 29 Dec 2020].

[32]   Bennet B. *Law and Medicine, Sydney, Holmes Beach, Fla: LBC Information Services*. W. Gaunt and Sons; 1997.

[33]   Concrete Constructions *(NSW) Pty Ltd v Nelson 92 ALR*. 1990. Available from https://www.australiancontractlaw.info/cases/database/concrete-constructions-v-nelson.

[34]   Manwaring K. 'Will emerging technologies outpace consumer protection law? The case of digital consumer manipulation'. *Competition and Consumer Law Journal*. 2018, vol. 26(2), pp. 141–81.

[35]   Lim L. 'Approaches to liability for breaches in data security'. *Macarthur Law Review*. 1999, vol. 3(8), pp. 81–99.

[36]   *Thornton v Shoe Lane Parking Ltd* [1971] 2 WLR 585, [1971] 1 All ER 686, [1970] EWCA Civ 2, [1971] RTR 79, [1971] 1 LLR 289, [1971] 2 QB 163, [1971] 1 Lloyd's Rep 289. 1971. Available from http://www.bailii.org/ew/cases/EWCA/Civ/1970/2.html.

[37]   Lippman A., Nchinda N., Retzepi K., Cameron A. *Medrec: Patient control of medical record distribution* [online]. 2018. Available from https://blockchain.ieee.org/technicalbriefs/july-2018/medRec-patient-control-of-medical-record-distribution [Accessed 29 Dec 2020].

[38]   Cousins J S.T. *What Is Business Process Design and Why Should I Care?* RivCom Ltd; 2002.

[39]   Regulation EU. *GDPR, adopted by the European Parliament* [online]. 2016. Available from http://eur-lex.europa.eu/legal-content/EN/TXT/?uri=celex%3A32016R0679 [Accessed 29 Dec 2020].

[40]   Ghorai K., Smits J.M., Ray P., Kluitman M. 'Business and legal framework for health data privacy assessment: example of ambient assisted living'. Amsterdam Platform for Privacy Research (APPR); Amsterdam; 2015.

[41]   Evans B.A., Beverly C.J., Tsai P.-F., Rettiganti M., Lefler L.L., Parks R.F. 'Older adults' live demonstration of electronic personal health record use: factors mediating initial proficiency'. *Computers, informatics, nursing : CIN*. 2018, vol. 36(12), pp. 603–9.

[42]   Turner A.M., Osterhage K., Hartzler A., *et al.* 'Use of patient portals for personal health information management: the older adult perspective'. *AMIA Annual Symposium proceedings. AMIA Symposium*. 2015, vol. 2015, pp. 1234–41.

Part II

Digital Health Services for Healthy Ageing

Chapter 7

Silvercare: a model for supporting healthy ageing services

Kasturi Bakshi[1], Jacqueline Blake[2], and Pradeep Ray[3,4]

7.1 Introduction

Ageing is a normal and inevitable physiological phenomenon. This is an age where people are urged to make this phase of life enjoyable and worth living. It has been recognised that improving the quality of life by focusing on issues such as social connections and maintaining mobility is as important as adding years to that life. In the twenty-first century, population ageing is one of the biggest social transformations underway (WHO). The present demographic transition of an ageing population is the consequence of declining fertility and mortality – an indicator of improving global health. The declining mortality rate can be attributed to better healthcare and is accompanied by a decline in fertility rates. Hence ageing need not be perceived in a negative way. According to a landmark report published by United Nations Population Fund (UNFPA) and HelpAge in October 2012, ageing in the twenty-first century is a celebration and a challenge [1].

A long and healthy life brings some great opportunities, like being able to pursue neglected passions, which may contribute to better mental health. Healthy elderly populations can contribute in many ways to their families and communities. One of the benefits of having healthy grandparents in close proximity is the provision of childcare, especially when both the parents are working. It has been seen that when grandparents and grandchildren spend time together, it can benefit both generations. For reaping the benefits of longevity, integration and participation of older persons in society is extremely important for potentially growing community capacity. Seniors provide an important and growing market for products and services if care is taken to meet their needs and requirements. Caring for the seniors

[1]Kalyani Institute for Study, Planning and Action for Rural Change (KINSPARC), Kalyani, India
[2]School of Science Technology and Engineering, USC, Australia
[3]Center for Entrepreneurship, University of Michigan-Shanghai Jiao Tong University Joint Institute, Shanghai, China
[4]School of Population Health, UNSW, Sydney, New South Wales, Australia

enables them to not worry about the things they cannot do anymore and celebrate the things that they can [2].

With this changing demography leading to an increase in demand for senior care, healthcare providers and all caregivers are looking for technologies and techniques for assistance. For a better quality of life for the seniors, social behaviour research and technological development need to work together.

This chapter presents an innovative human resource model of 'Silvercare', which implies care for seniors, thereby enabling economic care of ageing population (at emotional and intellectual levels) through the relatively younger seniors in the neighbourhood. Silvercare is a win-win (for both the seniors receiving the care and pensioners providing the care) solution for many services for the ageing population. The chapter starts with a background of aged care in various countries in Section 7.2, followed by the description of Silvercare model in Section 7.3. This is followed by case studies of Silvercare in India and Australia in Sections 7.4 and 7.5. The chapter ends with a discussion of our case study research in Section 7.6 and conclusions in Section 7.7.

7.2   Background of care for the elderly around the world

The ageing population worldwide is prompting people to look for solutions to address the needs of the elderly who have spent their lives serving others and are themselves in need of support now. 'We live in a society where care of young and old is increasingly segregated, with very limited opportunity for the two age groups to interact' [3]. If we tried to combine some of the activities of the two types of care centres, these could become great resources for each other. This model is being tried out with positive impact in Australia, UK, Japan and some other countries too. We will also discuss some good practices in different countries around the world.

7.2.1   Japan

Japan now has the oldest population in the world, and care for the elderly is no longer a matter of family concern alone but is a serious matter of social concern as well. 'Super-ageing is our destiny—it's the natural consequence of human evolution' said Hideyuki Okano, dean of Keio University's School of Medicine. He also argued that although Japan is the first super-ageing society, others will inevitably follow [4].

The impact of population ageing is huge and has many facets. Japan is an example of a rapidly growing population over 65 years old. A paper on Japan's ageing population and its silvercare industry by Eiichi and Hisakazu state, 'this dramatic change in the age structure of the population is already inducing profound changes to Japan's economy and society, with more set to come' [5]. In Japan, there has been a decrease in the working population and an increase in the non-working population since the late 1990s [5], with ageing of the population as the primary cause of the declining workforce. In the majority of Japan's organisations, a mandatory retirement age between 60 and 65 years old is in place leading to a pool of retired people who may not have been ready to cease paid work. Therefore, there is an increase in the number of retirees who do not work anymore but are eligible for pensions and other welfare schemes once they reach 65 years of age. They are usually fit and healthy and financially well off and covered by insurance and social security schemes. According to the 2011 Care Service Facilities and Business Study from the Ministry of Health, Labor and Welfare, Government of Japan, there are 20 000 providers of home visit care, day care, preventive home visit care and preventive day care; 6 000 senior care welfare facilities; 3 000 senior care public health facilities and 2 000 recovery and treatment facilities. These retirees are a rich source of skills and knowledge in affluent circumstances. To rejuvenate the Japanese society, a system could be developed which taps the skills and knowledge of senior citizens for the benefit of society and take the country forward.

Like all other consumer groups, seniors need to purchase the necessities of daily life, entertainment and other products; therefore, an increase in the number of seniors is increasing opportunities for organisations focused on this demographic. A market has already developed for assisted living for seniors and assistive technologies customised to make life easier for the seniors. In Japan, products and services focused on seniors that are provided by the private sector rather than the government are termed Silvercare [5] although Chéron calls this a Silver Market. Silvercare is a growing industry in Japan [6].

'Respect for the Aged Day' is a Japanese designated public holiday celebrated annually to honour elderly citizens. It started in 1966 as a national holiday and was held on every September 15. Since 2003, Respect for the Aged Day is held on the third Monday of September. On this National Holiday, people show respect to the elders by arranging feasts for the seniors, and children entertain their senior neighbours by singing, dancing, etc. Celebrating this day is a way of generating awareness regarding seniors in the community.

> Japan introduced a nursing care insurance system in April of 2000 which provided an opportunity for private businesses to enter a market formerly dominated by the government. The nursing care insurance system is a public, universal, and compulsory system in which all Japanese citizens over 40 years of age are registered and pay premiums. The insurance was originally introduced to allow Japanese citizens to freely choose and enter contracts with care service providers, and to be responsible for their own care [5].

Since then, senior care in Japan has become a full-fledged industry based on services paid for by nursing care insurance. With nursing care insurance benefits providing the needed funding, Japan's silvercare business can tap into the demand created by Japan's rapidly increasing elderly population.

7.2.2 Scotland

In 2011, 'Reshaping Care for Older People' [7] was a programme launched in Scotland to focus on the well-being of the seniors from 2011 to 2021 [8]. The clear vision of the programme is 'Older people in Scotland are valued as an asset, their voices are heard and older people are supported to enjoy full and positive lives in their own home or in a homely setting.'

The plan from the Government of Scotland is that they should move away from an overreliance on traditional 'institutional' care towards care and support in the home or a community setting that is designed around the needs of the individual, which encourages seniors to stay active and stay at home as long as possible. So the plan is to:

- prioritise preventive spending
- empower individuals and communities
- have organisations work closely together to deliver services
- have services to optimise quality of life.

However, in comparison to Japan's Silvercare model, this is primarily a policy for Government-provided services. The aim is to provide an inclusive community care model with a lot of importance given to 'personalisation', 'independence' and 'control', which play a significant role in living with dignity.

7.2.3   Netherlands

An innovative solution towards the increasingly depersonalised care in residential care facilities was taken by the Netherlands. This was also a time when a student housing issue existed; the programme provided free rent to university students in exchange for a minimum of 30 hours per month of good neighbour activities. These activities range from a simple visit to assist with technology and expeditions to shopping malls. The students sharing experiences from their lives and Arentshorst, Kloet and Peine stating that the seniors took a keen interest in the activities of the students, triggering reminiscences of their own activities that they had enjoyed. The progressive facility also welcomes people who need some day-to-day assistance from a local community into the facility. The philosophy of the facility was that healthcare delivery was a shared responsibility between staff and residents [9].

7.2.4   Germany

Germany in common with Japan qualifies as super-aged with more than 21% of their population over 65. Germany has been pursuing a range of policies to enable seniors to age, living independently in the community since 2009 [10]. This is another example of Silvercare accompanied with a long-term care insurance and healthcare providers using technology to improve access to services. Another innovation is the establishment of multigenerational homes. This innovative approach situates a building of senior-occupied apartments equipped with round-the-clock assistance right next door to a nursery school. The children enjoy recess in a yard shared with the seniors' building. The seniors continue to be part of the fabric of the community and enjoy the presence of the children in their everyday lives. The seniors in Germany have a high level of life satisfaction in comparison with the general population. One of the contributing factors may be the high levels of volunteering in the seniors at 34% [10].

7.2.5   Singapore

While Singapore is not currently a super-aged society, it is suggested that the sector of the population of people over 65 years old will become over 21% within the next decade [11]. The Singaporean government has taken a long-term strategic approach towards planning for an ageing society. This includes government-provided services in conjunction with the Silvercare model of private enterprises offering services. One of the strategies is to decrease the digital divide in seniors by promoting a programme where seniors with a high level of digital skills volunteer to pass on their skills to lower-skilled seniors using smaller self-help groups. For the person with a higher level of skill, they gain the altruistic benefits of volunteering [11].

7.3   Silvercare model

Ageing is associated with several kinds of problems. Ageing leads to deterioration of health conditions with impairment of vision, hearing, cognitive function, dementia and many other disabilities. Aged people are also more likely to suffer from diabetes, hypertension, osteoporosis, osteoarthritis and so on. Gradually seniors develop dependence and suffer from insecurity and loneliness. They long for care, support, company, respect and dignity.

Silvercare models serve to provide assisted living services. The Silvercare model has been used in several countries, such as Japan and Singapore [12]. Here we discuss the Silvercare model which is a win-win solution for two groups of people: elderly above 65 years (beneficiaries) and relatively young pensioners above 60 years (coordinators), retired from the workforce but willing to help older people in their neighbourhood. Typically one coordinator would serve about ten beneficiaries in the neighbourhood by visiting them and helping them over leisurely discussions and seminars/webinars on topics of interest, such as technology adoption (e.g., smartphones and their applications) and health/well-being.

The basic concept of this model is to utilise the resources available amongst the able seniors in the community for the benefit of those seniors who are in need. In other words 'by the seniors, for the seniors'.

The primary aims of Silvercare are:

- to improve the quality of life of elderly people by providing them with care and support in a community
- to increase awareness of the general population and sensitise the younger generation on the needs and issues of the aged
- advocacy for services for the elderly.

Community-based care can ensure the participation of the elderly in the process and not make them dependent completely on the care/service givers. A community-based model like Silvercare can help to sensitise the younger generation to the needs and issues of the elderly and motivate them to participate in ensuring the well-being of senior citizens.

Silvercare model is a win-win proposition for several stakeholders.

7.3.1   *Beneficiaries*

Seniors prefer living independently with dignity rather than in residential care nursing homes. Most of them have difficulty in adopting and using new technologies, such as smartphones and digital media. Consequently, they are deprived of many important communications coming over digital media from the government, banks, news organisations, etc. Besides, they yearn for frequent communication with children and grandchildren who are often in geographically remote locations. These people are not willing to pay for the latest technologies though their children are willing. Silvercare coordinators in the neighbourhood can visit their homes and help them overcome some of the difficulties with technology and information sources. They also need both emotional and physical support to move around and for home maintenance.

7.3.2   *Coordinators*

Those senior citizens who have retired but are very active and eager to volunteer, have ample free time, are financially stable and unencumbered (as mostly their children have settled down in life) form a team of volunteers to serve the seniors who need assistance. They possess better understanding of the problems of the aged and are in a position to empathise. Each coordinator identifies senior citizens in his/her neighbourhood and enrols them as beneficiaries provided those seniors are interested in getting assistance. Unpaid volunteer coordinators provide an excellent, economic way to help beneficiaries effectively as they can provide both physical and emotional support. However, these coordinators deserve full respect for their social contribution. Some NGOs for instance muktiweb.org are now tapping this resource through a streamlined process.

7.3.3   *Support group*

Medical professionals, lawyers, software engineers, sociologists and others step in as and when required. Medical professionals interact for medical emergencies and other medical care. Sociologists and some other members render their services in group activities to combat loneliness and generate awareness. Lawyers give legal advice and so on.

7.3.4   *Service providers*

The recognition of the over 65 years old demographic as a large and potential valuable market with different requirements has been growing since the 1990s. This market is served by government and non-government agencies with policies and services often aimed at allowing seniors to age within the community with suitable infrastructure. These services can range from support for reemployment or volunteering to utilise the senior's skills and knowledge to providing spaces where the community are encouraged to build relationships with seniors. An organisation in Germany calling this kinship by choice [10]. Private enterprise is also encouraged by governments to provide goods and services for this demographic focused on people who want to lead busy, productive and socially active lives that extend beyond the provision of residential care.

The next two sections (7.4 and 7.5) discuss the application of Silvercare in two countries India (Kalyani, West Bengal) and Australia (Sunshine Coast, Queensland) through two case studies on empowering the seniors (beneficiaries) on digital media technology which is discussed next.

7.3.5   Tablet-based well-being project

Bergström states that due to the increased importance of the Internet in the last 20 years, waiting until digital natives age into this demographic is not a valid strategy [13], finding that one of the biggest contributors to the digital divide is educational level. Without interventions to reverse this characteristic, inequality amongst seniors extends to quality of life and social connectedness.

The silvercare application case studies were conducted as part of the project called 'Tablet-Based Well-Being Check' led by Pradeep Ray [14]. In order to implement a practically feasible solution from the perspectives of all stakeholders (IT people, elderly, family members, healthcare providers and aged care providers), the project used a three-stage agile methodology to be able to capture and test the needs of the elderly in this design, as summarised in [14].

- The first stage involved the development and testing of a digital photo frame for well-being monitoring.
- In the second stage, the modification of the design was performed between November 2013 and February 2014 based on the feedback received from users and aged care service providers at the end of stage 1. Based on the revised prototype, a field trial was undertaken between April and June 2014 and involved a series of interviews with seven seniors and four healthcare staff (of an aged care provider) living in Sydney, Australia. The technology was simplified to standard drop-box-based software to facilitate a large-scale trial support outside Sydney.
- In the third stage, two case studies were conducted in KINSPARC of India and the University of Sunshine Coast, Australia, in 2015 as discussed in this chapter. The objective of the third stage was to examine users' experiences and attitudes towards the well-being technology in different economic and cultural settings, as described in this chapter.

This project promoted the use of tablets and two mature applications, Skype and Dropbox, for seniors to communicate and exchange photos with friends and family. Many seniors use photos to remain emotionally connected with their family members. The two applications had the benefit of being well-tested applications, with many skilled users in the community. Both applications also had the benefit of a free option, removing cost as a barrier for friends and family. Skype was introduced in 2003 and has millions of users worldwide of its voice and video call service. Dropbox provides a shared storage space for the exchange of photographs and other digital images. The use of technology has been found to maintain or facilitate building new social connections [15]. A mixed method study (qualitative as well as quantitative study) was used to gauge the acceptance and use of both Dropbox and Skype by the elderly to facilitate communication which will maintain and build social connections as they age. This study was conducted using two groups of participants one from Australia and the other from West Bengal, India [16].

The results of the project are discussed in Section 7.6 (Discussion).

7.4   Case study in India: Silvercare model of KINSPARC

The Indian aged population is currently the second-largest in the world. Like other countries, in India too, more and more old-age homes are being opened for the elderly. The government is also funding non-government organisations for senior care programmes, but it is not enough considering the huge population of the country. The Silvercare programme was launched in Kalyani, a city in the state of West Bengal, in India on 1 July 2013 by KINSPARC, a non-governmental organisation for research, training and development for improved quality of life. Kalyani is an ideal city for research and study on the elderly population. It is a small planned township built in the 1960s, where plots of land were given to senior government officials, university professors and other dignitaries by the government. At present, there is a sizeable ageing population in Kalyani in small nuclear families with children/younger family members migrating for livelihood. In India, as there is a lack of adequate social security and aged care service from the Government, there have been instances when these aged people were left in distress with nobody to lend a helping hand.

7.4.1   Local background

Before starting the programme, the needs of the elderly population was assessed by KINSPARC through individual interviews and group discussions. The Silvercare model was developed based on the needs and behaviour of the elderly, making sure that they were happy to participate in the programme and not find it annoying or interfering.

It was established that the main concern of the seniors was regarding health emergencies. Sushmita Devi (name changed), a 93-year-old lady confessed that during the night, she suffered from anxiety as she fears what would happen if she felt unwell in the middle of the night. She worries about what she would do and who she would call for help. Another common problem faced by this population is regarding visiting health clinics. In case of any health problem, they needed assistance regarding taking decisions about which doctor to consult, getting an appointment and having a caregiver go along with them. Many of the seniors also needed assistance to understand how to take the prescribed medicines. Forgetfulness is found to be very common and, as a result, forgetting to take the medicines on time is equally common.

The next important concern was their mental health. Almost everybody longed to see and spend time with their close ones like children and grandchildren and interact with them. A survey report by KINSPARC (100 senior citizens of Kalyani were interviewed in 2014) revealed the following important findings:

- 88% suffered from diseases for which senior citizens had to take medicines daily. (Diabetes, hypertension, arthritis and gastritis were the commonest problems.)
- 14% had no fixed family physician.
- 38% did not have medical insurance.
- Everyone suffered from loneliness, though in varying degrees or at least missed their loved ones.
- 80% had mobile phones and the remaining 20% had only landline phone connection.
- 100% preferred to stay in their own homes instead of staying in an old-age home.

KINSPARC decided to provide the following services to the seniors under the aegis of Silvercare:

- emergency medical care and providing assistance in accessing medical facility
- regular communication with beneficiaries to identify and address their needs and concerns
- group activities to combat loneliness and generate awareness
- promotion of active ageing.

7.4.2   Structure and function of the Silvercare team

For every 10 beneficiaries, there is one Silvercare coordinator. Each coordinator identified seniors in their neighbourhood who need support and communicated to them the details of the Silvercare model. The willing seniors signed up to become beneficiaries. Under normal conditions, coordinators communicated at least once in ten days with the ten beneficiaries and more frequently as and when needed.

Silvercare beneficiaries were senior citizens above 65 years of age (with the age relaxed in special cases) and lived alone or with a spouse above 65 years of age or with inmates who are also senior citizens. Only those senior citizens were enrolled who were interested in enrolling themselves as beneficiaries of the Silvercare programme and gave written consent.

Once the beneficiaries are identified, their following details were recorded:

- personal details like age, sex, address, phone number, email, other inmates, etc.

- medical history
- contact details of relatives/friends who could be contacted in case of emergency
- family physician's name and contact details
- medical insurance details.

The enrolled beneficiaries were provided with the following:

- one folder for keeping all medical (investigation and treatment) documents
- one folder for keeping all medical insurance-related documents
- one display board with contact numbers of coordinators/KINSPARC office, which were kept next to the landline telephone or in a prominent place like bedside table.

The Silvercare programme was launched on 1 July 2013. A seminar was organised by KINSPARC where senior citizens were invited to participate and interact with the Silvercare team. The concept of Silvercare programme was shared with the invitees, who highly appreciated it.

Initially, a total of ten service coordinators started working in the different sub-blocks of Kalyani township. Each service coordinator's target was to identify and enlist ten beneficiaries in his/her neighbourhood and collect necessary data for keeping records for smooth functioning of the programme. As more coordinators volunteered, more beneficiaries were enrolled.

7.4.3   Operations

Every month the coordinators submitted monthly reports which were used for a needs assessment of the beneficiaries and also monitoring of the programme. In the case of any emergency care provided to any beneficiary, the incidence reporting form was used for capturing the details of the operation and also feedback from beneficiaries. Coordinators and other management team members of Silvercare programme attended meetings once a week at KINSPARC, which also served as a platform for interaction and entertainment for them. As they too were retired seniors, they enjoyed spending time together in a meaningful way.

In case of any emergency, beneficiaries were advised to call their coordinators who were always ready to extend a helping hand and immediately take care of the situation. The coordinators also work as a team and assisted each other as and when needed. Besides medical care, a lot of attention was given to the mental health of the seniors. Loneliness among the elderly is a silent disease, but it can have serious consequences. Frequent visits by Silvercare coordinators and organised group activities have proved to be very useful.

7.4.4   Silvercare activities in Kalyani

7.4.4.1   Awareness programmes

KINSPARC organises awareness programmes on regular basis for seniors on topics relevant to them like diabetes, hypertension, osteoarthritis, osteoporosis, dementia, glaucoma, cataract, prevention of fall, common dental problems, nutrition for the elderly, mental health of the elderly, importance of exercise and physiotherapy, self-care for the elderly and so on. Topics were often decided based on demands from the seniors.

7.4.4.2 Recreational events

Picnics were organised for the seniors where lots of enjoyable activities were arranged and everyone was encouraged to participate. The seniors sang songs, recited poems, played games and had a great time. All seniors were not able to participate in outdoor activities due to restricted mobility or other disabilities. Moreover, such outdoor activities cannot be organised on daily basis and so KINSPARC tried to help seniors to combat loneliness by using information and communication technology.

7.4.4.3 Information and communication technology to combat loneliness

In 2014, very few elderly people used smartphones and most of them were not familiar with its use. KINSPARC participated in a joint project on mHealth with Asia Pacific Ubiquitous Health research Consortium (APuHC) which was android tablet-based Silvercare for the elderly in Kalyani. This was part of APuHC's WHO collaborating centre activities. The ten coordinators of Silvercare programme in Kalyani were provided with ten android tablets and ten dongles for WiFi connection. The coordinators took the responsibility to teach the beneficiaries how to use the tablets for communicating with their families and friends who were living miles away, using apps like 'Skype'. They also tried to train the seniors on social networking by using Facebook. The interested seniors were taught to play games like Solitaire and other interesting online games. Though some of them enjoyed such activities thoroughly, some others expressed no interest. Everyone was given two months' time after which, those who were interested were encouraged to buy their own tablets or smartphones and the coordinators used their tablets and dongles to train new candidates. The result of the process showed that everyone felt the well-being communication system was useful but 20% felt it was difficult for them to use it and found it cumbersome and 10% said they were not interested in getting trained. The rest 70% were happy with the newly acquired skill. Over the years, more and more seniors have begun using smartphones and now WhatsApp is the most popular app amongst them. Computer games and YouTube videos are also enjoyed by some.

7.4.4.4 Celebrating birthdays

Silvercare team celebrates the birthdays of their beneficiaries which makes the seniors very happy. Lately, the Silvercare team has begun 'Zoom meeting birthday celebrations' of the seniors where loved ones from all around the globe can join. This is very much appreciated by the family members of the beneficiary seniors and, interestingly, many times KINSPARC receives online surprise gifts from family members to be handed over to the concerned senior on the special day and the happiness experienced is overwhelming.

7.4.4.5 Active ageing

For promoting active ageing, KINSPARC has established a physiotherapy centre where interested seniors can come for therapy, exercise, balance training, etc. under the supervision of a qualified trainer/therapist. As the coordinators are also senior citizens, they too can avail this facility and the overall environment is friendly and comfortable. The caregivers/coordinators and the beneficiaries mingle well with each other and enjoy each other's company.

7.4.5 Project outcomes

The beneficiary seniors and their family members have often expressed their happiness and gratitude to the coordinators for all the support they enjoy. The organisation often receives messages of appreciation and donations from family members of the seniors.

As this programme provides voluntary service with no remuneration for the service provider, there is shortage of volunteers. This problem can be addressed by converting it into a business model.

7.5 Case study in Australia

In common with other countries that have an ageing population, Australia has a problem with the growing number of senior citizens. Currently, there is a sharp increase in public expenditure on care for people past the age of 80 and we can expect that to climb with continued improvements in medical care and other technologies to assist individuals to live longer. Currently in Australia, the policy is to keep seniors living independently in their own home supported by home care packages for as long as possible. In 2020, the funding for independent living home care packages has been increased by 1.6 billion or an extra 23 000 packages [17]. How can we support and teach skills to older people to live independently through the use of enabling technologies such as information technology? This support can be in the form of the provision of assistive tools to provide an environment for seniors that improves their quality of life in conjunction with reducing the demand for social services.

The aged care services in Australia are classified into two major categories: community-based (elderly residing at their homes) care and residential (elderly admitted to nursing homes) care. The recent increase in deaths of the elderly in care homes triggered a Royal Commission on aged care in Australia as reported in Dyer [18]. Since most elderly want to stay independently at their homes, community-based care services are now growing rapidly in Australia. The Silvercare model is most appropriate for community-based care, this chapter focuses mainly on this type of care [18].

7.5.1 Local background

In Australia, becoming a senior or retirement from paid work is a time of adjustment and change. It is at this time that people retire, move to retirement communities and may lose a partner. Decreasing physical mobility often increases the difficulty of maintaining existing levels of social connection with friends and family, while also reducing levels of incidental social encounters. This transition means that the skills, knowledge and experience gathered through active participation in the workforce and community can be lost resulting in a loss in community, social and human capital. One of the ways to unlock this social capital is by encouraging seniors to volunteer. Volunteering helps to overcome some of the problems associated with the transition to being a senior, that of loss of identity, loneliness and depression. People over the age of 75 reported as being the loneliest sector in Australia in 2018 [19]. Volunteering is one aspect of this project; Lumand Lightfoot found volunteering between 3 and 100 hours per month has positive effects on self-reported health and depression levels and with participants reporting better physical function than those who do not volunteer [20]. For the seniors working together in a volunteer organisation, acted to strengthen social ties with fellow volunteers [21, 22]. These social networks often outlasting the period of volunteering, with volunteers reporting higher quality of life.

7.5.2 Structure and organisation

In this project we approached people to participate, over 65, that attended a local University of the Third Age (U3A). Using the Silvercare model discussed above, a participant who was identified with higher-level technical skills and willing was given ten participants to look after and labelled a peer leader. Sixty-five participants started the project and thirty people completed the research. The demographics of the group who completed the research was 20 woman and 10 men, with an age range from 62 to 88 years old, with an average of 72.11. This is an organisation that promotes learning for fun and well-being, with the only requirement for entry is a willingness to participate and be interested in learning. The participants had to own a tablet and are willing to use and install the commercial applications Dropbox and Skype. The premise was that the participants would use the applications to maintain connections with existing friends and family, including younger people who may be resistant to using traditional communication methods such as telephones. Dropbox was promoted to exchange photographs to increase feelings of family participation in seniors, while Skype was used as a video calling platform.

7.5.3 Operations

The peer leaders emailed their group introducing themselves at the start of the project offering their assistance, while the researcher sent an instruction sheet on how to use the applications. After using the applications for three or four weeks, the participants were then phoned and asked to complete a questionnaire on their attitudes and experiences using the software, while the team leaders were interviewed in person about their experiences. A large number of participants were already familiar with and using some kind of electronic communication software to talk with friends and family with Apple's Facetime being noted as a popular communication mode among participants. While Dropbox proved more difficult with participants finding understanding of its mechanisms and usefulness challenging. The team leaders found that participants were slow to contact them preferring to drop out of the research if they found it difficult.

7.5.4   Outcomes

There were a few reasons participants drop out, a major reason being where it was perceived they lacked support. Other reasons included having difficulty getting applications to work and therefore they felt they could not answer the questionnaire, or they went away or were overwhelmed by events. One of the issues was that the participants had not met the peer leader and did not seem to feel comfortable asking for help. One of the strategies that could have made a difference to the participants' engagement was the arrangement of initial, in-person meetings between the peer leaders and their groups, which was missed out. Blake and Kerr in a similar demographic finding, note that participants expressed a desire for one-on-one in-person training [23]. The preference was for training to be provided by family members and failing that somebody that would sit with them in their own home.

7.6   Discussion

Quantitative data was collected and used to investigate how the Australian and Indian users viewed the applications and their usability at the end of the trial period. The survey was based upon the Unified Theory of Acceptance and Use of Technology (UTAUT) model [24]. While the UTAUT model was developed for an organisation, the dimensions used in the model fitted this project. Four questions were asked in the survey on the following constructs: performance expectancy, attitude towards using the system, social influence, facilitating conditions, self-efficacy, anxiety and behavioural intention [16]. The Indian participants gave a response combining their experience with both Skype and Dropbox; however, the Australian cohort gave separate responses for the two applications. These results and data were first reported in Blake and Ray as summarised below [16].

7.6.1   Performance expectancy

These questions were investigating how the seniors felt using the application would help them complete a task. Most users agreed or strongly agreed that the application was useful when used to contact their care coordinator or relatives more quickly (Skype Aust. = 55.55%, Dropbox Aust. = 51.85%, India = 90.0%) and enhanced their communication (Skype Aust. = 55.5%, Dropbox Aust. = 51.8%, India = 90.0%). The majority also agreed that the applications were useful (Skype Aust. = 62.9%, Dropbox Aust. = 38.4%, India = 80.0%) and that communicating their well-being status was easier (Skype Aust. = 51.8%, Dropbox Aust. = 48.1%, India = 95.0%).

7.6.2 Attitude towards using the system

This dimension investigated how the participants viewed using Skype and Dropbox. The results showed that they thought using the applications was a good idea (Skype Aust. = 88.9%, Dropbox Aust. = 85.2%, India = 95.0%), made communication more interesting (Skype Aust. = 66.6%, Dropbox Aust. = 62.9%, India = 85.0%) and using the applications to complete tasks was fun (Skype Aust. = 70.5%, Dropbox Aust. = 66.6%, India = 95.0%). The users also had positive responses to using the applications on the tablet (Skype Aust. = 62.9%, Dropbox Aust. = 59.2%, India = 90.0%).

7.6.3 Social influence

What the participants felt about their friends and family attitudes were towards them using Skype and Dropbox on a tablet was investigated in this section. The participants responded, particularly in India, that people who influenced their behaviour thought that they should use the applications (Skype Aust. = 59.2%, Dropbox Aust. = 55.5%, India = 95.0%); also positive was the question that people who are important to me think I should use these applications (Skype Aust. = 59.2%, Dropbox Aust. = 55.5%, India = 95.0%). For the question if the participants felt that they had been supported in their use of the application, there was a clear distinction between Australia and India. With the Indian cohort feeling more supported at 100% agreement, while in Australia 18.5% felt supported by the programme administrators and 29.6% feeling supported in general. This is a clear indication that the Silvercare system needed to be adjusted in Australia, perhaps to one with more emphasis on general support rather than support on demand.

7.6.4 Facilitating conditions

The participants were asked how their environment supported their use of Skype and Dropbox. When asked if they had the resources necessary to use the applications, there was a majority agreement (Australia = 88.9%, India = 100.0%); the participants also agreed that they had sufficient knowledge necessary to use the applications (Australia = 74.1%, India = 85.0%). The participants also agreed that using the applications on a tablet fitted in with their lifestyle (Australia = 66.6%, India = 80.0%) and that they could call on someone to help for system assistance (Australia = 59.2%, India = 20.0%).

7.6.5 Self-efficacy

The next dimension in the survey was investigating the participants' belief that they were capable of continuing to use the applications. The first question asked the participants to consider using the applications without anyone being available to tell them what to do, how confident were they that they could use the applications. The agreed and strongly agreed values were: Skype Aust. = 70.4%, Dropbox Aust. = 66.7%, India = 45.0%. If they had someone to call for help the values are: Skype Aust. = 81.5%, Dropbox Aust. = 70.0%, India=70.0%. If they had a lot of time to complete using the applications the agreed/strongly agreed values were: Australian = 44.4%, India = 50.0%, the last quest examined the participants' confidence in successfully using the application with online help only. Agreement values were: Skype Australian = 63.0.4%, India = 60.0% (agree only).

7.6.6   Anxiety

The anxiety dimension researched the participants' anxiety with using the applications affected their intention to use. The first question asked if they were anxious using the applications the agree/strongly agree values were: Australian = 7.4%, India = 25.0%; most of the respondents answered that they were not anxious with the disagree/strongly disagree responses (Australian = 85.2%, India = 60.0%). Fear of making mistakes they could not correct had negative results (Australian = 88.9%, India = 55.0%) with the agree/strongly agree values were: Australian = 11.1%, India = 25.0%. The same pattern of responses was also followed when asked if they found using the applications intimidating; the agree/strongly agree values were: Australian = 3.7%, India = 20.0% with most of the responses being disagree/strongly disagree as: Australian = 85.1%, India = 50.0%.

7.6.7   Intention to use the system

To test if the participants' intention was to continue to use the system in the future, the following set of questions was asked. The agreement responses were: Skype Aust. = 77.8%, Dropbox Aust. = 74.1%, India = 85.0%. The follow-up question was asking the participants to think about their intention to use the applications over the next six months with the agree/strongly agree responses were: Skype Aust. = 74.1%, Dropbox Aust. = 70.4%, India = 85.0%. Some participants stated that they wanted to use the application in order to be able to communicate with younger family members.

The questionnaire highlighted the key differences between Australian respondents and Indian, with the Indian experience being more positive with no withdrawals from the project. This highlights differences in how the project was run at each location; the Indian cohort had other activities in the project and there was a structured contact regime by Silvercare coordinators. In Australia, the participants had to ask for assistance and felt much less supported. The mode where assistance had to be requested could be contributed to the high withdrawal rate as participants felt they were being a nuisance or would rather wait for the family for assistance.

While the activities in Sunshine coast were restricted to the evaluation of the adoption of the social media applications Skype and Dropbox, the activities in Kalyani were of different types as described in Section 7.4.4. This was possible because the project lasted six months longer in Kalyani.

7.7   Conclusion

This chapter has discussed an innovative human resource model called Silvercare, where relatively younger retired people (coordinators) assist older seniors (beneficiaries) in their neighbourhood. This method provides effective help to seniors while keeping retired people engaged gainfully. Besides, it is a very cost-effective model as coordinators are unpaid volunteers and are able to help seniors quite patiently with matters related to changing mechanisms, such as technology.

One of the ways that seniors can be assisted in their desire for active ageing is to increase digital literacy as digital media plays a more and more significant role in all government (e.g., healthcare, pensions) and retail (e.g., shopping, cleaning) services. Digital literacy would mean seniors have confidence in finding use and creation of digital information/services. This confidence would mean that they could use digital means to undertake tasks such as banking, shopping, interacting with the government as well as communication giving equity of access despite decreased mobility. This chapter has discussed some case studies on digital literacy of the seniors using the Silvercare model across Australia and India undertaken as part of the Tablet-Based Well-being Check project led by Pradeep Ray on behalf of UNSW-Australia and partners including the University of Sunshine Coast and KINSPARC in India.

However, more studies are needed to illustrate the usefulness Silvercare model in many other types of services, e.g., from the government and businesses to the seniors, rapidly increasing in number in many countries of this world.

KINSPARC has plans to assist in the formation of cooperatives by senior citizens having common interests like creative arts (painting, knitting, stitching, etc.) and help them in doing business from home by selling their products online. To assist them in fighting against elder abuse, KINSPARC has plans to provide legal awareness and assistance in future.

References

[1]   UNFPA and HelpAge International. *Aging in the twenty-first century* [online]. 2012. Available from https://www.unfpa.org/publications/ageing-twenty-first-century [Accessed 08 July 2021].

[2]   Cornwall Care. 5 *reasons we love working with the elderly* [online]. 2017. Available from https://cornwallcare.com/about-us/news/5-reasons-we-love-working-elderly [Accessed 08 July 2021].

[3]   Jones C.H. 'Combining daycare for children and elderly people benefits all generations'. 2017.The Conversation. Available from https://theconversation.com/combining-daycare-for-children-and-elderly-people-benefits-all-generations-70724 [Accessed 08 July 2021].

[4]   McCurry J. 'Japan will be model for future super-ageing societies'. *The Lancet*. 2015, vol. 386(10003), p. 1523.

[5]   Eiichi O., Hisakazu M. Japan's aging population and its silver care industry. 2011. *Samsung Economic Research Institute (SERI) Quarterly*. Available from http://www.seriworld.org/16/qt_Section_list.html?mncd=0302&dep=2&year=2011&p_page=1 [Accessed 08 July 2021].

[6]   Chéron E. (eds.) '*Elderly consumers in Japan: the most mature "Silver market" worldwide*' in Haghirian P. (ed.). *Japanese Consumer Dynamics*. United Kingdom: Palgrave MacMillan; 2011. pp. 65–90.

[7]   The Scottish Government. *Reshaping Care for Older People 2011–2021.* Edinburgh: The Scottish Government; 2013. Available from https://www.gov.scot/publications/reshaping-care-older-people-2011-2021/ [Accessed 08 July 2021].

[8]   Jacobs S., Xie C., Reilly S., Hughes J., Challis D. 'Modernising social care services for older people: scoping the United Kingdom evidence base'. *Ageing and Society.* 2009, vol. 29(4), pp. 497–538.

[9]   Arentshorst M.E., Kloet R.R., Peine A. 'Intergenerational housing: the case of humanitas Netherlands'. *Journal of Housing for the Elderly.* 2019, vol. 33(3), pp. 244–56.

[10] American Association of Retired Persons. *The aging readiness and competitiveness report: Germany* [online]. 2017. Available from http://www.silvereco.org/en/wp-content/uploads/2017/12/ARC-Report-Germany.pdf [Accessed 08 July 2021].

[11] American Association of Retired Persons. *The 2018 aging readiness and competitiveness report: small innovative economics Singapore* [online]. 2018. Available from https://arc2018.aarpinternational.org/File%20Library/Countries/2018_Singapore.pdf [Accessed 08 July 2021].

[12] Cheron. Infocomm News (2013, 1 May). *Seniors help seniors through Silver IT Care* [online]. 2011. Available from https://www.ida.gov.sg/blog/insg/in-the-news/seniors-help-seniors-through-silver-it-care/ [Accessed 01 May 2013].

[13] Bergström A. 'Digital equality and the uptake of digital applications among seniors of different age'. *Nordicom Review.* 2017, vol. 38(s1), pp. 79–91.

[14] Ray P., Li J., Ariani A., Kapadia V., Shah V. 'Tablet-Based well-being check for the elderly: development and evaluation of usability and acceptability'. *JMIR human factors.* 2017, vol. 4(2),e12.

[15] Morris M.E., Adair B., Ozanne E., *et al.* 'Smart technologies to enhance social connectedness in older people who live at home'. *Australasian Journal on Ageing.* 2014, vol. 33(3), pp. 142–52.

[16] Blake J.N., Ray P. 'Facilitating digital communication in seniors'. Paper Presented at the IEEE International Symposium on Technology and Society. Trivandrum, India; 2016.

[17] Hermant N. *Governments $1.6 billion funding in federal Budget leaves 77 000 waiting* [online]. 2020, 17 December 2020. Available from https://www.abc.net.au/news/2020-10-08/aged-care-budget-funding-for-home-care-packages-falls-short/12736428 [Accessed 08 July 2021].

[18] Dyer S.M., van den Berg M.E.L., Barnett K., *et al. Review of Innovative Models of Aged Care.* Adelaide, Australia: Flinders University; 2019.

[19] Australian Institute of Health and Welfare. *Social isolation and loneliness* [online]. 2019. Available from https://www.aihw.gov.au/reports/australias-welfare/social-isolation-and-loneliness [Accessed 08 July 2021].

[20] Lum T.Y., Lightfoot E. 'The effects of volunteering on the physical and mental health of older people'. *Research on Aging.* 2005, vol. 27(1), pp. 31–55.

[21] McPherson M., Smith-Lovin L., Cook J.M. 'Birds of a feather: homophily in social networks'. *Annual Review of Sociology.* 2001, vol. 27(1), pp. 415–44.

[22] Taghian M., Polonsky M.J., D'Souza C. 'Volunteering in retirement and its impact on seniors subjective quality of life through personal outlook: a study of older Australians'. *VOLUNTAS: International Journal of Voluntary and Nonprofit Organizations*. 2019, vol. 30(5), pp. 1133–47.

[23] Blake J., Kerr D. 'Seniors use of social media'. Paper Presented at the 24th Asia-Pacific Decision Science Institute International Conference (APDSI); Brisbane, Australia; 2019.

[24] Viswanath V., Michael G.M., Gordon B.D., Fred D.D. 'User acceptance of information technology: toward a unified view'. *MIS Quarterly*. 2003, vol. 27(3), pp. 425–78.

Chapter 8

Safeguarding the elderly in a pandemic: role of lockdown policies and digital health technologies

Nazia Akter[1], Yan Hanrunyu[2], and Pradeep Kumar Ray[2,3]

8.1 Introduction

Since the coronavirus first surfaced in Wuhan of China, it has affected millions of people worldwide within a year. In December 2019, several patients with pneumonia of unknown cause were first detected in Wuhan. An unknown beta coronavirus was found in patients with pneumonia, later named 2019-nCoV [1]. At present, the new coronavirus (Covid-19) is affecting 213 countries and territories around the world.

Considering the fast spreading of the virus, and taking Wuhan as an example, different infected-ratio wise area zoning and shutdown of economic activities were implemented by different countries. Many countries have taken actions such as "strict-lockdown" that restricted human movement, border control, ban on import and export, the shutdown of educational and business organisations. Lockdown in Wuhan also included applying a ban on gathering activities, implementing regional traffic control, tracing out suspected patients, also managing suspected cases, confirmed cases and asymptomatic infections, and isolating them [2]. By the end of March 2020, over 100 countries worldwide had instituted either a full or partial lockdown, affecting billions of people [3]. And, in December 2020, many countries across the world are facing a second and deadly wave of the Covid-19.

However, the lockdown imposed to prevent coronavirus has brought not only economic shock but also an adverse effect on the health of the elderly. Almost every country is reporting the death of the elderly along with severe health complexity due to Covid-19. Therefore, there is a need to analyse the measures taken by governments in the name of lockdown, their effect on the elderly and their well-being, and the use of digital services to ease lockdown restrictions. Using the methodology of systematic literature review, this chapter aims to study the lockdown policies undertaken by various countries to analyse the impacts of lockdown on the aged people

[1]Synesis IT Limited, Bangladesh
[2]Center for Entrepreneurship, University of Michigan Joint Institute, Shanghai Jiao Tong University, China
[3]WHO Collaborating Centre on eHealth, School of Population Health, UNSW, Australia

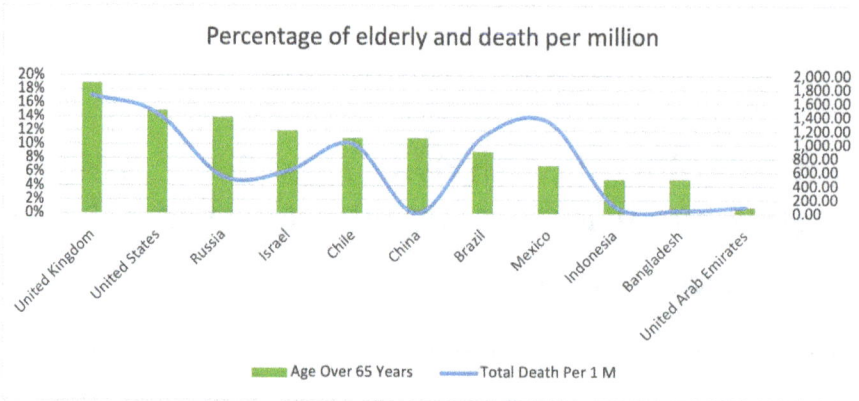

Figure 8.1   *Country-wise percentage of elderly in relation to death per million due to Covid-19 [6]. Source: [6] Our World in Data.* Coronavirus (COVID-19) vaccinations – statistics and research [online]. *2021. Available from https://ourworldindata.org/covid-vaccinations [Accessed Feb 13, 2021].*

and seek digital services that can help to ease current lockdown policies and restrictions to control Covid-19. Therefore, it is essential to make sure that these people get necessary healthcare services during the pandemic and can continue their daily activities.

The chapter starts with the research context in Section 8.2, followed by initial research questions in Section 8.3, followed by the research design in Section 8.4 based on a systematic literature review, followed by a summary of findings in Section 8.5 and a discussion in Section 8.6 and the conclusion in Section 8.7.

8.2   Research context

Due to Covid-19, the risk of death of people greater than 80 years old in high-income countries ranged from approximately 0.6 in a thousand in Florida to 17.5 in a thousand in Connecticut [4]. Though all human beings are at risk for contracting the Covid-19 virus, senior people are at a significant risk of developing severe illness due to physiological changes that come with ageing, limited outdoor activities and existing health condition [5]. Data show that nations with greater number of elderlies have observed a significant number of death due to Covid-19 (Figure 8.1). WHO states that worldwide older people are at a higher risk of developing severe illness with a fatality rate of 3.6% among 60–69 years old, which increases to 18% for people above 80 years. In addition, social disconnection is taking a toll on this age group as they are less used to digital technologies. So, lockdown may limit their social engagement, interfere with daily routines, enhance inactivity, increase drugs use and decrease sensory stimulation. All these circumstances together with isolation might have an adverse impact on the mental health of the elderly population [7].

On the other hand, many researchers stated that a national lockdown is not a cure suggesting that social distancing, self-isolation and quarantine are indispensable tools. South Korea, Singapore, Japan and Hong Kong approached these and managed to slow down the impact without taking strict lockdown measures [8]. South Korea got success with broad testing and strict quarantine measures and the Taiwan government relied on a ready emergency plan built upon the previous experience rather than implementing lockdown [9].

Most importantly, researchers are now exploring and recommending the use of existing digital health technologies and services that have the potential to better manage the outbreak of pandemic and thus can reduce the need for a stringent lockdown. The scope of digital health includes telehealth and telemedicine, mobile health, wearable devices for health, etc. Digital health tools have the potential to improve and enhance the delivery of healthcare in this pandemic. Following are some options of digital technologies and services that can play a role in pandemic.

8.2.1 Digital services and technologies for outbreak tracing

Remote detection of disease through objective measures is a possible way to improve timely escalation of care. On a larger scale, hospitals could use localised, de-identified data to track the spread and severity of the outbreak without violation of users' privacy to provide population-level care. This becomes more relevant when the asymptomatic carrier rate is estimated to be between 25% and 50% of the population. With a large population potentially carrying the virus, digital health technologies that measure physiologic parameters can be leveraged to help identify population clusters to identify an emerging Covid-19 outbreak [10].

8.2.2 Use of mobile applications for safe reopening

In many countries, mobile applications combined with other digital technologies are used for maintaining safe social distances, providing alert of a suspected area, providing remote health services, disseminating Covid-19-related information and so on. With the use of mobile application, wearables and Bluetooth Low Energy (BLE) technology, a school or university can be opened safely without posing health risk to the students (Figure 8.2).

8.2.3 Use of wearables with digital health services

Wearables can be used to maintain social distance. Many metrics derived from heart rhythm such as heart rate, heart rate variability and respiration rate could serve as potential markers of Covid-19 infection and are already measured by wearable devices such as the Apple Watch, Fitbit, etc. These wearables can be potential tools for maintaining social distance as well as distant tracking of patient's vitals [10].

8.2.4 Contact tracing tools and services

For digital contract tracing, WHO recommended an outbreak response tracker, symptoms tracing tools, proximity tracing tools, etc. However, the limitation is that

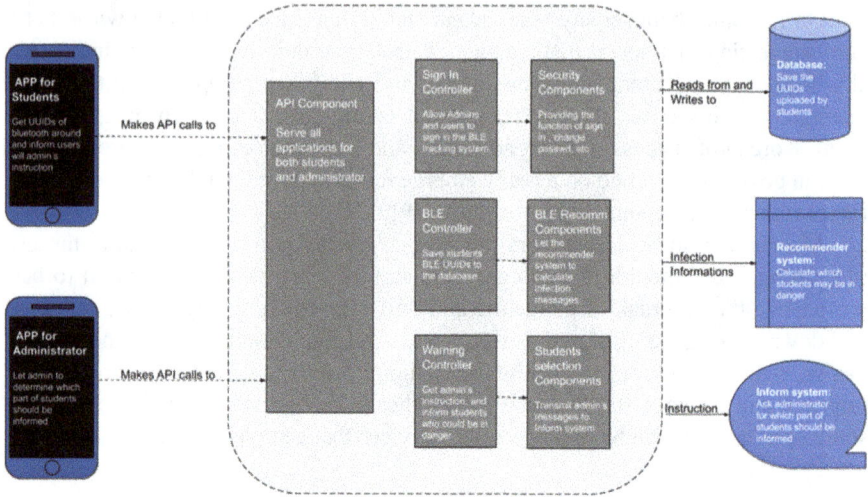

Figure 8.2   Example of combined digital services for contact tracing and opening schools safely [11]. Source: Geng R., Hu B., Li D. Safe back school APP smart tracing for school reopening [online]. JAZZ IT UP; 2020. Available from https://bingcheng.openmc.cn/blog/en/2020/Safe-Back-School-App.html [Accessed Jan 06, 2021].

although testing and contact tracing capacity have been ramped up, these are only effective when the number of cases is small enough [12]. China has shown the world that if well tracked, early introduction of an emerging pathogen provides a unique opportunity to characterise its transmission, natural history and the effectiveness of screening.

8.2.5   Use of AI and big data in digital health services

The use of emerging technologies has the potentials to mitigate the impact of the Covid-19 pandemic, such as Internet of Things (IoT), Unmanned Aerial Vehicles (UAVs), block-chain, Artificial Intelligence (AI), 5G, etc. Till the time a cure for this disease surfaces, these technologies have the potential to alleviate the lockdown [13].

In summary, the new-normal that arose due to Covid-19 made people to adopt changes in lifestyle, travelling and communication, and also changes the way how people seek health services, communicate or use technologies. It has shown us the potential that digital health services and technologies can be a major contributor in providing safe reopening of economic and other daily activities, thus safeguarding the elderly people in a pandemic.

There is available research focusing on the economic and other aspects of lock-down. Some research discusses about the alternative to lockdown approaches and very few researches focused on the impact of lockdown on the health of the elderly based on different geographical context. This research is aiming to provide a com-prehensive analysis of the lockdown measures taken worldwide, their consequences on the health of the elderly and also to discuss alternative approches to strict lock-downs and the potentialities of digital health services and technologies.

8.3   Research questions

To meet the objectives mentioned, we pose the following research questions:

1. What are the actions taken by different countries to implement lockdown due to Covid-19?
2. What are the impacts of such actions on the health of the elderly and how much they are affected?
3. What digital services and alternative approaches could be effective, and what are the possible improvement suggestions to strict lockdown?

For the research methodology, we have used a systematic literature review method based on "Procedures for Performing Systematic Reviews" by Barbara Kitchenham [14]. Understanding the effectiveness of strict lockdown, partial lock-down, and alternative approaches to lockdown and their consequences might lead us to new ways to manage such a pandemic. The systematic review also identifies gaps in current research.

8.4   Research design

We have conducted a systematic search of peer-reviewed articles to find relevant literature on lockdown for Covid-19 management, its impact on the health of the elderly and its provable alternative approaches. When selecting the articles, com-pleteness and the number of articles is also taken into account. All full-text papers that met the research design criteria were included in the analysis.

8.4.1   Database and keywords

To search the impact of coronavirus and its alternative approaches, our choices on the electronic databases include EBSCO, JSTOR, Google Scholar, PubMed, Elsevier Science Direct and Scopus. During the search of the electronic databases, three search categories were combined based on the issues, which are given below:

1. coronavirus (coronavirus or Covid-19 or 2019-ncov or covid19 or covid-19 or corona virus or pandemic)
2. lockdown (lockdown or quarantine)
3. elderly (health of elderly or elderly or old age or senior citizens or seniors)
4. digital services (digital health services, telehealth, digital health).

8.4.2   Criteria for inclusion and exclusion

- Primarily, the research only focused on the journal articles whose research abstracts were clearly defined and included the economic information of Covid-19. In addition, we consciously excluded articles with other focus areas.
- Articles are excluded as per the mentioned criteria to match with our defined search strategy:

  i.   published before December 2019
  ii. research objectives do not contain the health impact of the Covid-19 on the elderly and lockdown.

8.4.3   Limitations

- Time: Since the study was on the impact of Covid-19, to ensure the integrity of timeliness, we have selected articles that were published from December 2019 to 2020.
- Keywords: The keywords chosen for searching articles are the word strings mentioned above.
- Literature type: To ensure information integrity, we have selected only the journal articles with full text to extract data.
- Language: English is chosen for the convenience of the reader and to reach a larger audience. Therefore, we used the language choice function of the databases.
- Peer-review: To achieve higher quality and information authenticity, we have chosen peer-reviewed articles.

8.4.4   Screening results

Based on the article selection strategy and criteria selection mentioned above, article screening for this study was performed and 20 articles were selected for this chapter. These initial results included a total of 3 673 articles. A total of 3 488 articles were excluded based on the inclusion and exclusion criteria. We identified 185 published papers, and their abstracts were reviewed for potential relevance. Finally, 56 full texts were reviewed, of which 36 articles were excluded. We finally selected 20 articles for systematic analysis (Figure 8.3).

The next section presents a systematic analysis of shortlisted papers based on our three research questions listed in Section 8.5.

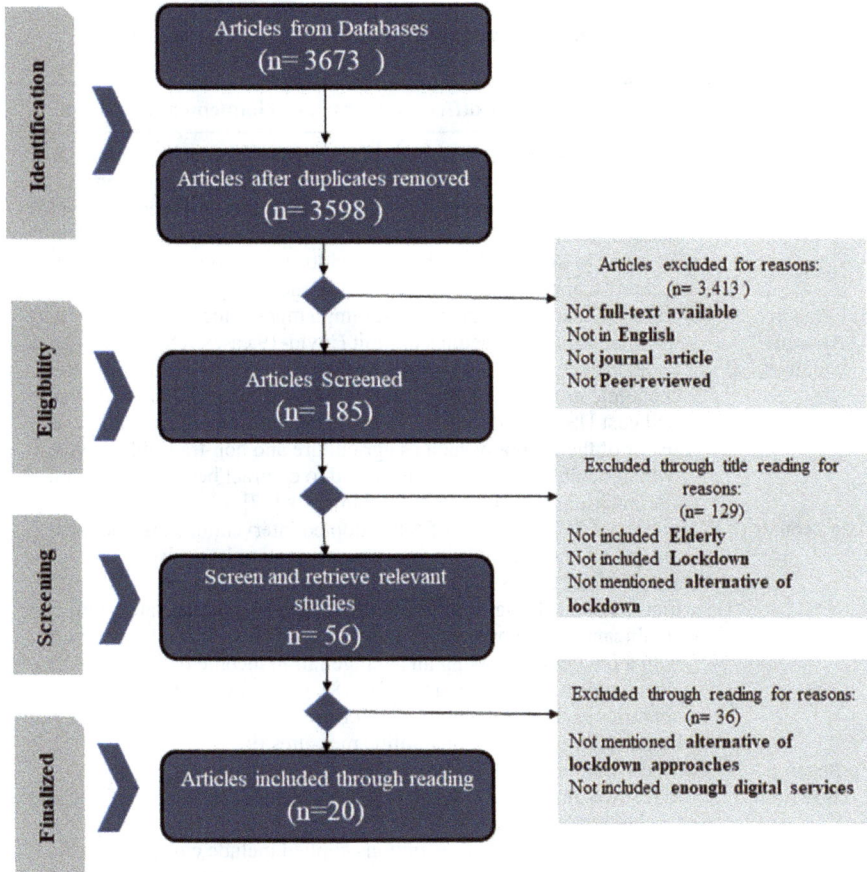

Figure 8.3   Article screening result

8.5   Findings

8.5.1   Actions taken by different countries to implement lockdown

To prevent and restrain the outbreak of the pandemic, governments worldwide have taken some stringent actions. Following are the actions taken for implementing lockdown in different countries in Table 8.1.

8.5.2   Impacts of such actions on the health of the elderly and how much they are affected

Though many countries have imposed strict lockdown to save people from the pandemic, this measure has adverse effects on the health of the elderly as well as on other general people. Table 8.2 presents the severe effects of lockdown on seniors worldwide.

Table 8.1   Actions taken by different countries to implement lockdown

Research Question 1: Actions taken by different countries to implement lockdown	
United States	To control the spread of the virus, partial shutdown was implemented in New York and a few more cities, and the stricter government lockdown in many other cities along with a "stay-at-home" order [15]. During the first wave of the pandemic, around 316 million people in 42 states in the USA have been asked to stay at home as part of the lockdown approach to slow down the pandemic [16].
Sub-Saharan African countries	Some sub-Saharan African countries implemented lockdown following the international guidelines to limit Covid-19 cases. The pandemic could trigger a recession in the sub-Saharan African region with the economic growth declining from 2.4% in 2019 to −5.1% in 2020 and will cost USD 37–79 billion. It will also adversely affect nearly every sector of the economy such as agriculture and non-tradeable services, with agricultural production expected to contract between 2.6% and 7% and a 13–25% decline in food imports [17].
Asian countries	Countries of different parts of Asia adopted interventions that included mitigation and suppression measures, e.g., case-based isolation, school closures, restricting public events and lockdowns to minimise transmissions. Long-term lockdown measures are associated with significant unemployment, economic hardship and social disruption with a prediction showing an average fall in income by 70% and consumption expenditure by 30% [18]. In contrast, some Asian countries such as Singapore, South Korea and Taiwan got success with broad testing and strict quarantine measures [9].
European countries	European countries had gone for both strict lockdown and partial lockdown implemented with measurements like cancelling of flights, closing borders, closing down shops, restaurants, schools, churches, etc. [8]. The significant restrictions applied include closing borders, restriction on labour mobility and public gathering as part of the lockdown activity [19].
Global perspective	Many of the countries implemented strict lockdowns, such as restrictions on borders, transportations and public gatherings. Lockdown measures also included international tourism contraction with the closing of hotels, restaurants, etc. [9]. Many governments took stringent measures ranging from closing down educational institutions to imposing a ban on public gatherings [20]. All non-essential services have been forced to shut down, restricting the trade of a majority of goods across country borders [13].

8.5.3   Digital health and other approaches to strict lockdown and their effectiveness

By maintaining social distancing, self-isolation and quarantine methods, many Asian countries have managed to slow down the impact without taking strict lockdown measures. While South Korea got success with broad testing and strict quarantine measures along with digital health tools and services, the Taiwan government relied on a ready emergency plan built upon the previous experience rather than

Table 8.2   Impacts of lockdown on elderly

Research Question 2: Impacts of lockdown and restriction on the health of elderly	
Risk due to the sedentary lifestyle of the elderly during the lockdown	Quarantine reduced physical activity levels of elderly people, and nearly 70% of the respondents of the study reported an increase in time spent sitting or lying down and over 35% reported weight gain during the lockdown period [21]. A higher rate of thromboembolic events (blood vessel clot) and in-hospital mortality are seen during the pandemic. Also, a higher rate of acute embolic events (blockage inside a blood vessel), associated with prolonged immobility due to rigid quarantine dispositions or strict lockdown policies has been observed. Extended confinement times for lockdown led to reduced physical activity and family care, which might have exacerbated sedentary behaviours and indirectly contributed to thromboembolic events in an already vulnerable elderly population [22]. There is a prediction that the effects of the Covid-19 lockdown on patients and a linear association existed between the length of lockdown and the worsening of lockdown and diabetes-related complications [23].
Impacts on mental well-being	Emotional distress due to lockdown to prevent Covid-19 is placing the elderly into a psychological crisis. About 4% of the rise in anxiety, a 3% rise in depressive scores, and a 7% rise of acute stress disorder are associated with economic losses due to lockdown. Besides, an increase in the use of anxiolytic substances, alcohol or other drugs has been observed in those over 60 with higher levels of anxiety, depression and acute stress while stuck in the middle of lockdown [7].
Risk of dementia	Due to reduced social activities during the lockdown, nearly 60% of senior citizen mentioned that they now spent more time in passive recreational activities, such as watching television. On the other hand, one in six elderly people at risk of dementia also decreased production and mental-stimulating activities. Increased sedentary lifestyle, unhealthy diet and lower engagement in non-passive recreational activities during the lockdown have increased the risk of dementia. Furthermore, fewer social interactions, small social networks, and a low level of physical activity are increasing depressive symptoms in community-dwelling seniors [21].

implementing lockdown. Table 8.3 presents the alternative suggestions for the traditional lockdown approach.

8.6   Discussion

To fight the Covid-19 pandemic, different governments across the globe have taken several initiatives to stop spreading the virus. However, these decisions and activities severely impacted the economic sectors. The literature aimed to find out (i) the actions taken by the different countries to implement lockdown (ii) the impact of such actions on the health of the elderly who are most affected and (iii) the alternative approaches to strict lockdown.

Table 8.3   Digital health and alternative approaches to strict lockdown

Research Question 3: Alternative approaches to strict lockdown

Contact-tracing wristband or wearable	Traditional contact tracing, widely adopted across the world, found to be time-consuming and resource-intensive. Many experts are now suggesting smartphone-based mobile apps to automate the contact-tracing process as an alternative to it. Unfortunately, older people around the world are more likely to use older smartphones. And even in a country like the UK, only 40% of over 65 used smartphones to connect to the internet in 2019. Therefore, to support vulnerable people contact-tracing wristband or wearable, and social distancing alert mechanism and wearable to monitor symptoms could be good alternatives rather than imposing strict lockdown [24].
Mobile applications-based contact tracing	App-based contact tracing has found to be effective irrespective of age, gender, region or even country of residence. The data reveal that concerns about cybersecurity and privacy, coupled with trust in government, are important determinants of support [25]. So far, mobile applications have been proven beneficial for citizens, health professionals and decision-makers in facing the Covid-19 pandemic. Mobile applications can help provide reliable information to citizens and health professionals, decreasing misinformation and confusion, tracking symptoms and mental health of citizens, home monitoring and isolation, discovering new predictors, optimising healthcare resource allocation, and reducing the burden of hospitals [26].
Test–trace–isolate strategy	Gradually relaxing the lockdown combining with an intense test–trace–isolate strategy could prevent onward transmission. This approach would be an alternative to strict lockdown measures while awaiting an effective vaccine against Covid-19 [27]. Lockdown combined with universal testing with case isolation, contact tracing and facemask use by the general population is the only scenario with the potential for higher effectiveness in reducing infections, number of deaths and lockdown duration than ongoing lockdown with no additional interventions. This strategy can reduce the number of deaths up to 48%, leading to the early elimination of the infection [28].
Partial lockdown with social distancing	An age-structured mathematical model in France shows a full lockdown that achieves 60% isolation in the whole population remains the most effective strategy for minimising both the morbidity and mortality burden of the epidemic. But targeting one or several age groups with higher efficiency could achieve comparable reductions while allowing important societal and economic activities. The strategies involving isolation of the elderly showed significant potential to reduce mortality rates [29]. Another study proposed a dynamic cycle of 50-day suppression followed by a 30-day relaxation for 18 months, or until a suitable treatment or vaccination become available to reduce the health impact of Covid-19 [18]. If this pandemic lasts for a year or two as projected, then a recession is inevitable in the USA and other countries due to long-term lockdown approaches. That is why experts are suggesting implementing steps like partial lockdowns as an alternative to strict full lockdown [20].

To restrict the outbreak of Covid-19, most countries have implemented the highest-level emergency response plan, used control measures and imposed restrictions on multiple systems and public gatherings across the country. Strategies also include community-based control, transport limitation and restriction, isolation, and personnel quarantine. In the lockdown response stringency index, it can be seen that most of the countries took strict measures to implement lockdown. Along with the economic and social threats, the imposed restrictions for controlling the pandemic pose the greatest threats to the health of the elderly. An aggressive effort such as lockdown provided a temporary decline in new cases, but the actions taken to implement lockdown have badly impacted senior citizens' physical and mental health worldwide.

The mortality rate of Covid-19 among elderly people is much greater than other common diseases. The number of deaths in patients more than 65 years old without any underlying conditions for France, Italy, Mexico, the Netherlands, Sweden, Georgia, and New York City show that the proportion of these deaths ranged from 0.7% to 3.6% of all Covid-19 deaths. However, Mexico had a much higher percentage of (17.7%) death rate [4]. The social consequences of quarantine and lockdown must also be taken into account. Social disconnection is detrimental for this age group because isolation may limit their social engagement, interfere with daily routines, enhance inactivity, increase drugs use and decrease sensory stimulation. All these circumstances together with isolation might have an adverse impact on the mental health of the elderly population [7].

On the other hand, alternative approaches to lockdown are taken by these Asian countries (South Korea, Hong Kong, Singapore and Japan) such as mass testing, contact tracing, isolation, quarantine, etc., have been successful in preventing the virus from spreading further and preventing the community transmission. These countries have been able to keep most of their factories, malls and restaurants open when nations around the world are shutting down. Another alternative proposed is a dynamic cycle lockdown until a suitable treatment is available to reduce the health impact of Covid-19 [18]. Other solution could be Bluetooth-based contact tracking technology to prevent the outbreak of coronavirus. Contact tracing based on Bluetooth technology with the smart alert system can replace the traditional contact-tracking based on manual screening and paperwork because it is a simpler, quicker and more accurate way [11].

As the world needs to find a way to get back to normal life or accept the new normal for Covid-19, the world leaders should look forward to the alternative approaches to lockdown along with more use of digital health services which would also help sustain the growth of world economy. Data privacy and effective contact-tracing technologies can be implemented to identify the Covid-19 positive population cluster and mitigate the risk. Data from initial outbreaks, when detailed contact tracing is possible and sources of infection can still be reliably inferred, are particularly powerful in estimating critical values pertinent to describing transmission and the natural history of a disease. On the other hand, wearable technologies suggesting a risky zone of Covid-19 can provide people more safety, and people will feel more confident and risk-free to resume regular economic and business activities. There is

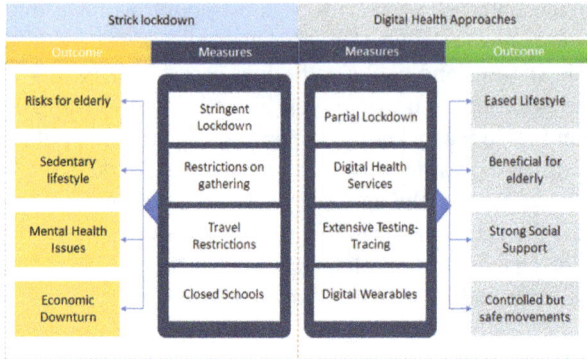

Figure 8.4   Comparison of lockdown approaches and their provable outcome

a comparison illustrated in Figure 8.4 depicting lockdown approaches versus use of digital health services with the potential outcome.

In summary, a combined strategy of universal testing, efficient and faster contact tracing and general population's personal hygiene and social distance mechanism, and the use of digital health services with a partial lockdown could potentially lead to the elimination of coronavirus. Successful implementation of this approach would require effective testing infrastructure and contact-tracing strategies along with isolation and quarantine facilities. These would not save the lives of the elderly but the entire humankind as well as the world economy.

The primary limitation of this chapter is that it requires a more comprehensive picture of the digital health approaches of a lockdown and further analysis of success stories of partial lockdown measurements taken by different countries. In addition, further research is required to find out how digital health services can be effectively used more innovatively to avoid future prolonged lockdowns, as the world is now facing the second wave of Covid-19.

8.7   Conclusion

Our systematic literature has shown that the governments worldwide took several strategies to save the countries from pandemic using lockdown and partial lockdown policies. The study provided information about the severe impacts of the lockdown policies and their limitations in terms of the health of the elderly and found how these severely impacted their lives due to disruption in movement and social gatherings. If Covid-19 stays for long (and even for future pandemics), the policy-makers are required to come up with more innovative, granular approaches than complete lockdown to safeguard the older people. These measures could be different in different countries/communities based on their economic, social and cultural needs. Moreover, the use of digital services and technologies in contact tracing and health service delivery can be useful for maintaining social distancing and resuming economic activities. The challenge is to develop a unified, global high-level policy framework with an integrated digital approach, which would require substantial research in the foreseeable future.

References

[1] Zhu N., Zhang D., Wang W., *et al.* 'A novel coronavirus from patients with pneumonia in China, 2019'. *New England Journal of Medicine.* 2020, vol. 382(8), pp. 727–33.

[2] China CDC Weekly. *Tracking the epidemic (2021)* [online]. 2020. Available from http://weekly.chinacdc.cn/news/TrackingtheEpidemic.htm [Accessed Dec 26, 2020].

[3] BBC News. *Coronavirus: the world in lockdown in maps and charts* [online]. 2020. Available from https://www.bbc.com/news/world-52103747 [Accessed Dec 20, 2020].

[4] Ioannidis J.P.A., Axfors C., Contopoulos-Ioannidis D.G. 'Population-Level COVID-19 mortality risk for non-elderly individuals overall and for non-elderly individuals without underlying diseases in pandemic epicenters'. *Environmental Research.* 2020, vol. 188, 109890.

[5] WHO/Europe | Coronavirus disease (COVID-19) outbreak. *Health care considerations for older people during COVID-19 pandemic* [online]. 2020. Available from https://www.euro.who.int/en/health-topics/health-emergen-cies/coronavirus-covid-19/publications-and-technical-guidance/vulnerable-populations/health-care-considerations-for-older-people-during-covid-19-pandemic [Accessed Dec 26, 2020].

[6] Our World in Data. *Coronavirus (COVID-19) vaccinations – statistics and research [online].* 2021. Available from https://ourworldindata.org/covid-vac-cinations [Accessed Feb 13, 2021].

[7] García-Fernández L., Romero-Ferreiro V., López-Roldán P.D., Padilla S., Rodriguez-Jimenez R. 'Mental health in elderly Spanish people in times of COVID-19 outbreak'. *The American Journal of Geriatric Psychiatry.* 2020, vol. 28(10), pp. 1040–5.

[8] Comite U. 'Businesses and public health between using lock down as a tool against Covid-19 pandemic in Italy: the impact in a global perspective'. *Advances in Management.* 2020, vol. 13, pp. 41–7.

[9] Welfens P.J.J. 'Macroeconomic and health care aspects of the coronavirus epidemic: EU, US and global perspectives'. *International Economics and Economic Policy.* 2020, vol. 17(2), pp. 295–362.

[10] Seshadri D.R., Davies E.V., Harlow E.R., *et al..* ' 'Wearable sensors for COVID-19: a call to action to harness our digital infrastructure for remote patient monitoring and virtual assessments". *Frontiers in Digital Health.* 2020, vol. 2,8.

[11] Geng R., Hu B., Li D. *Safe back school APP smart tracing for school reopening* [online]. JAZZ IT UP; 2020. Available from https://bingcheng.openmc.cn/blog/en/2020/Safe-Back-School-App.html [Accessed Jan 06, 2021].

[12]   World Health Organization. *Digital tools for COVID-19 contact tracing: an-nex: contact tracing in the context of COVID-19, 2 June 2020.* WHO/2019-nCoV/Contact_Tracing/Tools_Annex/2020.1v. Geneva: World Health Organization; 2020. Available from https://apps.who.int/iris/handle/10665/332265 [Accessed Feb 13, 2021].

[13]   Chamola V., Hassija V., Gupta V., Guizani M., *et al.* 'A comprehensive review of the COVID-19 pandemic and the role of IoT, drones, AI, block-chain, and 5G in managing its impact'. *IEEE Access.* 2020, vol. 8, pp. 90225–65.

[14]   Kitchenham B. *Procedures for Performing Systematic Reviews.* Keele, UK: Keele University; 2004.

[15]   Stawicki S.P., Jeanmonod R., Miller A.C., *et al.* 'The 2019-2020 novel coro-navirus (severe acute respiratory syndrome coronavirus 2) pandemic: a joint American College of academic international medicine-world academic coun-cil of emergency medicine multidisciplinary COVID-19 working group con-sensus paper'. *Journal of Global Infectious Diseases.* 2020, vol. 12(2), pp. 47–93.

[16]   Kim R.Y. 'The impact of COVID-19 on consumers: preparing for digital sales'. *IEEE Engineering Management Review.* 2020, vol. 48(3), pp. 212–18.

[17]   Renzaho A.M.N. 'The need for the right socio-economic and cultural fit in the COVID-19 response in sub-Saharan Africa: examining demographic, eco-nomic political, health, and socio-cultural differentials in COVID-19 mor-bidity and mortality'. *International Journal of Environmental Research and Public Health.* 2020, vol. 17(10), 3445.

[18]   Chowdhury R., Heng K., Shawon M.S.R., *et al.* 'Dynamic interventions to control COVID-19 pandemic: a multivariate prediction modelling study com-paring 16 worldwide countries'. *European Journal of Epidemiology.* 2020, vol. 35(5), pp. 389–99.

[19]   Pacces A.M., Weimer M. 'From diversity to coordination: a European ap-proach to COVID-19'. *European Journal of Risk Regulation.* 2020, vol. 11(2), pp. 283–96.

[20]   Mamoon D. *Economic and social thought health and economic outcomes of COVID 19* [online]. 2020. Available from www.kspjournals.org [Accessed Dec 26, 2020].

[21]   Di Santo S.G., Franchini F., Filiputti B., Martone A., Sannino S. 'The effects of COVID-19 and quarantine measures on the lifestyles and mental health of people over 60 at increased risk of dementia'. *Frontiers in Psychiatry.* 2020, vol. 11, pp. 578–628.

[22]   Slullitel P.A., Lucero C.M., Soruco M.L., *et al.* 'Prolonged social lockdown during COVID-19 pandemic and hip fracture epidemiology'. *International Orthopaedics.* 2020, vol. 44(10), pp. 1887–95.

[23]   Önmez A., Gamsızkan Z., Özdemir Şeyma., *et al.* 'The effect of COVID-19 lockdown on glycemic control in patients with type 2 diabetes mellitus in tur-key'. *Diabetes & Metabolic Syndrome: Clinical Research & Reviews.* 2020, vol. 14(6), pp. 1963–6.

[24] Anderez D.O., Kanjo E., Pogrebna G., *et al. A* modified epidemiological model to understand the uneven impact of COVID-19 on vulnerable individuals and the approaches required to help them emerge from lockdown [online]. 2020. Available from http://arxiv.org/abs/2006.10495 [Accessed Jan 20, 2021].

[25] Altmann S., Milsom L., Zillessen H., *et al.* 'Acceptability of app-based contact tracing for COVID-19: cross-country survey study'. *JMIR mHealth and uHealth.* 2020, vol. 8, p. e19857.

[26] Kondylakis H., Katehakis D.G., Kouroubali A., *et al.* 'COVID-19 mobile apps: a systematic review of the literature'. *Journal of Medical Internet Research.* 2020, vol. 22(12), p. e23170.

[27] Panovska-Griffiths J., Kerr C.C., Stuart R.M., *et al.* 'Determining the optimal strategy for reopening schools, the impact of test and trace interventions, and the risk of occurrence of a second COVID-19 epidemic wave in the UK: a modelling study'. *The Lancet Child & Adolescent Health.* 2020, vol. 4(11), pp. 817–27.

[28] Goscé L., Phillips P.A., Spinola P., Gupta D.R.K., Abubakar P.I., *et al.* 'Modelling SARS-COV2 spread in London: approaches to lift the lockdown'. *Journal of Infection.* 2020, vol. 81(2), pp. 260–5.

[29] Roche B., Garchitorena A., Roiz D. 'The impact of lockdown strategies targeting age groups on the burden of COVID-19 in France'. *Epidemics.* 2020, vol. 33, 100424.

Chapter 9

Digital mental health in Bangladesh "MonerDaktar": caring seniors during COVID-19

Tanjir Rashid Soron[1], Md Moshiur Rahman[2], and Zaid Farzan Chowdhury[1]

9.1 Introduction

Mental health matters and there is "No Health Without Mental Health." However, mental health care has long been neglected in health care policy, receives a tiny fraction of the health care budget, and is stigmatized [1]. As a result, about 85% of people who are living in low- and middle-income countries (LMICs) received no treatment even for serious mental health disorders [2]. However, this long-standing crisis in health care deepened during the recent coronavirus (COVID-19) pandemic due to bereavement, isolation, loss of income, fear of death, substance abuse, and/ or exacerbating pre-existing mental illness, and all-round helplessness [3]. Although the mental health crisis is accelerating, there are inadequate solutions to meet this crisis. The situation is more severe for seniors in LMICs as they have limited and in most cases no access to expert mental health professionals [4].

However, the explosive growth of digital technology and the use of different digital methods and tools may reduce the wide mental health treatment gap in Bangladesh [5]. The emerging different forms of digital methods and tools are connecting people and ensuring access to care throughout the year and during a lockdown [6]. A new digital mental health intervention (DMHI) called "MonerDaktar" (https://monerdaktar.health/) was launched in 2020 and is providing holistic online mental health care in Bangladesh.

This chapter presents the mental health care crisis of seniors during COVID-19, and how digital methods and tools ensure access to mental health care in LMICs with a case study of "MonerDaktar" service in Bangladesh. The chapter is organized into different sections. In Section 9.2, the authors discuss the mental health problem and its causes in different contexts. Section 9.3 focuses on the mental health crisis of the senior citizens as observed during the COVID-19. We share a brief introduction regarding the DMHI in Section 9.4, which will help the readers to have an idea about

[1]Telepsychiatry Research and Innovation Network Ltd, Dhaka, Bangladesh
[2]Graduate School of Biomedical and Health Sciences, Hiroshima University, Hiroshima, Japan

the digital health intervention in Bangladesh. Section 9.5 specifically discusses the DMHIs for senior citizens. In Section 9.6, the authors share the experience of developing the first and largest digital mental health platform "MonerDaktar," which connects psychiatrists and psychologists with clients directly and offers freedom of mutual selection for both patients and professionals. After this section, we describe the operation of "MonerDaktar" as a digital health intervention (Section 9.7) and its evaluation (Section 9.8). The chapter concludes in Section 9.9. We believe sharing the experience and the lesson from "MonerDaktar" will help other researchers, innovators, and entrepreneurs to develop better user-centered, affordable, and sustainable digital mental health care services for the elderly population.

9.2   Aging and mental health problems

World Population Prospects 2019 projected 1 in every 6 people will be over the age of 65 years by 2050 [7], and the number of senior citizens is increasing more rapidly in developing countries than the developed countries [8]. This rapid increment of senior citizens is imposing multilayer and multidimensional challenges for the families, communities, and countries [9] which necessitate multifaceted coordinated chronic health care [10].

Mental health care is neglected in most of the developing countries [11] and the access to quality mental health services is limited, and the problem is more intense in the LMICs [12]. Moreover, the situation is more disappointing for senior citizens in LMICs due to their unique additional biological and psychosocial vulnerable factors [13]. A bidirectional relationship exists between mental health and most of the chronic medical conditions. For example, people with diabetes are more likely to develop depression and depression is a risk factor for diabetes [14]. A similar relationship is also observed in cerebrovascular disorders, chronic respiratory disorders, chronic renal disorders, and cancer [15]. Moreover, socioeconomic factors, lifestyle, and social networks play important role in mental health and well-being of elderly people [16]. According to World Health Organization (WHO), more than 20% of senior citizens suffer from a neuropsychiatric disorder, and it costs 6.6% of all disabilities [17]. Dementia and major depressive disorder are the two leading contributors of all disability-adjusted life years (DALYs) in the old age group [18]. Andreas *et al.* [19] reported that 50% of the population aged 65 to 84 years experienced at least one mental disorder in their lifetime and 33% encountered the symptoms within the past year. The anxiety-related disorder is one of the most common mental disorders among the elderly, and it is assumed that the actual burden of the problem is much higher than that was previously reported [20]. The rate and number of substance use disorders and sleeping disorders are also increasing among them. Though suicide in late life is hardly discussed in the LMICs, many studies documented suicide rate is highest in the elderly age group [21].

Mental health received low priority in most countries of the South East Asia region and most of these countries lack national mental health policies, strategies, and mental health legislation, and receive low budgets for mental health services

[22]. However, the burden of mental disorders is increasing in the region. A study in India reported the contribution of mental disorders to the total DALYs in the country increased from 2·5% in 1990 to 4·7% (3·7–5·6) in 2017 [23]. Bangladesh is expecting 17.2 million elderly people by 2025 [24] with a prevalence of depression ranging from 36.9% to 45% among the elderly [25, 26]. However, the country is yet to have any national strategic plan or policy for their mental health and well-being.

9.3 COVID-19 and mental health crisis of elderly people

More than 75% of individuals aged 65 years or more have one or more chronic conditions [27]. The comorbid medical condition makes the elderly population vulnerable to mental health disorders and the complication of the COVID-19 infection. Moreover, the social restriction and lock-down imposed due to the COVID-19 pandemic increases the risk of anxiety and depression in the elderly [28]. Besides the loss of income, inactivity, limited access to basic services, and decreased family and social support are known risk factors for developing the mental disorder in a pandemic. Meng *et al.* [29] found about 37.1% of the elderly faced depression and anxiety during the pandemics and a rapid surge of acute exacerbation of pre-existing mental health disorders was also noticed [28]. Though most of the studies revealed the mental health problem among the older age group increased during the COVID-19 crisis, a contradictory finding was also reported [29]. However, they were less likely than younger adults to seek mental health help [30] as many of them considered seeking help for mental illness as a sign of weakness or it may cost their freedom, and they considered the problems as normal age-related changes [31]. In addition, the lack of self-motivation, mental health literacy, and formal and informal support acts as significant barriers for seeking help for mental health [32].

According to WHO, the COVID-19 pandemic has disrupted or halted critical mental health services in 93% of countries worldwide [33]. The mental health care service has been neglected for a long time in developing countries, and during this COVID-19 pandemic, the crisis deepened and the situation became more complicated than at any other time. For example, more than 92% of people in Bangladesh are deprived of the necessary mental health care [34], and when the first lockdown was imposed most of the hospitals stopped delivering mental health services. Our senior citizens were most vulnerable. A study reported about 50% of people age 65 and above were suffering from depression [35]. Although only 8% of the total patients with COVID-19 were elderly persons, they account for almost 42% of total deaths in Bangladesh [36]. The anxiety, panic, and phobia spread rapidly among the elderly when every print, electronic, and social media continuously highlight their vulnerability.

9.4 Digital mental health services in Bangladesh

Bangladesh is a country of 170 million people where fewer than 230 psychiatrists and 52 clinical psychologists are fighting to address the increased mental health burden in the country. Moreover, most of these mental health professionals are living in the capital city Dhaka, which limits access to mental health care [37]. As a result, less than 8% of people in Bangladesh received mental health care [38]. Moreover, the government's total expenditure on mental health was 0.5% of total government health expenditure [39]. However, the rapid growth of information communication technologies brought new hope to ensure access to health care for all. The wide mobile network coverage and internet interconnected all the corners of the country. At present, almost every family poses a mobile phone in Bangladesh due to the wide range of availability and rapid reduction in price. Moreover, mobile network connections became stronger. This rapid growth of technology has opened the opportunity to serve with DMHs to reduce the wide mental health treatment gap [40]. The DMHIs use different digital tools and methods including smartphone applications, remote monitoring and tracking devices, wearable computers, and virtual/augmented reality headsets [41].

The effectiveness of digital mental health care has been documented in multiple systematic reviews and meta-analyses [40]. Digital health care is transforming health care in both developed and developing countries, and the acceptance of this service is increasing in both developed and developing countries. Bangladeshi rural communities were willing to accept digital health services due to their easy access, time-saving nature, and low cost [42]. Nevertheless, we should acknowledge that access to the internet and digital tools are not equal to every stratum in the country [43]. However, the Bangladesh government introduced "Union Digital Centers" to ensure access to the internet and digital communication for all.

The rapid digital transformation facilitated the growth of digital health services including various digital mental health services such as Mind Tale, Maya Apa, MonerDaktar, Monershastho, and Kaan Pete Roi [44]. A brief compartive analysis among the serives was done in Table 9.1 Bangladesh's first emotional support and suicide prevention helpline "Kaan Pete Roi" has been working since 2013, which provides emergency, suicide-related support through a group of volunteers after a short training program [45]. It does not provide 24/7 suicide support at this moment. Mind Tale is the first nationwide mobile phone call-based mental health service that was launched in 2016 and served more than 8000 clients [46]. Maya Apa [47] is serving people with different physical and mental health problems with the chat option from their mobile application. In addition, LifeSpring and MonerBondhu are working to increase awareness through regular and social media programs.

Many volunteers stepped forward to form Facebook groups and pages to increase awareness and provide psychological support. However, the information should be reliable, and it should be shared on social media following the standard ethical standards. Telepsychiatry Research and Innovation Network (TRIN; https://trin.ltd) [48] is working as the leading digital mental health service and research organization in the country to reduce the wide mental health treatment gap with different digital mental health initiatives. These digital mental health services attracted mental health professionals, clients, and companies in Bangladesh.

Earlier, most of the digital mental health services in Bangladesh aimed to provide counseling and initial primary care rather than delivering holistic mental health

Table 9.1 A brief comparison of the current existing digital mental health services in Bangladesh

Criteria	Mind Tale	Moner Jotno Mobile E	Kaan Pete Roi	Maya Apa	MonerDaktar
Platform	Mobile phone call-based service http://www.mind-tale.com/# https://www.synesisit.com.bd/detailsVas?id=29	Mobile phone call based mental health support. http://www.brac.net/latest-news/item/1277-telecounselling-service-moner-jotno-mobile-e-for-anxieties-related-to-covid-19	Mobile phone-based emergency support http://shuni.org/	Mobile application to provide short message based services (SMS) https://www.mayaiswithyou.com/notfound	Mobile app and website https://monerdaktar.health/.
Nature of service	Both psychological therapy and in referred cases psychiatric consultations	Psychological support	suicide prevention-related emergency support	Suggestions by the trained psychologists and also other physical health-related support	Psychiatric consultation, psychotherapy and counseling, and mental health assessments
Method and communication of service delivery	Only audio call	Audio call	Audio call	Chat message	Audio call, video, and chat
Service delivery time	24/7 hours (in most of the time)	8 am till 12 midnight	Friday to Wednesday 3 pm to 9 pm, Thursday 3 pm to 3 am	24 hours chat message	24/7 matching the schedule of client and expert
Experts	Psychologist and psychiatrists	Only psychologists	Trained volunteers in psychological support in emergency situation, volunteers	Trainee psychologist and other health professionals	Clinical psychologists and psychiatrists

(Continues)

Table 9.1   Continued

Criteria	Mind Tale	Moner Jotno Mobile E	Kaan Pete Roi	Maya Apa	MonerDaktar
Freedom of selection of expert	No	No	No	No	Yes
Dashboard and session reminder	Only the professional has the dashboard. No reminder option	Organization dashboard. But no dashboard for clients No session reminder	Organization dashboard. But no dashboard for clients	Dashboard for both clients and organization point of view with limited features	Both clients and professionals have the dashboard to track the progress of the service, store information, appointment reminder and be an active part of the management
ePrescription and mental health resources	No	No	No	No	Yes
Unique features	A specific helpline 7899 or 27899 can be reached at a minimal cost	Counselling support platform	First suicide-prevention helpline	Short message services (SMS)-based service—both physical and mental health	Integrated both smartphone and website-compatible platform deliver holistic mental health services from expert professionals

(Continues)

Table 9.1 Continued

Criteria	Mind Tale	Moner Jotno Mobile E	Kaan Pete Roi	Maya Apa	MonerDaktar
Types of services	Counselling and Psychotherapy sessions, psychiatric consultations only when referred	Short-term psychological support	Suicide-prevention helpline, mainly emergency support	Suggestion on mental health issues, health-related consultations	Mental health service, psychiatric consultations, psychotherapy and assessment of different mental health issues

care through connecting psychiatrists and psychologists directly with the clients. "MonerDaktar" fills this gap in the digital mental health service in Bangladesh with the following features:

Integrated digital mental health care from one platform: All the necessary mental health services like psychiatric consultation, psychotherapy, and mental health assessments are available from the "MonerDaktar." Moreover, the system allows referral from one type of service to another, and interdisciplinary service can also be delivered to a client whenever necessary. This type of integrated digitalized service has been missing prior to "MonerDaktar."

Service delivery only by reputed experts: "MonerDaktar" delivers its service only by the reputed clinical psychologists and psychiatrists. The platform does not allow the registration of trainee psychologists or psychiatrists, thus ensure the quality of service. Moreover, the experts provide evidence-based interventions and ePrescriptions.

Freedom of choice: "MonerDaktar" gives the freedom to select a professional and take the service at their convenient time. The professionals were also allowed to fix and edit their consultation schedules according to their convenience. This freedom of selection from senior mental health experts was first introduced in "MonerDaktar" in Bangladesh.

9.5   DMHI for senior citizens

With the advancement of digital health methods and tools, DMHIs are now considered promising intervention programs to address the mental health burden in LMICs, where there are few mental health providers [49]. Moreover, digital methods and tools have transformed health care, and many researchers believe that digital mental health care will lead to mental health intervention and service researches for the older population [50] both in diagnostics [51–53] and in treatment [54–56]. Moreover, the recent trend showed older adults are increasingly using digital technologies for health care purposes [57, 58]. Many digital methods and tools have been implemented in mental health in a different context [59], and the engagement of the elder population substantially increased [60–62]. The DMHI evades the mental health stigma and removes the geographical barrier and travel cost, which were a few important concerns of older people [63].

Despite the huge opportunity and scope to help senior people with digital mental health care, we should consider the challenges of successful implementation and scale-up of the DMHIs such as technological backwardness and lower internet penetration [64–67]. Developers, practitioners, researchers, and entrepreneurs should consider this digital inequality, the background knowledge, and the needs of older people, who are not "digital natives" [68]. We observed increased attention and unprecedented growth of DMHI all over the world during this COVID-19 crisis. Thousands of doctors, psychiatrists, psychologists, and other professionals from LMICs shared their personal phone numbers and social media profiles to provide the service rather than developing a secured dedicated standard hotline and mobile application [69]. These incidents raised several ethical and legal issues, which should be addressed for scaling the service. However, the growth and enthusiasm should receive national and international support in the LMICs as it potentiates the scope of bridging the treatment gap.

9.6 The development and testing of "MonerDaktar"

"MonerDaktar" was developed through literature search, in-depth interview, focus group discussion (FGD), user journey analysis, heuristic evaluation, and post-evaluation modification. The literature review was conducted focusing on the recent trends of digital mental health innovations, existing guidelines of digital methods and tools, user-centered designing, implementation theories, and barriers of digital mental health implementation in LMICs.

9.6.1 Design of "MonerDaktar"

"MonerDaktar" was developed by a multi-disciplinary team led by a qualified and experienced psychiatrist Dr. Tanjir Rashid Soron. This digital service was intended to be a complete virtual mental health platform with all necessary mental health services including (1) psychiatric consultation, (2) psychotherapy and counseling, and (3) psychological assessments. Moreover, in the system, we uploaded multiple audios, videos, and written materials to promote mental health literacy and prevent mental health problems. During the conceptional framework of designing, the following features and services were considered to ensure access to mental health for all and providing holistic digitalized mental health care in Bangladesh:

1. Psychiatric Consultation: Through secured audio or video communication from the most reputed psychiatrists in the country.
2. Psychotherapy and Counseling: "MonerDaktar" would allow only the clinical psychologist to register in the system and provide evidence-based psychotherapy and counseling through secured audio or video platform.
3. Mental Health Assessment: Multiple self-rated or clinician-rated valid mental assessment tools would be available to measure the severity of the problems, confirm a diagnosis, or monitor the progress of the interventions.
4. Online self-material and resources: We would regularly upload articles, audio, video materials for the user to practice at home.
5. List of all available experts and a search option by name, degree, affiliation, and geographical distribution of the professionals.
6. Dashboard for both clients and professionals: All the necessary information for the client management is available in the professional dashboard and the clients are also able to see their previous and upcoming appointments, notifications, and so on.
7. Online electronic medical record (EMR): An EMR will be generated over the course of time.
8. ePrescription and referral.

Based on these initial features and concepts, Dr. Soron conducted six FGDs with the different mental health professionals, including psychiatrists from the National Institute of Mental Health (NIMH), Dhaka, Bangabandhu Sheikh Mujib Medical University, members of Bangladesh Child and Adolescent Psychiatry Society, and clinical psychologists of Bangladesh Clinical Psychology Society (BCPS), and Department of Clinical Psychology of the University of Dhaka. The duration of the FGDs ranged from 60 to 80 minutes, and 6–9 expert professionals joined each FGD. We shared our initial design and service blueprint of the website and mobile application using an initial 10 minutes presentation and possible user journey. During the discussion, the experts shared their feedback about the homepage design, the dashboard content, the issue related to privacy, and ePrescription. They also shared their concern of acceptability among senior health care professionals and people living in lower socioeconomic status. The mental health professionals shared their thoughts to make the website usable for all and discussed the key features that would help to increase acceptability.

"MonerDaktar" team conducted two FGDs with the potential user of "MonerDaktar" and those who have already received any of the currently existing digital health services in Bangladesh. We tried to find out their experience of using any existing digital methods and tools, the challenges of using the digital tool, their expectations, and suggestion for developing a complete digital mental health solution. All these FGDs were audio-recorded, transcribed, and the manuscript has been written. However, it was not published yet and the detailed finding of the chapter is not in the scope of this chapter. Despite that, we would like to share there was a significant difference in the design acceptance and color preference between the age group under 20 years and those 65 years and above. There was a suggestion to use multiple pages to accommodate large volumes of information without squeezing them in the small screen, which may hamper the reading of seniors. Based on the suggestions and comments from these discussions, the "MonerDaktar" IT team developed the initial website and mobile application. The first version of the website and mobile application was evaluated through a systemic process.

9.6.2   Testing and assessment of "MonerDaktar"

We completed the user journey analysis of both the clients and professionals followed by heuristic evaluation [70]. Twenty volunteers participated in our initial assessment process where more than 80% of the users considered the system easy to operate. However, there was a significant variation in the aesthetic issues, login fields, and user profile visibility between the under-20 years age group and the above-65 years group. Moreover, the respondents reported difficulty in reading the resource materials on their mobile phones. A few users asked to clarify the difference between psychiatric consultation and psychotherapy. Based on the feedback of the expert professionals and users, a slight modification was done.

9.7 "MonerDaktar" as a DMHI

"MonerDaktar" was launched on March 5, 2020 with several unique features such as the availability of consultation from the most reputed professionals, freedom of selection of experts and time, and availability of all sorts of mental health services from one digital platform. The movement restriction for the COVID-19 and the closure of the private chamber of health professionals including mental health professionals accelerated the popularity of "MonerDaktar" [71]. Though the service was not specifically designed for senior citizens, we found they were interested in "MonerDaktar" and continuously taking the service from this digital tool.

Within a month after launching the "MonerDaktar," BCPS (http://bcps.org.bd/) and the Department of Clinical Psychology of the University of Dhaka expressed their interest to collaborate with "MonerDaktar." We agreed to provide free mental health services during the peak of the COVID-19 infection. Almost 90% of the members of the Bangladesh Society for Clinical Psychology joined "MonerDaktar" and provided psychotherapy and counseling. The members of the Bangladesh Association of Psychiatrists (https://www.bapbd.org/) also joined and 112 mental health professionals registered in "MonerDaktar" by the end of August 2020. During the peak of COVID-19 infection, the seniors in Bangladesh also faced a panicky situation due to the overload of information and misinformation [72]. Their mental health condition deteriorated and the severity of preexisting psychiatric disorders increased. However, the scope of treatment squeezed as private chambers and many mental health hospitals stopped providing direct face-to-face service. Moreover, the risk of infection was high in the few institutions where the service was available. All these factors motivated older people to seek mental health services from "MonerDaktar." The availability of consultation from the senior mental health experts in the country and the option of receiving the service from home were important factors to ensure acceptability and trust from the seniors. Another big advantage was the cost efficiency of the service. "MonerDaktar" provided psychiatric consultation and psychotherapy free of cost during the COVID-19 pandemic. MonerDaktar was able to provide that confidence and trust among them. We served more than 350 senior people with 743 individual psychotherapy sessions, 104 psychiatric consultations, and 169 basic mental health information and assessment from the platform.

9.7.1 A real case example

Mr. X (pseudonym) is a 68-year-old retired government officer who broke down into tears after hearing the news that his son who was living in New York, USA, got infected with COVID-19 and hospitalized. His daughter-in-law, who was a doctor, also got infected and there was none to take care of their 3-year-old grandson. The mental health condition of Mrs. X was more severe. Both of them were unable to sleep, crying most of the time, and there were agitation and panic in the family. Their relatives considered taking them to the nearest mental health hospitals. However, most of the hospitals were unwilling to provide face-to-face regular consultations. Mr. and Mrs. X were also afraid of being infected with COVID-19 and putting their life and others at risk. Moreover, they could not detach themselves from the societal stigmas and were worried about how their acquaintances would react when they will come to know about their psychiatric consultation. At that time, he watched the news of "MonerDaktar" on Ekattor TV and came to know that "MonerDaktar" was providing online psychiatric consultation and psychotherapy free of cost. He was relieved and immediately called one of the reputed psychiatrists and started taking antidepressants and anxiolytics. Furthermore, the psychiatrist asked both of them to start psychotherapy and referred to one of the senior clinical psychologists of "MonerDaktar." They received online Cognitive Behavior Therapy (CBT) sessions from the psychologist weekly during the next three months and continued the antidepressant medicine. Both of them were also regularly reading and watching our articles and videos from the platform. The severity of depression of Mr. X was reduced. The depression was measured using a valid depression assessment tool for the Bangladeshi population called "Bangla Montgomery Asberg Depression Rating Scale" (MADRSB). The MADRSB score for Mr. X dropped from 46 to 13 (higher score indicates, higher severity) [72] and in the case of Mrs. X, the depression score was reduced from 38 to 9. They continued a regular monthly follow-up for another three months from their respective psychiatrist and psychologist from "MonerDaktar." They expressed thanks and gratitude to "MonerDaktar" for helping them in a very critical situation and making both psychiatric consultation and psychotherapy available from the platform that was not available from any other digital health providers.

9.8   Evaluation and challenges

"MonerDaktar" aimed to ensure access to mental health experts through a digital platform with other components such as providing information to reduce stigma related to mental illness and a self-care guide to practice at home. "MonerDaktar" is still in the early stages and formal research about its impact and effectiveness has been designed. However, it is yet to be completed as we have extended the research area. Considering this limitation, we conducted a couple of surveys and evaluated our service delivery information and clients' feedback assessment. One of the main objectives behind the development of "MonerDaktar" was increasing access to mental health care from expert professionals for all. This innovative digital tool was able to connect and serve 2,537 people till December 2020 from all the 64 districts where more than 42% of the clients contacted from the rural areas. This indicated "MonerDaktar" was successful in removing the geographic barriers. Furthermore, it served people from 16 years to 74 years old for different mental health issues. Within six months of launching the service, more than 100 psychiatrists and clinical psychologists registered in "MonerDaktar" platform that made it the largest mental health platform in Bangladesh. With the help of 100 professionals, "MonerDaktar" was able to provide expert mental health service 24/7. In addition to the direct audio or video communication with the mental health expert, "MonerDaktar" also provided various audio, video, and other written materials to increase mental health awareness and learn self-help skills [73].

The data from our service delivery register system revealed among the total 2 537 clients 63% of them were female and 58% of the users were between 18 and 35 years old. We found 357 clients were over 60 years old. The common mental health problems were anxiety and stress-related, depression, sleep disturbance, concentration, relationship, fear of being infected, and exacerbation of preexisting mental health issues such as obsessive-compulsive disorder. During this COVID-19 crisis, "MonerDaktar" served the seniors with 104 psychiatric consultations, 743 individual psychotherapy sessions, and 169 basic mental health information and assessments. There were no such digital methods and tools in Bangladesh, where both psychiatric consultation and psychotherapy in audio and video format from the expert professionals till the end of January 2021.

We also conducted an online quick survey to find out more structured feedback from the professionals. More than 84% of respondents (professionals) of the study considered this platform gave them the alternative and convenient way to communicate providing mental health care, 73% of them considered the platform has reduced the dropout rate, which for the senior was lower than traditional face-to-face sessions [74]. However, a few of them reported that the internet connection issues hampered the quality of the video conference. Based on the result of the study and the feedback of the professionals, we launched the updated website in January 2021, https://monerdaktar.health/. The different levels of technological proficiency of the professionals and clients and the unequivocal internet speed in different locations are the major challenges for us to ensure uniform high-quality service. We found increased interest and active participation from the senior citizens for "MonerDaktar"; this observation was supported by a couple of recent research findings where the authors concluded elderly population becoming interested to use the internet for health [75, 76]. However, many of them had limited access to digital health services [77, 78] and the crisis deepened in the LMICs. Mobile phone sharing among family members is not a rare phenomenon in Bangladesh especially among the poor and seniors who also seek help from the young for smooth operations of their smart devices. The seniors reported problems in registration and sharing their previous health documents. The problem is related to their lack of familiarity using online virtual platforms, reduced visual acuity, and cognitive declines.

The electronic and print media highlighted the activities of the "MonerDaktar" [71], and we faced difficulties to meet the need of the people despite having more than 100 professionals. The professionals preferred to provide the service using a website from their desktop or laptop devices. On the other hand, clients preferred mobile applications for the service. When a large number of people started using the "MonerDaktar" platform, we faced a few new challenges specifically with the mobile applications. Another challenge was serving people who have low internet speed. The team of "MonerDaktar" was very concerned about privacy, data security, and ensuring ethical evidence-based care in the digital platform. We followed the standard protocols to maintain data security, privacy, and quality of care. Having that challenge at hand, "MonerDaktar" effectively served a wide range of the population who are in need in the crisis period of COVID-19, especially the old-age people.

Though we have a lack of research-based effectiveness, efficiency, and impact of "MonerDaktar" in the mental health care system in Bangladesh, we can claim that the digital mental health service is well accepted by the clients of all age groups and professionals. Moreover, it is documented the senior citizens are interested in taking service from the digital platform.

"MonerDaktar" plans to integrate into this the existing fragile health care system in Bangladesh and explore the feasibility of scaling up in the other LMICs to ensure access to mental health care anytime from anywhere in their local language. Another factor that "MonerDaktar" aims to address is the digital divide. This service is currently funded by TRIN Ltd (www.trin.ltd), and the collaboration with other multinational organizations or government support will help its future scale-up plan.

9.9   Conclusion

"MonerDaktar" documented how a low-cost digital tool played a critical and important role in ensuring access to mental health care for all including the seniors during an emergency. Not only the timely mental health intervention is important to reduce the disease burden but the lack of appropriate support may also destroy the process of healthy aging. We believe the success of MonerDaktar in connecting senior citizens with the mental health professionals during this COVID-19 will motivate entrepreneurs, researchers, or academics from other LMICs to develop similar innovative digital solutions to reduce the mental health treatment gaps in their community. We consider the experience and learning of "MonerDaktar" will motivate future researchers to explore the different aspects of the service and find out the evidence-based guidelines to design future digital methods and tools for healthy aging of seniors and connecting them with the digital mental health tools more efficiently.

References

[1]   The Parliament Magazine. *Mental health – the hidden epidemic* [online]. 2020. Available from https://www.theparliamentmagazine.eu/news/article/mental-health-the-hidden-epidemic [Accessed 14 Jan 2021].

[2]   Demyttenaere K., Bruffaerts R., Posada-Villa J., Gasquet I., Kovess V., Lepine J.P. 'WHO world mental health survey consortium'. *JAMA*. 2004, vol. 291, pp. 2581–90.

[3]   World Health Organization. *COVID-19 disrupting mental health services in most countries, WHO survey* [online]. 2020. Available from https://www.who.int/news/item/05-10-2020-covid-19-disrupting-mental-health-services-in-most-countries-who-survey [Accessed 21 Feb 2021].

[4]   Rathod S., Pinninti N., Irfan M., *et al.*. ' 'Mental health service provision in low- and middle-income countries". *Health Services Insights*. 2017, vol. 10, pp. 117863291794_35–7.

[5] Soron T.R. 'Telepsychiatry for depression management in Bangladesh'. *International Journal of Mental Health*. 2016, vol. 45(4), pp. 279–80.

[6] Torous J., Jän Myrick K., Rauseo-Ricupero N., Firth J. 'Digital mental health and COVID-19: using technology today to accelerate the curve on access and quality tomorrow'. *JMIR Mental Health*. 2020, vol. 7(3), p. e18848.

[7] United Nations, Department of Economic and Social Affairs, Population Division. *World population prospects 2019: highlights (ST/ESA/SER.A/423)* [online]. 2019. Available from https://population.un.org/wpp/Publications/Files/WPP2019_Highlights.pdf [Accessed 12 Feb 2021].

[8] World Health Organization and National Institute on Aging, U.S. Department of Health and Human Services. *Global health and aging. NIH publication no. 11-7737* [online]. 2011. Available from https://www.who.int/ageing/publications/global_health.pdf [Accessed 11 Feb 2021].

[9] United Nations. *World population prospects: the 2017 revision* [online]. 2017. Available from https://population.un.org/wpp/ [Accessed 19 Feb 2021].

[10] Shrivastava S.R.B.L., Shrivastava P.S., Ramasamy J. 'Health-care of elderly: determinants, needs and services'. *International Journal of Preventive Medicine*. 2013, vol. 4(10), pp. 1224–5.

[11] Roberts T., Miguel Esponda G., Krupchanka D., Shidhaye R., Patel V., Rathod S. 'Factors associated with health service utilisation for common mental disorders: a systematic review'. *BMC Psychiatry*. 2018, vol. 18(1), p. 262.

[12] Wainberg M.L., Scorza P., Shultz J.M., *et al.*. ' 'Challenges and opportunities in global mental health: a research-to-practice perspective". *Current Psychiatry Reports*. 2017, vol. 19(5),p. 28.

[13] Fernandes L., Paúl C. 'Editorial: aging and mental health'. *Frontiers in Aging Neuroscience*. 2017, vol. 9, p. 25.

[14] Anderson R.J., Freedland K.E., Clouse R.E., Lustman P.J. 'The prevalence of comorbid depression in adults with diabetes: a meta-analysis'. *Diabetes Care*. 2001, vol. 24(6), pp. 1069–78.

[15] Karim M.E., Firoz A.H.M., Alam M.F. 'Assessment of depression in Parkinson's disease, psoriasis, stroke, and cancer patients'. *Bangladesh Journal of Psychiatry*. 2001, vol. 15(2), pp. 11–18.

[16] Ohrnberger J., Fichera E., Sutton M. 'The dynamics of physical and mental health in the older population'. *The Journal of the Economics of Ageing*. 2017, vol. 9(4), pp. 52–62.

[17] World Health Organization. *Mental health of older adults* [online]. 2017. Available from https://www.who.int/news-room/fact-sheets/detail/mental-health-of-older-adults [Accessed 15 Feb 2021].

[18] Murray C.J.L., Lopez A.D. *The Global burden of disease: a comprehensive assessment of mortality and disability from diseases, injuries, and risk factors in 1990 and projected to 2020: summary [online]*. Geneva: World Health Organization, World Bank & Harvard School of Public Health; 1996. Available from https://apps.who.int/iris/handle/10665/41864 [Accessed 22 Feb 2021].

[19] Andreas S., Schulz H., Volkert J., *et al.* 'Prevalence of mental disorders in elderly people: the European MentDis_ICF65+ study'. *British Journal of Psychiatry*. 2017, vol. 210(2), pp. 125–31.

[20] Kirmizioglu Y., Doğan O., Kuğu N., Akyüz G. 'Prevalence of anxiety disorders among elderly people'. *International Journal of Geriatric Psychiatry*. 2009, vol. 24(9), pp. 1026–33.

[21] Centers for Disease Control and Prevention and National Association of Chronic Disease Directors. *The state of mental health and aging in America issue brief 1: what do the data tell us [online]?* Atlanta, GA: National Association of Chronic Disease Directors; 2008. Available from https://www. cdc.gov/aging/pdf/mental_health.pdf [Accessed 24 Feb 2021].

[22] Sharan P., Sagar R., Kumar S. 'Mental health policies in south-east Asia and the public health role of screening instruments for depression'. *WHO South-East Asia Journal of Public Health*. 2017, vol. 6(1), pp. 5–11.

[23] India State-Level Disease Burden Initiative Mental Disorders Collaborators. 'The burden of mental disorders across the states of India: the global burden of disease study 1990-2017'. *The Lancet Psychiatry*. 2020, vol. 7(2), pp. 148–61.

[24] Bangladesh Bureau of Statistics (Bangladesh). *Elderly population in Bangladesh: current features and future perspectives* [online]. 2015. Available from http://203.112.218.65:8008/WebTestApplication/userfiles/ Image/PopMonographs/elderlyFinal.pdf [Accessed 17 Jan 2021].

[25] Wahlin Åke., Palmer K., Sternäng O., Hamadani J.D., Kabir Z.N. 'Prevalence of depressive symptoms and suicidal thoughts among elderly persons in rural Bangladesh'. *International Psychogeriatrics*. 2015, vol. 27(12), pp. 1999–2008.

[26] Disu T.R., Anne N.J., Griffiths M.D., Mamun M.A. 'Risk factors of geriatric depression among elderly Bangladeshi people: a pilot interview study'. *Asian journal of psychiatry*. 2019, vol. 44, pp. 163–9.

[27] Canadian Institute for Health Information. *Seniors and the health care system: what Is the impact of multiple chronic conditions?* [online]. 2011. Available from https://secure.cihi.ca/free_products/air-chronic_disease_aib_ en.pdf [Accessed 29 Jan 2021].

[28] Mehra A., Rani S., Sahoo S., *et al.* 'A crisis for elderly with mental disorders: relapse of symptoms due to heightened anxiety due to COVID-19'. *Asian Journal of Psychiatry*. 2020, vol. 51, pp. 1–3.

[29] Meng H., Xu Y., Dai J., Zhang Y., Liu B., Yang H. 'Analyze the psychological impact of COVID-19 among the elderly population in China and make corresponding suggestions'. *Psychiatry Research*. 2020, vol. 289(5), pp. 112983–3.

[30] Fontes W.H de .A., Gonçalves Júnior J., de Vasconcelos C.A.C., da Silva C.G.L., Gadelha M.S.V. 'Impacts of the SARS-CoV-2 pandemic on the mental health of the elderly'. *Frontiers in Psychiatry*. 2020, vol. 11, p. 841.

[31] González-Sanguino C., Ausín B., Castellanos Miguel Ángel., *et al.* 'Mental health consequences during the initial stage of the 2020 coronavirus

pandemic (COVID-19) in Spain'. *Brain, Behavior, and Immunity.* 2020, vol. 87, pp. 172–6.

[32] Mackenzie C.S., Scott T., Mather A., Sareen J. 'Older adults' help-seeking attitudes and treatment beliefs concerning mental health problems'. *The American Journal of Geriatric Psychiatry.* 2008, vol. 16(12), pp. 1010–19.

[33] de Mendonça Lima C.A., Ivbijaro G. 'Mental health and wellbeing of older people: opportunities and challenges'. *Mental Health in Family Medicine.* 2013, vol. 10(3), pp. 125–7.

[34] National Institute of Mental Health (Bangladesh). *National mental health survey of Bangladesh, 2018-19, Provisional Fact Sheet* [online]. 2019. Available from https://www.who.int/docs/default-source/searo/bangladesh/pdf-reports/cat-2/nimh-fact-sheet-5-11-19.pdf?sfvrsn=3e62d4b0_2 [Accessed 02 Jan 2021].

[35] Mehra A., Rani S., Sahoo S., *et al.* 'A crisis for elderly with mental disorders: relapse of symptoms due to heightened anxiety due to COVID-19'. *Asian Journal of Psychiatry.* 2020, vol. 51,102114.

[36] World Health Organization. *COVID-19 disrupting mental health services in most countries, WHO survey* [online]. 2020. Available from https://www.who.int/news/item/05-10-2020-covid-19-disrupting-mental-health-services-in-most-countries-who-survey [Accessed 01 Feb 2021].

[37] Soron T.R. 'Telepsychiatry—from a dream to reality in Bangladesh'. *Journal of the International Society for Telemedicine and eHealth.* 2017, vol. 5(2017), pp. e53–5.

[38] National Institute of Mental Health (Bangladesh). *National mental health survey of Bangladesh, 2018-19, Provisional Fact Sheet* [online]. 2019. Available from https://www.who.int/docs/default-source/searo/bangladesh/pdf-reports/cat-2/nimh-fact-sheet-5-11-19.pdf?sfvrsn=3e62d4b0_2 [Accessed 07 Jan 2021].

[39] World Health Organization. *Global spending on health: a world in transition* [online]. Geneva, WHO/HIS/HGF/HFWorkingPaper/19.4. License: CC BY-NC-SA 3.0 IGO. 2019. Available from https://www.who.int/health_financing/documents/health-expenditure-report-2019.pdf?ua=1 [Accessed 05-01-2021].

[40] Soron T.R. 'Psychopathology of violence against doctors'. *Acta Psychopathologica.* 2016, vol. 2(3), p. 3.

[41] Hollis C., Falconer C.J., Martin J.L., *et al.* 'Annual research review: digital health interventions for children and young people with mental health problems – a systematic and meta-review'. *Journal of Child Psychology and Psychiatry.* 2017, vol. 58(4), pp. 474–503.

[42] Khatun F., Heywood A.E., Ray P.K., Bhuiya A., Liaw S.-T. 'Community readiness for adopting mHealth in rural Bangladesh: a qualitative exploration'. *International Journal of Medical Informatics.* 2016, vol. 93, pp. 49–56.

[43] Ahmed S.I., Jackson S.J., Zaber M., Morshed M.B., Ismail M.H.B., Afrose S. 'Ecologies of use and design: individual and social practices of mobile phone use within low-literate rickshawpuller communities in urban Bangladesh'.

Proceedings of the 4th Annual Symposium on Computing for Development (ACM DEV'13). Association for Computing Machinery; New York, NY, USA; 2013. pp. 1–10.

[44]   Wootton R., Yellowlees P., McLaren P. *Telepsychiatry and E-mental Health.* London: Royal Society of Medical Press Ltd; 2003.

[45]   Kan Pete Roi. *Kan Pete Roi. Bangladesh: info@shuni.org* [online]. 2020. Available from http://shuni.org/ [Accessed 11 Jan 2021].

[46]   Akter N., Chowdhury R., Soron T. 'Mental health in COVID-19 – an e-health service to provide tele-mental health support in pandemic'. *Asian Hospital and Healthcare Management.* 2020, vol. 2(1), pp. 60–3.

[47]   Maya apa. *Maya apa. Bangladesh* [online]. 2020. Available from https://www.mayaiswithyou.com/ [Accessed 18 Feb 2021].

[48]   Telepsychiatry Research and Innovation Network Ltd. *Telepsychiatry Research and Innovation Network Ltd. Bangladesh* [online]. 2020. Available from https://sites.google.com/view/trinltd/home [Accessed 28 Jan 2021].

[49]   Rahmadiana M., Karyotaki E., Passchier J., *et al.* 'Guided internet-based transdiagnostic intervention for Indonesian university students with symptoms of anxiety and depression: a pilot study protocol'. *Internet Interventions.* 2019, vol. 15, pp. 28–34.

[50]   Fortuna K.L., Torous J., Depp C.A., *et al.* 'A future research agenda for digital geriatric mental healthcare'. *The American Journal of Geriatric Psychiatry.* 2019, vol. 27(11), pp. 1277–85.

[51]   Depp C., Torous J., Thompson W. 'Technology-based early warning systems for bipolar disorder: a conceptual framework'. *JMIR Mental Health.* 2016, vol. 3, p. e42.

[52]   Ben-Zeev D., Kaiser S.M., Brenner C.J., Begale M., Duffecy J., Mohr D.C. 'Development and usability testing of focus: a smartphone system for self-management of schizophrenia'. *Psychiatric Rehabilitation Journal.* 2013, vol. 36(4), pp. 289–96.

[53]   Depp C.A., Mausbach B., Granholm E., *et al.* 'Mobile interventions for severe mental illness: design and preliminary data from three approaches'. *The Journal of Nervous and Mental Disease.* 2010, vol. 198(10), pp. 715–21.

[54]   Aschbrenner K.A., Naslund J.A., Gill L.E., Bartels S.J., Ben-Zeev D. 'A qualitative study of client-clinician text exchanges in a mobile health intervention for individuals with psychotic disorders and substance use'. *Journal of Dual Diagnosis.* 2016, vol. 12(1), pp. 63–71.

[55]   Rus-Calafell M., Gutiérrez-Maldonado J., Ribas-Sabaté J. 'A virtual reality-integrated program for improving social skills in patients with schizophrenia: a pilot study'. *Journal of Behavior Therapy and Experimental Psychiatry.* 2014, vol. 45(1), pp. 81–9.

[56]   Naslund J.A., Aschbrenner K.A., Marsch L.A., McHugo G.J., Bartels S.J. 'Facebook for supporting a lifestyle intervention for people with major depressive disorder, bipolar disorder, and schizophrenia: an exploratory study'. *Psychiatric Quarterly.* 2018, vol. 89(1), pp. 81–94.

[57] Jefee Bahloul H., Mani N. 'International telepsychiatry: a review of what has been published'. *Journal of Telemedicine and Telecare*. 2013, vol. 19(5), pp. 293–4.

[58] Soron T.R. 'Acceptance of a mobile APP for autism assessment in Bangladesh'. *Journal of intellectual disability research : JIDR*. 2019, vol. 63(7), pp. 661–2.

[59] Quinn C.C., Staub S., Barr E., Gruber-Baldini A. 'Mobile support for older adults and their caregivers: dyad usability study'. *JMIR Aging*. 2019, vol. 2(1), p. e12276.

[60] Communications Market Report (United Kingdom). *Adults' Media use and Attitudes: Report 2015*. London, UK: Ofcom; 2015.

[61] Communications Market Report (United Kingdom). *Adults' Media use and Attitudes: Report 2017*. London, UK: Ofcom; 2017.

[62] Astell A. 'Technology and fun for a happy old age' in Sixsmith A., Gutman G. (eds.). *Technologies for Active Aging. International Perspectives on Aging*. Vol. 9. Springer: Boston, MA; 2013. pp. 169–87.

[63] Fortuna K.L., Lohman M.C., Gill L.E., Bruce M.L., Bartels S.J. 'Adapting a psychosocial intervention for smartphone delivery to middle-aged and older adults with serious mental illness'. *The American Journal of Geriatric Psychiatry*. 2017, vol. 25(8), pp. 819–28.

[64] Hollis C., Morriss R., Martin J., *et al.* 'Technological innovations in mental healthcare: harnessing the digital revolution'. *British Journal of Psychiatry*. 2015, vol. 206(4), pp. 263–5.

[65] Hunsaker A., Hargittai E. 'A review of internet use among older adults'. *New Media & Society*. 2018, vol. 20(10), pp. 3937–54.

[66] Seifert A., Schlomann A., Rietz C., Schelling H.R. 'The use of mobile devices for physical activity tracking in older adults' everyday life'. *Digital Health*. 2017, vol. 3,2055207617740088.

[67] Pew Research Center. *Tech adoption climbs among older adults* [online]. 2017. Available from http://www.pewInternet.org/wp-content/uploads/sites/9/2017/05/PI_2017.05.17_Older-Americans-Tech_FINAL.pdf [Accessed 05 Jan 2021].

[68] Prensky M. 'Digital natives, digital immigrants: Part 1'. *On the Horizon*. 2001, vol. 9(5), pp. 1–6.

[69] Soron T.R., Shariful Islam S.M., Ahmed H.U., Ahmed S.I. 'The hope and hype of telepsychiatry during the COVID-19 pandemic'. *The Lancet Psychiatry*. 2020, vol. 7(8), p. e50.

[70] Yáñez Gómez R., Cascado Caballero D., Sevillano J.-L., Gómez R.Y., Caballero D.C. 'Heuristic evaluation on mobile interfaces: a new checklist'. *The Scientific World Journal*. 2014, vol. 2014, pp. 1–19.

[71] Ekattor TV. *Mental health news: Ekattor TV. Bangladesh* [online]. 2020 [Accessed 02 Jan 2021].

[72] Hasan M.T., Hossain S., Saran T.R., Ahmed H.U. 'Addressing the COVID-19 related stigma and discrimination: a fight against "infodemic" in Bangladesh'. *Minerva Psichiatrica*. 2020, vol. 61(4), pp. 184–7.

[73] Soron T.R. 'MONERDAKTAR – the journey of developing a digital platform for mental health care in Bangladesh'. *20th World Congress of Psychiatry*; Virtual, 10/03/2021–13/03/2021; 2021. pp. 1–3.

[74] Soron T.R. 'Monerdaktar: a large online mental health service to improve access to care in Bangladesh during the COVID-19 pandemic'. *29th European Congress of Psychiatry*; Virtual, 10/04/2021–13/04/2021; 2021. pp. 1–4.

[75] Salovaara A., Lehmuskallio A., Hedman L., Valkonen P., Näsänena J. 'Information technologies and transitions in the lives of 55–65-year-olds: the case of colliding life interests'. *International Journal of Human-Computer Studies*. 2010, vol. 68(11), pp. 803–21.

[76] Zhu S.B., Deng X.Z. 'Study on influence factors of older health information seeking'. *Library and Information Service*. 2015, vol. 5, pp. 60–7.

[77] Zheng R., Spears J., Luptak M., Wilby F. 'Understanding older adults' perceptions of internet use: an exploratory factor analysis". *Educational Gerontology*. 2015, vol. 41(7), pp. 504–18.

[78] Sun X., Yan W., Zhou H., *et al*. 'Internet use and need for digital health technology among the elderly: a cross-sectional survey in China". *BMC Public Health*. 2020, vol. 20(1), p. 1386.

Chapter 10

Digital health for aged care from a service perspective

Yuan You[1,2], Yan Hanrunyu[3], and Pradeep Kumar Ray[1,3]

10.1   Introduction

Aged care requires a variety of professional services, such as general practitioners, specialists, pharmacists, nurses, physiotherapists, home helpers, social workers, dietitians, hairdressers, and cleaners. These service providers usually belong to different clinics, medical centers, hospitals, or other profit or non-profit organizations, dispersed geographically.

The care for the elderly is provided in different settings, such as nursing home-based (residential care), home-based for elderly living independently, or a combination. An aged care service is a complex operation involving a chain of service providers. For example, a digital health service provides health-care service remotely through the collaboration of multiple organizations, such as the telecom/mobile network provider, hospital of health-care provider, nursing home or aged care provider, radiology or CT scan provider, pathology (blood test) provider, etc. as shown in Figure 10.1. This complexity of aged care operation is an important consideration for both residential and home-based care.

Given the fact that medication errors are more fatal compared to road accidents and the increasing urgency of efficient and effective management of medication (e.g., vaccines during COVID-19, which is now the #1 killer of the elderly), it is important to get the service process of medication management right. Unlike in residential care (where the medication administration is managed by care workers) medication is mostly administered by the individual in home-based care and is more vulnerable to human errors. Hence medication management in home care is the focus of our case study in this chapter.

[1]School of Population Health, UNSW, Sydney, NSW, Australia
[2]Services Greater China Region, Customer Success, SAP SE, Germany
[3]Center for Entrepreneurship, University of Michigan-Shanghai Jiao Tong University Joint Institute, Shanghai, China

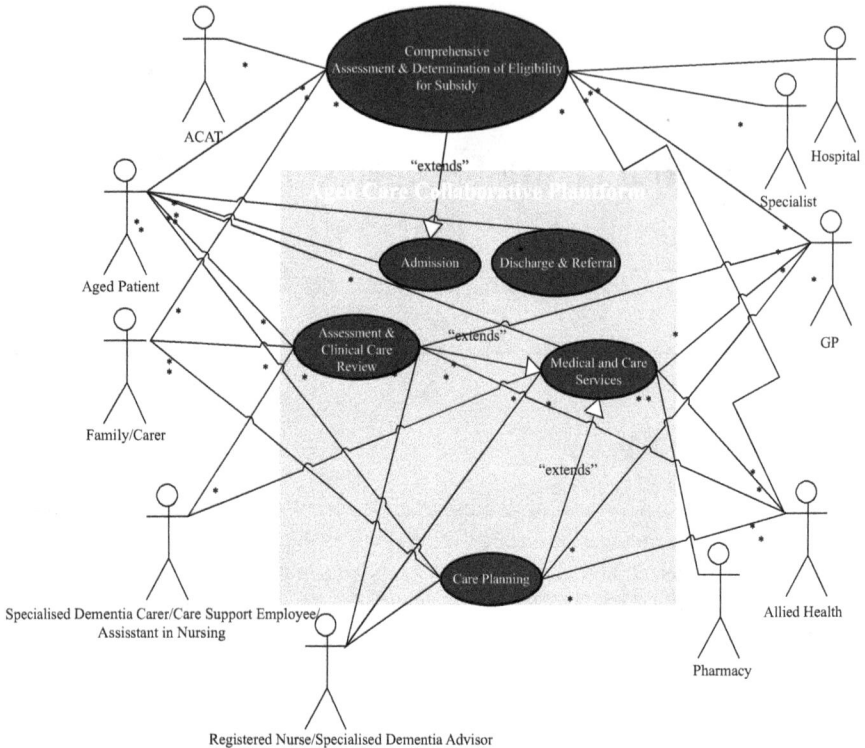

*Figure 10.1   Residential aged care as a multi-party collaboration environment
[1]. Source: Asia Pacific Ubiquitous Healthcare Research Centre,
UNSW – Australia, Presentation on Smart Services CRC Foundry
Project Presentation "Aged Care Collaborative Platform," March
2013.*

Currently, many types of software platforms, tools, and techniques are available
for aged care. The aims of the chapter are to illustrate digital methods and tools with
examples at different levels as follows:

1. Section 10.2 identifies the services and scenarios of aged care including the
   providers of those services;
2. Section 10.3 models the workflow of service request and delivery based on
   the sub-process of medication, e.g., drug request and delivery and medication-
   adherence/patient-compliance monitoring;
3. Section 10.3 examines the processes from the perspective of supply chain management and maps the processes of drug request and delivery to a service supply
   chain model;
4. Section 10.5 discusses the role of technology and tools, such as Radio Frequency
   Identification (RFID) and automatic pill dispensers.

Section 10.6 discusses how all these four elements contribute to effective medication management, an important aspect of aged care. Section 10.7 concludes the chapter with pointers to the limitations of the chapter and possible future work.

10.2 Aged care services and providers

According to the problems and development requirements in the field of medical and health care, the health-care services should be gradually transformed to prevention-oriented comprehensive medical model combining hospitals, communities, families, and individuals from the current hospital-centered treatment-based model. They can provide services including remote health consultation, remote real-time monitoring, remote diagnosis, personal health record, network-based health-care education, and other personalized services for the public through personalized medical information management and services configuration and integration [2].

We briefly describe examples from different parts of the world, namely Asia, Australia, and Europe in Sub-sections 10.2.1–10.2.3. It may be noted that there are now a variety of aged care providers in the world managed by the government, semi-government, fully private, non-government/charity organizations (NGOs). Also, they operate for-profit and not-for-profit modes.

10.2.1   Asia

A national health study conducted in Taiwan introduced three models for long-term care: home care, community care, and residential care. After the implementation of the home care model for 50 families and 200 participants, "the hospital readmission rate was reduced from 8.19% to 3.17%, and the hospital visit rate was reduced from 2.95% to 2.90%" [3]. Chapter 11 discusses the situation in China, where aged care is provided by the government, private sector, and NGOs. However, traditionally the elderly in Chinese and Asian families (including in India and Thailand) spend their old age at the family homes and hence their care is not in an organized form unlike in most western countries though the situation is changing due to the migration of younger family members overseas for work and career. Also the scarce resources of the governments of many developing countries in Asia require the private sector to play a more and more active role in aged care.

10.2.2   Australia

The aged care services in Australia are classified into two major categories: community-based (elderly residing at their homes) care and residential (elderly admitted to nursing homes) care. The recent increase in deaths of the elderly in care homes triggered a Royal Commission on aged care in Australia as reported in [3]. Since most elderly want to stay independently at their homes, community-based care services are now growing rapidly in Australia [4].

In Australia, aged care is highly organized as in many western countries. Although the actual care is managed by a variety of organizations (churches, NGOs,

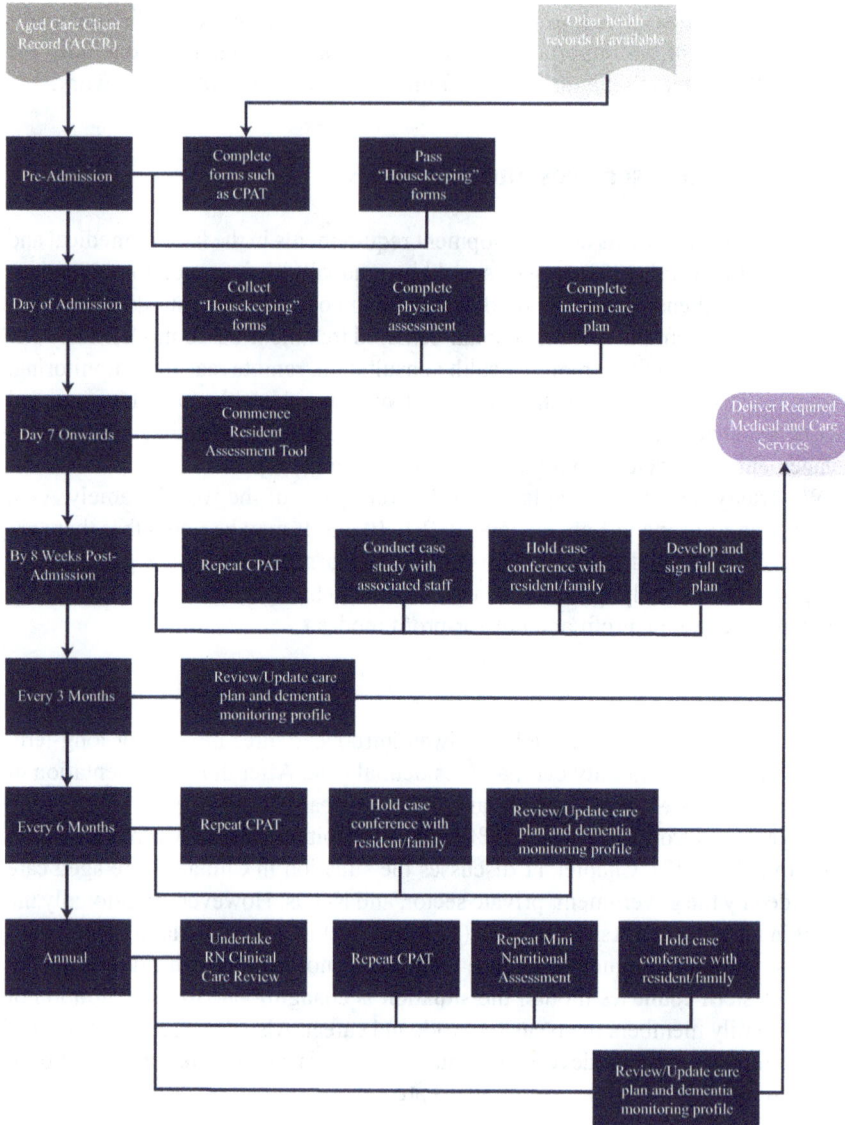

*Figure 10.2   Aged care processes for admission, assessment, and care planning
[1]. Sources: Asia Pacific Ubiquitous Healthcare Research Centre,
UNSW—Australia, Presentation on Smart Services CRC Foundry
Project Presentation "Aged Care Collaborative Platform," March
2013.*

for-profit businesses, etc.), the government plays a very major role by funding
the care of the vulnerable (e.g., less affluent elderly). Figure 10.2 shows the typi-
cal service processes in residential care in Australia. They involve some essential

compliance requirements of the government agencies Care Planning Assessment Tool (CPAT) to decide on the eligibility and reimbursement levels of aged care clients in Australia. Figure 10.2 shows some major business processes at a residential care facility at different stages of residential care, such as pre-admission, admission day, day 7 onwards, every 3 months, every 6 months, and annually. Each of these processes can then be expanded and implemented through digital methods and tools on aged care platforms [1]. Although some of these processes (e.g., day of admission, day 7 onwards) are not required for home-based care, there are similar processes for others (e.g., pre-admission including CPAT, and monitoring on regular basis, such as quarterly and annually).

10.2.3   Europe

Many European countries implement the welfare state principle in a big way and hence aged care is a major responsibility of the governments as in Australia and other western countries. More detailed scenarios of aged care in European countries are discussed in Chapters 12 and 13. A study in the Netherlands identified four different types of home-based care networks among community-dwelling older adults: 19% the partner network (care was mainly provided by partners, with little care from private caregivers or professionals), 25% the mixed network (care was provided by a combination of children, professionals, and/or other family members), 15% the privately paid network (privately paid care was provided), and 40% the professional network [5].

In another research undertaken by Hägglund *et al.* [6], a 3-year project "OLD@ HOME" [7] was used to analyze the scenarios in home care. Three groups of healthcare service providers were identified: (1) general practitioners, (2) district nurses, and (3) home help service personnel. General practitioners "prepare a house call, examine and diagnose, consult other healthcare professionals ... prescribe or change medication, plan follow-up visit, refer to other clinics ..." District nurses conduct all the activities that general practitioners do and also delegate tasks to home help service personnel, who "... handle medication perform healthcare tasks (delegated by DN), receive and handle alarms, consult the DN ..."

Toivanen *et al.* [7] used an "activity-theoretical approach" to explain the requirements gathering in the problem domain of home care for information system analysis. They used the "activity analysis and development" framework to find the actors involved in the domain: "registered and auxiliary nurses, physicians, medical, nursing and system administrators, home helpers, physiotherapists, home help coordinators, social workers, various actors in the NGOs and, naturally, the customers themselves." And some functions or services of home care were identified: "planning visit," "domestic aid," "home health care," "transport services," "meal services," "on-call help services," "physical rehabilitation," "social security guidance," etc.

In addition, a study on user requirements for home care system [8] identified several stakeholders in the "network of home care." These stakeholders were categorized into (1) "the cared": people who receive care at home; (2) "carers": spouse

Table 10.1   Service providers

Professional service provider	Secondary service provider	Service organizer
General practitioners	Social workers	Care coordinators
Hospitals	Dietitians	
Nurses	Hairdressers	
Pharmacists	Cleaners	
Physiotherapists	Logistics	
Specialists		
Home helpers (caregiver)		

or family member; (3) visitors: social workers, community nurses, paramedics, and general practitioners; (4) remote users: general practitioners; (5) technology providers; (6) institutional stakeholders; and (7) other stakeholders: family who live elsewhere, neighbors.

Based on the research mentioned above, major health-care service providers are general practitioners, specialists, pharmacists, nurses, physiotherapists, home helpers, social workers, dietitians, hairdressers, cleaners, and logistics service providers.

As shown in Table 10.1, different types of service providers are categorized into three categories: professional service provider, secondary service provider, and service provider. However, this chapter only focuses on the professional service providers who are involved in the medication use process, namely general practitioners, pharmacists, third-party logistics, and the care coordinator. The service organizer or care coordinator acts as an administrator, or a service hub, of all the service providers, and interfaces with the subject of care. The care coordinator usually belongs to an aged care facility, e.g., a nursing home.

10.3   Service workflows

Service integration for the coordinated care could be approached from three levels: (1) system/sector-based service integration from a macro level, focusing on integrating services provided by different organizations, (2) agency-based service integration, focusing on integrating services provided by one agency, and (3) client/family-based service coordination, focusing on assisting the subject of care to obtain services provided by different service providers [4]. This chapter approaches the analysis from a macro level, describing the business processes/workflows for the cooperation of different aged care service providers. Nevertheless, one party has to become the integrator of different aged care service providers and administrate the delivery of services, therefore becoming the focal unit of aged care.

There are many services provided by aged care service providers, making the complexity quite high. To simplify the analysis, the scope in this chapter is limited to the medication use process which includes the "drug request and delivery process," and the "medication adherence-monitoring process."

The process of medication management includes a number of elements, thereby necessitating a collaboration across supply chains involving multiple countries, as highlighted during the vaccine management of COVID-19. Here are the elements with the names of primary organizations and countries:

1. drug raw materials development and processing (e.g., China)
2. transfer of drug raw materials for mass production by the pharmaceuticals to many countries (e.g., India, Australia, Europe, USA)
3. manufacture of the drugs/vaccines in many countries (including India, Australia, Europe)
4. transfer of drugs across countries to the recipient population, sometimes needing extreme environmental control (e.g., Pfizer BioN Tech vaccine storage at −70°C)
5. administration of the drugs/vaccines by individual pharmacies, care providers, and homes (as evidenced in the massive operation of COVID-19 vaccination in individual countries with priority for the elderly)
6. monitoring and management of drug/vaccine reactions among individuals (through local general practitioners, pharmacies, and hospitals).

The above supply chain operation provides some idea about the complexity of the tasks and hence risks involved that need to be mitigated using robust processes of medication management. However, Sections 10.3.1–10.3.4 of this chapter focus mainly on points 5 and 6 mentioned above to address the issues of home-based care, though the entire process is quite fascinating and the literature is also evolving both in academic and popular media.

10.3.1 Drug request and delivery process

From the order fulfillment perspective, the drug-ordering process could be considered as a multi-agent system, where coordination is needed. Information sharing, by reducing uncertainty and facilitating coordination, can improve the performance. In a process model of medication management focused on outpatient prescribing [9], five major activities are identified: "Prescribe," "Transmit," "Dispense," "Administrator," and "Monitor." And four major actors are directly involved in the process: patient, general practitioner (prescribing clinician), pharmacist, and information systems (e-prescribing system, paper-based, or electronic medical record, etc.). Both the General Practitioner (GP) and pharmacist need to have access to certain information, such as drug information, patient information, and drug restrictions, which could be provided by Electronic Health Record and other health information systems. "Problematic prescriptions may require a call to the clinician; as a result, prescriptions may be changed or cancelled rather than being dispensed." In home-based aged care, one needs to consider the delivery of drugs, drug reminders and the monitoring of dispensing, using evolving medication-dispensing devices.

The Australian Digital Health Agency [10] released several documentations of the Electronic Transfer of Prescription. These documentations, from the perspective of Information Technology (IT) solution, covered the concept of operations, business requirements, detailed requirements, and other aspects of the "prescribing-dispensing process" (PDP). Electronic Transfer of Prescription (ETP) from National E-Health Transition Authority (NEHTA)-Australia proposed three processes: the "electronic prescribing and dispensing" process, the "facility-managed supply" process, and the "dispensing on prescriber's instruction" process, which is also known as the "script owing" scenario. These three processes involve different participants and different protocols of medication management. Based on the ETP described above, this chapter integrates the three processes mentioned above and suggests a "drug request and delivery" process. And some adjustments have been made to make it fit the scenario of home-based aged care.

10.3.2   Participants

The drug request and delivery process (Figure 10.3) involves four actors or participants: (1) the aged care facility, to which the subject of care has given consent to obtain medication on his or her behalf [10], acting as a home care coordinator; (2) the general practitioner, who acts as a prescriber; (3) the pharmacy, which is the dispenser of medication, and (4) the third-party logistics provider, who performs the logistics functions of the process.

10.3.3   Scenarios

The drug request and delivery process could start in three scenarios: (1) GP starts the process by creating a prescription. The consultation with the subject of care occurs prior to this stage of this process [10]. (2) Aged care facility requests drug with prescription that has remaining dispenses. (3) Aged care facility requests drug without prescription. The drug would be dispensed on the prescriber's instruction.

10.3.4   Sub-processes

The drug request and delivery process consists of two sub-processes: (1) PDP [10] and (2) the logistics process. The aged care facility coordinates all the parties involved and connects the two sub-processes.

The PDP involves activities including drug requesting in one of the three scenarios mentioned above, prescription issuing, medication dispensing, medication supplying, etc. (1) If the general practitioner initiates the process by creating and issuing prescription, the prescription will be electronically sent to the aged care facility, which will then confirm consent given by the subject of care and send the prescription to pharmacy. The pharmacist will perform the dispensing task and notice the aged care facility that the dispensing has been finished. After that, the aged care facility will request the third-party logistics provider to pick up the drugs from a certain pharmacy and deliver them to the home of the subject of care. After the delivery is completed, the third-party logistics provider will inform the aged care facility, which will then confirm details with the subject of care and record

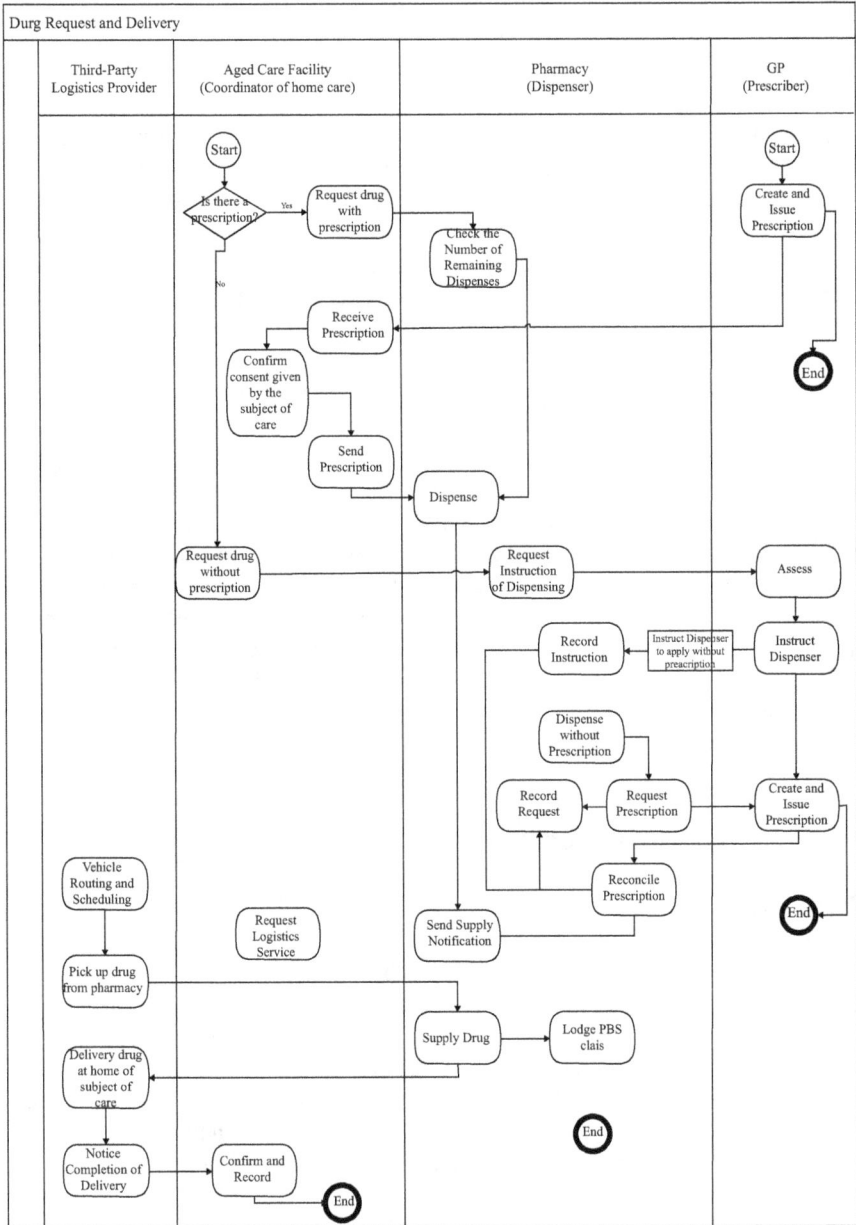

Figure 10.3   The business process of medication request and delivery

the delivery. (2) If the aged care facility, on behalf of the subject of care, requests medication from the pharmacy with the provision of prescription, the pharmacy will check the number of remaining dispenses of the prescription. If there are still dispenses left, the pharmacist will dispense the drug and record the related informa-tion. (3) A more complex situation is that the aged care facility, on behalf of the subject of care, requests drug from the pharmacy without providing the prescription. If that happens, the pharmacist will ask the general practitioner for instruction on which the pharmacist can dispense drugs. After receiving the request for instruction, the general practitioner will assess whether or not an instruction can be created. If the assessment is passed, the general practitioner will instruct the pharmacist to dispense the drug without prescription. The pharmacist will then record the instruc-tion and dispense medication. After that, the pharmacist will request the prescription from the general practitioner. Next, the general practitioner will create and issue prescription to the pharmacist, who will reconcile prescription and notice the aged care facility to request for logistics services.

The logistics activities in the process are performed by third-party logistics pro-viders. The major logistics activity in the drug-ordering process is picking up the drugs from the pharmacies and delivering them to care receivers' homes. Picking and delivery practices have already been used in health-care industry. In a case study of Metrohealth Medical Center, a similar operation was introduced: patients could be picked up by vehicles and sent to the medical center and then returned to their homes [11]. Efficient vehicle routing and scheduling are required for such opera-tions. Therefore, the detailed location information of the pharmacies and care homes should be available for the third-party logistics providers. And the pharmacies and the subjects of care should be informed of the pick-up and delivery time, requiring that (1) the third-party logistics providers are capable of scheduling efficiently and (2) information is shared effectively.

10.4   Supply chain model: Jidoka

The Japanese automobile manufacturer Toyota is well known for its Toyota produc-tion system. One of its guiding principles is called Jidoka, which can be loosely translated as "automation with a human touch," which means "as when a problem occurs, the equipment stops immediately, preventing defective products from being produced" [12]. This mechanism aims at detecting quality problems at sources. Activities involved in Jidoka are "detecting the problem," "stopping the process," "restoring the process to proper function," "investigating the root cause of the prob-lem," and "installing countermeasures." And these practices have been applied in the health-care sector [13]. The same practice could be used in aged care as well, especially in drug request and delivery.

Quality problems in the drug request and delivery process could cause medical errors. A project [14] aimed at reducing medical errors using lean six sigma princi-ples identified several sources of medical error: (1) "additional instructions" that are not recorded by the pharmacy; (2) "wrong dose"; (3) "wrong drug"; (4) "duplicate order entry"; (5) different frequency on the "Medication Administration Record" and the "medication order"; (6) omissions; (7) "discontinuation order not carried out when received"; (8) "order not received"; (9) "medication order" recorded on the "wrong patient"; and (10) "route." All these sources of medication error should be detected by a mechanism built in the drug request and delivery process. The proposal of this chapter is to implement "Jidoka" for aged care, illustrating with the example of Medication Management.

Information inaccuracy and inconsistency are defined as "defects." All the parties involved in the process should make efforts in finding defects all the time. When a defect is detected in any steps of the process, the participant in that process should report this information immediately. Once a defect is reported, the whole drug request and delivery process involving specific patient and drug should be stopped. The error should then be corrected and the process should be restored, followed by the investigation of the root cause of the defect. Finally, specific countermeasures should be institutionalized to improve the quality of the process.

Shared knowledge based on an information platform thus becomes critical to the detection of defects that could cause medication errors. Mechanism of reporting could be implemented through the functions of IT system that facilitates the drug request and delivery process, based on mobile and web technology. A dedicated group of professionals should be formed by the aged care facility, being responsible for communicating with different parties to investigate quality problems.

10.4.1   Medication adherence as a supply chain management problem

Medication non-adherence is recognized as one of the most important and costly worldwide health-care problems in the twenty-first century. The literature on the prevalence of non-adherence is challenging in that estimates vary widely by country, the methodologies employed, and the criteria used to define low adherence [15]. Reasons for non-compliance include "forgetfulness," "side effects," "difficulty in keeping medication to hand," "difficulty in storing medication," "complex treatment regimen," "cost of the drug," "patient sees no benefit from treatment," "patient decides to try non-prescription alternatives," "patient does not understand the need for medication," "patient struggles with self-administration," "long-term treatment 'fatigue'," and "short-term benefit" [16].

"It is proposed that improvements to the medication use system will improve medication adherence and, by so doing, will also improve patient health outcomes" [17].

10.4.2   Measuring quality using RFID

RFID is a technology used for the identification of objects and information transfer from a distance through radio waves. Object identification standards enable tracking an object in the global range [18]. RFID technology has been developed for inpatient medication use, which consists of two processes: (1) "the inpatient and pharmacy process" and (2) "the inpatient medication administering process" [19]. These two processes correlate to the "drug request and delivery process" and the "medication adherence-monitoring process," respectively, in the scenario of home-based aged care. This section focuses on the "medication adherence-monitoring process" and examines how information exchange happens when the elderly take medicine using RFID-based medication adherence-monitoring system.

In medication administration, the "five rights" guidance has been widely used, which includes "the right patient, the right drug, the right dose, the right route, and the right time" [20]. The "five rights" could also be used as a framework to guide the information exchange in such RFID-based medication adherence-monitoring system.

Several existing medication monitoring-related solutions are as follows:

Community pharmacists performing Continuous Medication Monitoring (CoMM) systematically monitor each new prescription and refill dispensed for medication-related problems. CoMM complements medication management performed by pharmacists, as well as claims-based reviews performed by health plans, and positions pharmacists to monitor the safety and effectiveness of medication therapy [21].

ePrescription potentially represents the digitization of both prescribing and dispensing. ePrescribing solutions can also support medication reconciliation, remote monitoring of adherence through refill tracking, and issuing of automatic refill alerts [22].

The Medication Event-Monitoring System (MEMS V TrackCap, AARDEX Ltd., Zug, Switzerland) is one popular electronic monitoring of adherence solution (http://www.aardexgroup.com), which "has been reported on in >250 peer-reviewed publications" [17].

Having discussed the supply chain perspective of medication management, we now discuss in Section 10.5 the tools perspective, which is important to avoid human errors (that could be fatal) in medication administration at homes of the elderly.

10.5   Tools for medication adherence monitoring

There are now several automated pill dispensers to monitor medication adherence and comparison is available at [23]. Some of them work as follows. The pill bottle is attached to an RFID tag, which was associated with prescription information. The prescription was filled by pharmacists and stored in an XML database. Prescription information included the time to take medicine, special warning, prescription duration, and customized alert. The "stand" consisted of an RFID reader, network connection, and other reminder-related parts. The RFID reader was used to read the RFID tags. Through the network connection to the XML database, queries could be run. Patients only had to (1) place the bottle in the stand and (2) remove the bottle from the stand. "When a pill bottle is removed from the stand, it assumes that the person is taking their pills." In addition, a medication monitor could be located in a relative's home to monitor the medicine-taking behavior of the patient.

Another solution using RFID was introduced by McCall *et al.* [24]. The RFID-based Medication Adherence Intelligence System had five components: RFID reader, scale, microcontroller, LCD panel, and rotation platform. Pill bottles were

Table 10.2   Access to information enabled by RFID for medication management

Information	Access to information
Patient	RFID tags that identify unique patient and are distributed to the subject of care for long-term use, along with the medication adherence-monitoring system/device
Drug	RFID tags that identify prescription information, which is stored in the central database, where pharmacists, GP, or other aged care service providers could run query to monitor patient compliance
Dose	Sensor components of the medication adherence-monitoring system/device
Time	Timer
Behavior	Behavior/action sensor components

attached by RFID tags that identified the "medicine name," schedule," "dosage," and "specific instruction." Pill bottles were placed on the rotation platform and weighed by the scale. Thus the dosage taken by the patient could be measured and compared with the regimen. The RFID tag "does not require any other alteration in the current manufacturing and pharmacy operating procedures. Just like a regular printed label on a medicine bottle."

Typically, such medication adherence-monitoring system using RFID technology involves two sub-processes: the prescription regimen reading sub-process and the medication use-monitoring sub-process. In the first sub-process, prescription information is stored in a remote information repository, which could be reached through network connections. Specific information is identified by RFID tag. An RFID reader, by scanning the tags, captures a unique identifier to run the query in the central database. In the second sub-process, a sensor system monitors patients' behaviors. The behaviors to be sensed could be opening and closing the lid, placing the pill bottle on certain places, or how much dosage has been taken out of the pill bottle, etc. But the ultimate purpose of monitoring all kinds of behaviors is to ensure patient compliance. However, assumptions always have to be made that if expected behaviors of the subject of care are detected the medication is considered to have been taken.

Based on the research of existing solutions and the "five rights" guideline mentioned above, the proposed RFID-based medication adherence-monitoring framework (Table 10.2) includes the exchange of five types of information (1) patient information, which could be stored in Electronic Health Record system or any other types of patient database; (2) medication information, which is consistent with the information mentioned in the drug request and delivery process; (3) dose information, which could be captured by some sensor system, e.g., weight sensor; (4) the time when medication is taken, which is available from a timer; and (5) behavior information, which could be detected by some sensor system in order to ensure the behavior of taking medicine has indeed happened. The first four types of information correspond to the "the right patient," "the right drug," "the right dose," and "the right time" in the "five rights" guidance, respectively. "The right route" could not yet be ensured by the framework. However, it could be assumed that the medicine in this scenario is all pills taken by mouth, not involving other methods such as injection.

An "RFID tagging system" has been proposed that used the RFID tags "simply as a means to uniquely identify the patient, before retrieving the data from a centralized server," instead of storing patient information on the tag. The same solution is applied to the framework proposed in this chapter for not only patient tags but tags attached to the drug (pill bottle). "Various techniques are available to read them all sequentially. These techniques, grouped under the name of 'singulation', identify tags by allowing only the tags with specific serial numbers to respond" [25].

Information not only flows from the patient side to the aged care service provider side but also flows vice versa. When it is time for a certain patient to take medicine, the system should be able to send patient information, drug information, and dose information to the patient or his/her family through the medication adherence-monitoring system/device, providing the function of reminder.

10.6   Discussion

This section discusses the role of digital methods and tools for improving aged care from a workflow and process perspective. As discussed in Sections 10.4 and 10.5, we have focused on the context of medication management from a supply chain management viewpoint. Figure 10.4 presents medication management from a client's perspective, and Figure 10.5 presents from supply chain process' (Jidoka) perspective. As discussed in Sections 10.4 and 10.5, the digital tools (automatic pill dispensers) based on RFID technologies play an important role in achieving the five rights of medication discussed in Section 10.4.2.

It may be noted that the discussion covers both residential and home-based care processes of the elderly. We have explained the four major aspects of digital

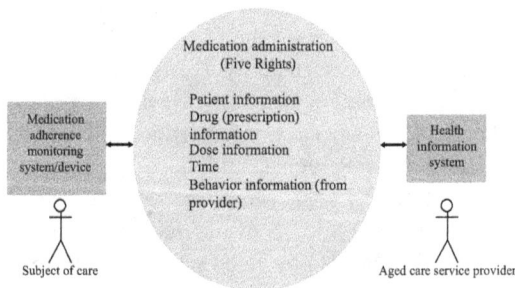

Figure 10.4   Client's perspective of medication management

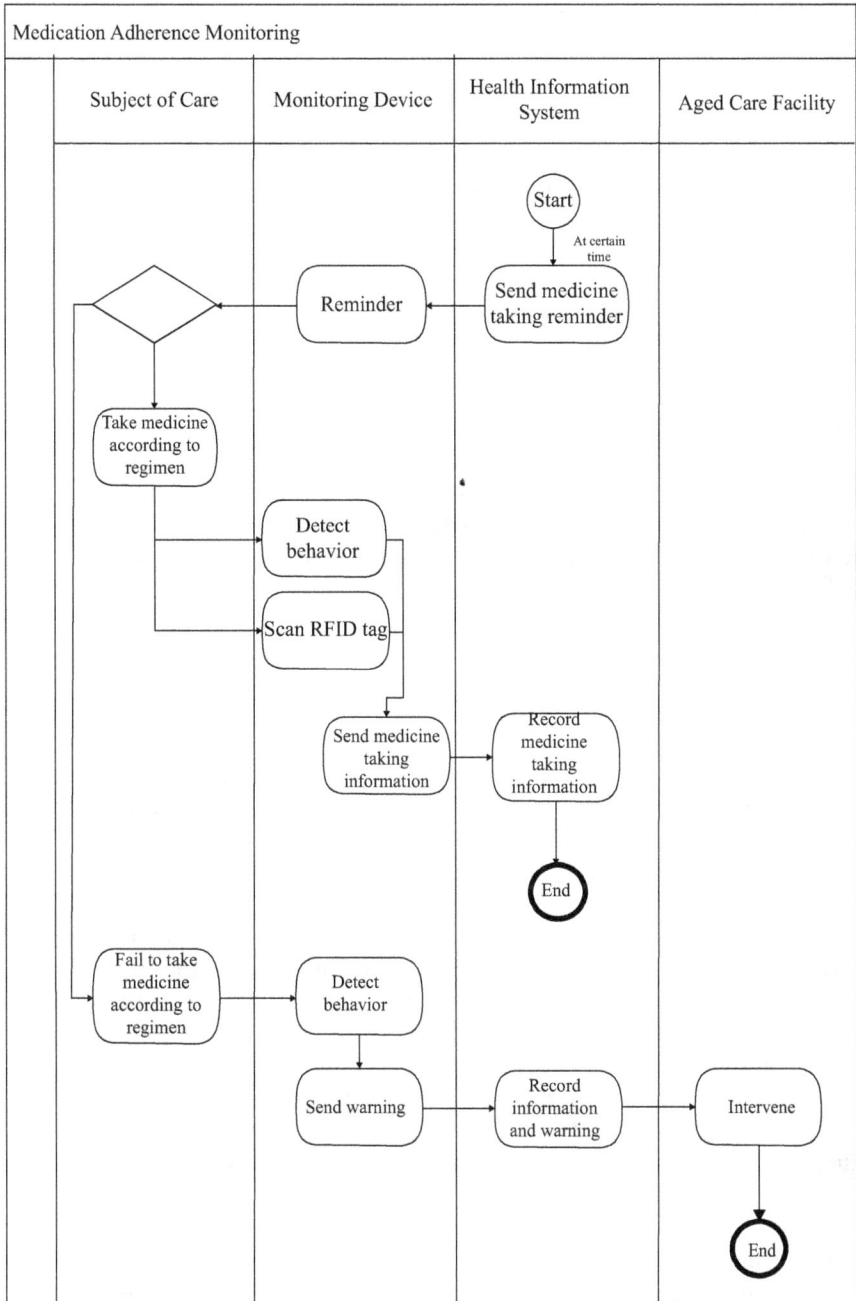

Figure 10.5   Supply chain management's perspective of medication management

methods (processes) and tools (including technology) for healthy aging from the perspective of aged care:

- services and providers
- service workflows and processes
- case study of medication management for aged care from the perspective of

  - supply chain processes
  - tools and technologies (pill dispenser using RFID).

The flowchart in Figure 10.5 shows the workflow of RFID-based medication adherence-monitoring system.

It may be noted that this chapter has focused on the service management of medications in the context of home-based care. However, similar methodology can be used to describe other service management scenarios in both residential and home-based care. Also home-based care processes overlap with telehealth, eHealth, and mHealth described in [26].

10.7   Conclusion and future work

This chapter has provided an overview of the principles of digital methods and tools for enabling aged care services, as explained in the context of medication management (important aspect of aged care) from the perspective of supply chain management. The discussion has been organized at three major levels: service level, process level, and technology/tools level. The same methodology is applicable for other types of aged care services, such as admission, assessment, and care planning shown in Figure 10.2 in the Section 10.2 "Aged Care Services and Providers". We have omitted details of any other processes in this chapter for brevity. More details are available in Ref. [1] and other literature. Also we have not been able to discuss the complexities of business and legal processes of multi-party collaboration shown in Figure 10.1. Interested readers may look up our work as part of the European Union project AU2EU (see [27]). The adoption of digital methods and tools for health care has grown substantially during COVID-19 due to a large number of deaths of the elderly worldwide and the ability of digital methods and tools to reduce infection between patients and care professionals (due to remote operation). Hence we believe digital health has a bright future in the field of aged care and health care. Chapters 11–16 of this book discuss the growing use of digital technologies, such as Internet of Things (IOT), mobile apps, and other robots for healthy aging. This topic has many facets as described in the book [28].

References

[1]   Asia Pacific ubiquitous Healthcare Research Centre. *Presentation on Smart Services CRC Foundry Project Presentation Aged Care Collaborative Platform*. Australia: UNSW; 2013.

[2]   Wang P., Ding Z., Jiang C., Zhou M. 'Design and implementation of a web-service-based public-oriented personalized health care platform'. *IEEE Transactions on Systems, Man, and Cybernetics: Systems*. 2013, vol. 43(4), pp. 941–57.

[3]   Hsu M.-H., Chu T.-B., Yen J.-C., *et al.* 'Development and implementation of a national telehealth project for long-term care: a preliminary study'. *Computer Methods and Programs in Biomedicine*. 2010, vol. 97(3), pp. 286–92.

[4]   Dyer S.M., van den Berg M.E.L., Barnett K., *et al. Review of Innovative Models of Aged Care*. Adelaide, Australia: Flinders University; 2019.

[5]   Bijnsdorp F.M., Pasman H.R.W., Francke A.L., Evans N., Peeters C.F.W., Broese van Groenou M.I. 'Who provides care in the last year of life? A description of care networks of community-dwelling older adults in the Netherlands'. *BMC Palliative Care*. 2019, vol. 18(1), p. 41.

[6]   Hägglund M., Scandurra I., Koch S. 'Scenarios to capture work processes in shared homecare – from analysis to application'. *International Journal of Medical Informatics*. 2010, vol. 79(6), pp. e126–34.

[7]   Toivanen M., Hakkinen H., Eerola A., Korpela M., Mursu A. *Gathering, Structuring and Describing Information Needs in Home Care: A Method for Requirements Exploration in a 'Gray Area'." MEDINFO 2004, Fieschi et al.* Amsterdam: IOS Press; 2004. pp. 1398–402.

[8]   McGee-Lennon M.R., Gray P.D. 'Including stakeholders in the design of homecare systems: identification and categorization of complex user requirements'. INCLUDE Conference; 2007.

[9]   Bell D.S., Cretin S., Marken R.S., Landman A.B. 'A conceptual framework for evaluating outpatient electronic prescribing systems based on their functional capabilities'. *Journal of the American Medical Informatics Association*. 2004, vol. 11(1), pp. 60–70.

[10] The Australian Digital Health Agency. *Electronic prescriptions [online]*. Available from https://www.digitalhealth.gov.au/initiatives-and-programs/electronic-prescriptions [Accessed Feb 2021].

[11] Miller T., Matthew J. *Liberatore, Logistics Management: An Analytics-Based Approach*. Business Expert Press; 2020.

[12] Toyota Production System. *Company information vision & philosophy, toyota [online]*. 2020. Available from https://global.toyota/en/company/vision-and-philosophy/production-system/ [Accessed 07 Dec 2020].

[13] Grout J.R., Toussaint J.S. 'Mistake-proofing healthcare: why stopping processes may be a good start'. *Business Horizons*. 2010, vol. 53(2), pp. 149–56.

[14] Esimai G. 'Lean six sigma reduces medication errors'. *Quality Progress*. 2005, vol. 38(4), pp. 51–7.

[15]   Feehan M., Morrison M.A., Tak C., Morisky D.E., DeAngelis M.M., Munger M.A. 'Factors predicting self-reported medication low adherence in a large sample of adults in the US general population: a cross-sectional study'. *BMJ Open*. 2017, vol. 7(6), p. e014435.

[16]   Fagan T., Crowley A., Jayasinghe S., Allt-Graham J., Brown L. *Australian Health Services Supply Chain, GRA Supply Chain [online]*. Available from https://www.gra.net.au/uploads/resource/167-GRA-Aged-Care-Supply-Chain.pdf [Accessed Feb 2021].

[17]   Murray M.D., Morrow D.G., Weiner M., *et al*. 'A conceptual framework to study medication adherence in older adults'. *The American Journal of Geriatric Pharmacotherapy*. 2004, vol. 2(1), pp. 36–43.

[18]   Fescioglu-Unver N., Choi S.H., Sheen D., Kumara S., *et al*. 'RFID in production and service systems: technology, applications and issues'. *Information Systems Frontiers*. 2015, vol. 17(6), pp. 1369–80.

[19]   Lai C.L., Chien S.W., Chang L.H., Chen S.C., Fang K. 'Enhancing medication safety and healthcare for inpatients using RFID'. Management of Engineering and Technology, Portland International Center, 5-9 Aug 2007; 2007. pp. 2783–90.

[20]   Delaune S.C., Ladner P.K. *Fundamentals of Nursing: Standards and Practice*. New York: Delmar; 1998.

[21]   Goedken A.M., Huang S., McDonough R.P., Deninger M.J., Doucette W.R. 'Medication-related problems identified through continuous medication monitoring'. *Pharmacy*. 2018, vol. 6(3), p. 86.

[22]   Car J., Tan W.S., Huang Z., Sloot P., Franklin B.D. 'eHealth in the future of medications management: personalisation, monitoring and adherence'. *BMC Medicine*. 2017, vol. 15(1),73.

[23]   Medipense. *A comparison of IoT-connected, automated pill dispensers [online]*. Available from https://medipense.medium.com/2017-the-year-of-the-iot-automated-pill-dispenser-ca1d41f0592b [Accessed Feb 2021].

[24]   McCall C., Maynes B., Zou C.C., Zhang N.J. 'RMAIS: RFID-based medication adherence intelligence system'. Engineering in Medicine and Biology Society (EMBC), 2010 Annual International Conference of the IEEE; 2010. pp. 3768–71.

[25]   Asif Z., Mandviwalla M. 'Integrating the supply chain with RFID: a technical and business analysis'. *Communications of the Association for Information Systems*. 2005, vol. 15(1), p. 24.

[26]   Motamarri S., Akter S., Ray P.K. 'The status of healthcare service delivery systems: comparison, mobile health, and healthcare service design, Chapter 20' in Ray P.K., Nakashima N., Ahmed A., Ro S.-C., Soshino Y. (eds.). *Mobile Technologies for Delivering Healthcare in Remote, Rural or Developing Regions, IET Book Series on Health Technologies*. UK: IET Press; 2020. pp. 323–234.

[27]   Ghorai K., Smits J.M., Kluitman M., Ray P.K. 'Business and legal framework for the exchange of mHealth data for aged care across countries, Chapter 22' in Ray P.K., Nakashima N., Ahmed A., Ro S.-C., Soshino Y. (eds.). *Mobile*

Technologies for Delivering Healthcare in Remote, Rural or Developing Regions, IET Book Series on Health Technologies. UK: IET Press; 2020. pp. 357–80.

[28]   Ray P.K., Nakashima N., Ahmed A., Ro S.-C., Soshino Y. (eds.). *Mobile Technologies for Delivering Healthcare in Remote, Rural or Developing Regions, IET Book Series on Health Technologies.* UK: IET Press; 2020.

Chapter 11

Role of digital technology in aged care in China

Zhiyu Hao[1], Chao Xu[2], Lina Li[2], and Pradeep K Ray[1,3]

11.1 Introduction

Chinese society is ageing fast 'as the elderly population outnumbers the newborn' [1]. This process of population ageing was partly caused by the one-child policy that was issued in 1980 [2]. Although the universal two-child policy was implemented in 2015, the ageing trend cannot be changed significantly [3]. People aged older than 60 in China has reached a number of 250 million and the growth every year is approximately 20–30 million in the following 20 years [1]. According to a report by World Bank, people older than the age of 65 will represent 26% of China's population, and those aged 80 and older are expected to represent 5% by 2050 [4].

The 'State Plan for Active Response to Population Ageing' issued by the State Council defined technological innovation as the first power and strategic support of a positive response to the ageing of population [5]. There is an increasing number of elderly people who live alone in China (Table 11.1).

The new model of support for the aged thus emphasizes the role of digital technology in aged care in China. Because of the intensified mismatch between demand and supply currently at play, a variety of services and products of digital technology in aged care is expected to surge.

The development of science and technology in China is very rapid. Currently, China has well established mobile communication and Internet service. The network construction was promoted by 'the rapid development of e-commerce' in China (Table 11.2) [8].

The high penetration rate of mobile devices and communication networks showcase the rapid development of technology in China. The advancing technology provides an excellent foundation for Mobile Health (mHealth) development, which aids in aged care in China. mHealth refers to the use of information and communication technology to deliver medical service and information [9]. Therefore, the application of digital technology in aged care is very important and helpful.

[1]University of Michigan Joint Institute, Shanghai Jiao Tong University, China
[2]Shanghai Haiyang Internet Elderly Services Co. LTD, China
[3]School of Population Health, University of New South Wales, Australia

Table 11.1   Increasing number of elderly people who live alone in China

Resource	Details
Sixth National Demographic Census	The number of aged Chinese citizens living alone 'has risen 40% from 1990 to 2010' [1].
China Family Development Report in 2015	Elderly people living alone account for nearly 10% of the total, and those living with only spouses account for 41.9% [6].
iiMedia Research	By 2020, there will be 30 million aged people living alone [7].

By the end of 2018, mobile phones were used by 98.6% of Internet users accessed it in China. 'The Internet penetration rate in China was 57.7%' [10]. However, by December 2017, Internet users aged 60 and older accounted for 5.2% of all Internet users and only 16.7% of the total population of the elderly [7]. Therefore, although some researches show that the new Chinese seniors are embracing digital development [1], learning to use it is still challenging for many of the elderly.

Compared with other age groups, the elderly are more interested in the Internet for health reasons such as searching for health information [11]. Social participation is an important reflector of their quality of life [10]. Better aged care involves a better quality of life. It is thus essential for aged care to have the digital technology that provides social participation to the elderly.

This chapter presents the role of digital technology in aged care in China. It starts with a background and necessity of aged care in China in Section 11.1, followed by explaining the methodology of literature review in Section 11.2. This is followed by the demonstration of the market potential in healthy ageing, the existing digital technologies in aged care in China and their development prospect in Section 11.3. The case study of Haiyang Group is then presented in Section 11.4. The chapter ends with a discussion of our case study research in Section 11.5, a statement of study limitations in Section 11.6 and conclusions in Section 11.7.

Table 11.2   Network development summary in China

Time	Details
2016	'The 4G broadband penetration rate has reached 80% and mobile broadband has entered the era of 4G' [8].
Present	More and more areas in China are moving into the 5G era. Most of the stations, airports and shopping malls provide free Wi-Fi in China [8].

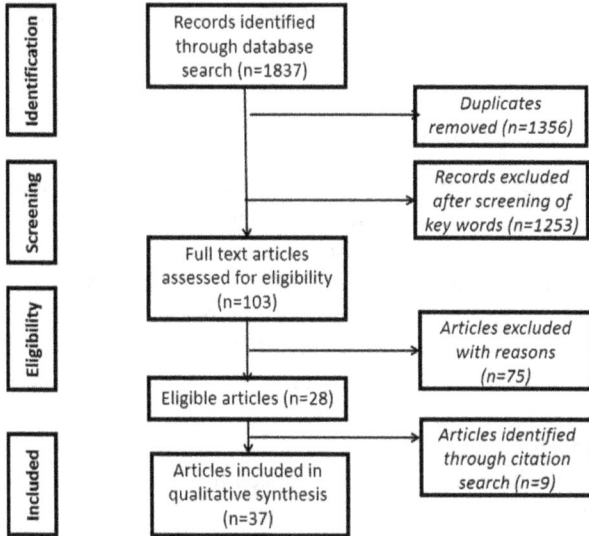

Figure 11.1   Literature search methodology summary

11.2   Methodology

This systematic review complied with the Preferred Reporting Items for Systematic Reviews and Meta-Analyses (PRISMA) statement and guidelines [12]. The methodology is summarized in Figure 11.1.

11.2.1   *Identification of resources and search strategy*

For this study, we selected articles from three sources: electronic databases, citation searches of selected articles and official government policy website. A total of nine databases (CNKI, NCBI, ScienceDirect, BMC, SpringerLink, Hitachi Review, SAGE, Hindawi and IEEE Xplorer) were selected as being the most frequently used in our research community, providing access to research with an in-depth understanding of the digital technology in aged care in China, defined as a large number of citation retrieved from those databases. In order to conduct an extensive and comprehensive search of the literature, we selected the following keywords closely related to digital technology in aged care in China: 'digital technology', 'aged care', 'healthcare', 'elderly', 'China', 'mHealth', 'mobile health', 'smart-phone based', 'digital product' and 'digital platform'. The search was carried out by using the identified keywords above in combination with Boolean connectors ('OR', 'AND').

In the meantime, three official government policy websites (Central People's Government of the People's Republic of China, Department of Ageing Health and China National Committee on Ageing) were selected to find out the plans and promotion policies of the government and industry. At the end of this process, a total of 1 837 articles were retrieved, and 1 356 articles were selected after removing 481 duplicate articles (as shown in Figure 11.1).

11.2.2   Selection of relevant articles

When searching in the database, we only consider articles written in English. When searching for government policies and plans, we also accept Chinese documents. Articles were selected by scanning for keywords in the titles, abstracts and list of keywords. At the end of this process, 103 articles were included for further review. Next, the full text of articles was independently browsed by Zhiyu Hao for their relevance to the aims of the study, that is, 28 articles were included as they discussed the issues related to digital technology in aged care in China. The reference lists of these 28 selected articles were used to locate other relevant articles, which may not have been identified in the initial database search. A total of 37 articles were selected for review, including 6 articles selected from the citation search (as shown in Figure 11.1).

11.2.3   Data extraction and analysis

Zhiyu Hao worked to extract the following information from the 37 papers included in the systematic review: (1) aims and objectives of the study; (2) types of digital technology used in aged care in China; (3) chosen study methodologies and (4) any challenges associated with the adoption of digital technology among the elderly in China. Those extracted data were entered into spreadsheets. Identified issues and results were clustered and labelled on the basis of their similarities. The clusters were labelled and reviewed again for consistency. These reassessment and relabelling steps were repeated until consensus was reached on cluster labels. According to similarities, identified issues were grouped into four categories reflecting the following perspectives: (1) government policies; (2) market for technology in aged care; (3) existing technology in aged care in China and (4) challenges and prospects.

11.3   Results

11.3.1   Plans and promotions of the government and the industry

11.3.1.1   Promotions of development of elderly care services

Various policy documents were promulgated in China these years to promote the development of elderly care services. Table 11.3 presents some of the policies released from 2019.

These plans help significantly to improve the environment for elderly care services and promote the industry.

Table 11.3   Policies to promote elderly care services

Time	Issuing organization	Policy
2019	General Office of the State Council of China	'Suggestions on promoting the development of elderly care services', which indicated the problems such as unbalanced development, insufficient effective supply and low quality of services [13]. It aimed at the establishment of a long-term care service system for the elderly, the improvement of the quality of elderly care services and the effective meeting of diversified elderly care needs on the basis of guaranteeing everyone's access to basic elderly care services by 2022 [13].
2019	Ministry of Civil Affairs	'Suggestions on further expanding the supply of elderly care services and promoting the Consumption of elderly care services' [14].
November 2020	Ministry of Civil Affairs	'Measures for the Management of Pension Institutions' [15].
May 2020	Xinjiang Uygur Autonomous Region	'Measures for the Construction of the Health Service System for the Elderly in the Autonomous Region' [16].

11.3.1.2   Solving the difficulty of using intelligent technology for the elderly

The government released several policies to help the elderly overcome the difficulty of using intelligent technology. Table 11.4 shows some of the recent policies.

The policy documents help popularize information technology accessibility and ease the anxiety of older people about new technologies, thus solving the difficulty of using intelligent technology for the elderly. Removing the barriers to consumption by the elderly in the digital world will help unlock the potential of consumption and greatly promote the development of e-commerce and the digital economy in turn.

11.3.1.3   Internet plus nursing services

After a pilot project of 'Internet plus nursing services' was launched in 2019, it was further advanced and expanded to all provinces in China in 2020 [20]. It emphasized the home care services that the elderly can receive by digital technology [20]. The elderly can thus achieve personalized and differentiated nursing services. The project can help to deepen ideological reform and improve institutional supply for digital technology in aged care services.

Table 11.4   Policies to overcome the difficulty of using technology for the elderly

Time	Issuing organization	Policy
11 September 2020	Ministry of Industry and Information Technology; China Disabled Persons Federation (CDPF)	Guidelines to speed up the building of barrier-free information facilities in China, bridge the 'digital divide' and contribute to inclusive social development [17].
November 2020	State Council	A notice indicating the 'digital divide' faced by the elderly with the rapid growth of the elderly population in China [18]. It aims to solve the difficulties encountered by the elderly in the application of intelligent technology, thus enabling them to better adapt and integrate into smart society [18].
December 2020	National Office on Ageing	'Wisdom to help the elderly' campaign was launched according to the notice [19]. Voluntary training services, popularization of intelligent technology applications and technical guidance are provided to the elderly [19].

11.3.1.4   Encouraging participation in the elderly care service industry

'Suggestions on promoting the development of elderly care services' were put forward by the State Council to encourage the participation in the elderly care service industry (Table 11.5).

Since the 'Implementation plan of encouraging private capital to participate in the development of elderly care service industry' came into force in 2015 [21], the

Table 11.5   Details of 'suggestions on promoting the development of elderly care services'

Objective	Relevant content and analysis
Reduce the burden of taxes and fees for the elderly care services	Support policies for tax reduction and exemption given to the elderly care service institutions that provide day care, rehabilitation care, meal assistance and travel assistance services in the community [13]. The elderly care service institutions can enjoy resident price policies for electricity, water, gas and heat, which is relatively lower [13].
Attract people to enter the elderly care service industry	The policy emphasizes expanding investment and financing channels for elderly care services and expanding employment and entrepreneurship for elderly care services [13].

elderly service industry has prospered. This plan emphasizes multiple ways for private capital to participate in the development of the industry, promoting the integrated development of medical care, improving investment and financing policies and strengthening the guarantee of talents [21].

11.3.2 Case of technology in aged care in China

China's digital technology for elderly care is more like quasi-public goods [22]. As shown in Section 3.1, the government plays an important role in developing and promoting elderly care services. In the meantime, other non-government aspects can also show that the market potential for digital technology in aged care in China is huge.

11.3.2.1 Acceptance by the elderly

A field study on the elderly in Qingdao found that when the elderly perfectly understand the features of 'smart home care service', 63% of the repliers will consider this service as a way to their better life [23].

In China, ageing at home, usually together with family, is 'the most popular living arrangement for' the elderly [24]. With the development of market economy, a new model containing 'community care' and 'institution care' has been introduced [25].

According to the analysis of 198 news reports on smart elderly care industry (Table 11.6), the highest frequency, 59.1%, is to improve the level of institutional modernization services [26]. The main opportunity is to meet the spiritual and health needs of the elderly, accounting for 56.8%, while the satisfaction of physiological needs and safety needs is relatively low [26].

Table 11.6   Opportunities for Chinese elderly care industry in the smart environment [26]

Category	Code	Opportunities	Frequency (%)
Elderly user needs	1	Meet the spiritual needs of the elderly	56.8
	2	Meeting the health needs of the elderly	56.8
	3	Meeting the physiological needs of the elderly	40.9
	4	Meeting the safety needs of the elderly	22.7
Product service offering	5	Improve the level of institutional modernization services	59.1
	6	The service organization is easy to manage	22.7
	7	Improve service information integration	20.5
	8	Provide precision and customized services	20.5
Government promotion	9	Support for government decision-making	13.6

Market size of the silver economy in China
(trillion RMB)

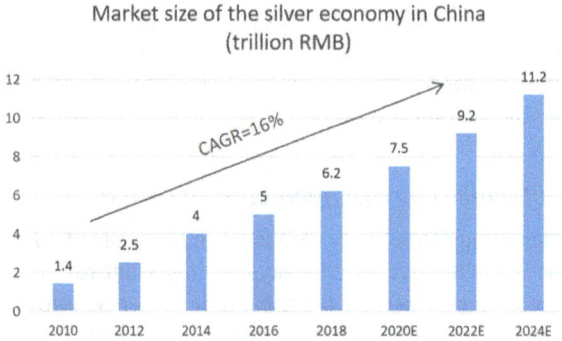

Figure 11.2   Market size of the silver economy in China [2]

11.3.2.2   The 'silver economy' prosperity

'Silver economy' refers to the industry that serves for the elderly consumption with the ageing of the society. With the ageing Chinese population, the market size of the 'Chinese silver economy' almost 'doubled from 2015 to 2020' [1]. Based on the report of FORWARD Research Institute [27], the Compound Annual Growth Rate (CAGR) of 'silver economy in China' is estimated to be about 16% (Figure 11.2) [1].

As the 'China National Committee on Ageing' forecasted, people over 60 would contribute to one-third of the GDP in China by 2050 [1]. As the number of middle class increases, the average income for seniors increases too [1]. According to iiMedia Research, more aged people will have income above 4 000 RMB (Figure 11.3) [3].

According to iiMedia Research, 30 million seniors will live alone by 2020 [7]. Because of the mismatch between demand and supply, a variety of services and products of digital technology in aged care is expected to surge (Figure 11.4). The market size of elderly care in China is expected to reach about 385 billion yuan in 2020 with a broad market prospect [7] (Figure 11.4).

Number of senior citizens (million) grouped by
income level

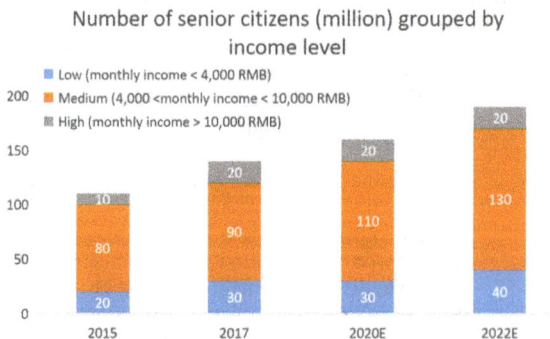

Figure 11.3   Growing number of senior citizens grouped by income level [3]

Market Size of the elderly care in China
(billion RMB)

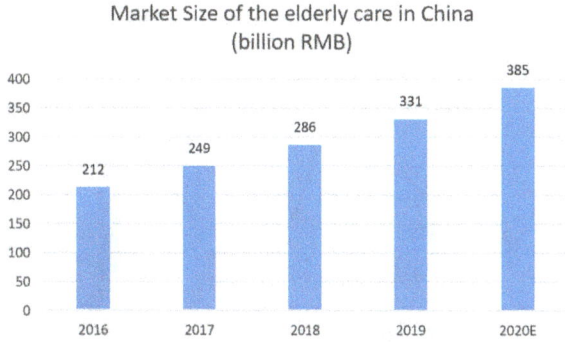

Figure 11.4   Market size of the elderly care in China [7]

11.3.2.3   Large scale of the mobile medical industry

According to FORWARD Research, the mobile medical market in China will exceed 50 billion RMB by the end of 2020 [28]. Internet giants like Alibaba and Baidu have planned to enter the market [8]. Since there are about '1.17 billion phone users in China', the scale of smartphone medical applications has a large room for further development [8]. By using digital platforms on a smartphone, there can be a easy connection between healthcare provider and users, 'which not only saves time and travelling fees but also allows doctors to' give their patients a more efficient treatment [8]. A survey by Cube Labs finds that healthcare application are estimated to be used by 30% of smartphone users by 2015 [8].

The scale of China's mobile medical market is growing rapidly, not only with thousands of mobile medical apps but also with the market scale increasing from 1.98 billion yuan in 2013 to 20.1 billion yuan in 2017, with a compound annual growth rate of 78.48% [28] (Figure 11.5). According to the development situation of mHealth since 2018, the overall scale of the industry is estimated to exceed 50 billion yuan in 2020 [28] (Figure 11.5).

The scale of China's mobile medical market

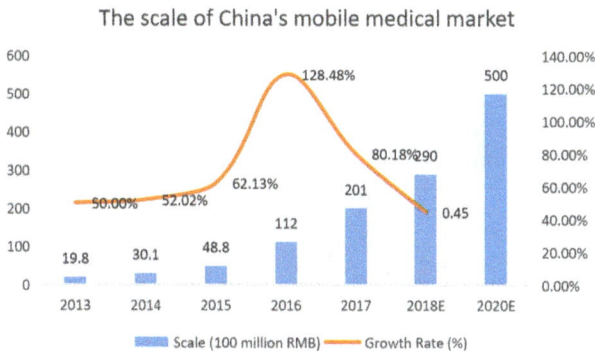

Figure 11.5   The scale of China's mobile medical market [27]

The user scale of China's mobile medical and health market

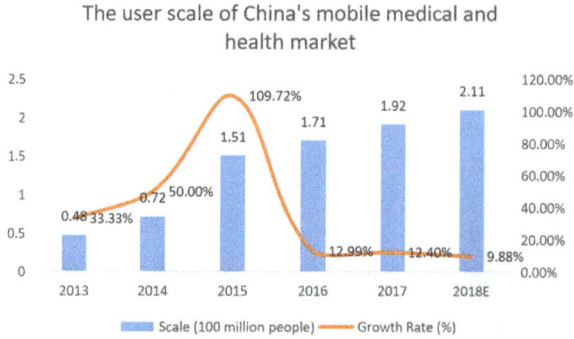

Figure 11.6   *The user scale of China's mobile medical market [27]*

The number of mobile medical users has been growing year by year, exceeding 100 million in 2015 and reaching 192 million in 2017 [27] (Figure 11.6). Although the growth trend of the number of mobile medical users is slowing down, users have gradually formed the habit of using mobile terminals to access medical services [27] (Figure 11.6).

11.3.2.4   'New Chinese seniors': more educated and open to digital technologies

'The improved human capital, a better quality of life and a more reliable social welfare system all contribute to forging the new Chinese seniors' [1]. According to the Chinese Research Center for Ageing [29], the percentage of Chinese senior citizens never being in school has dropped 43.9% from 2000 to 2015 (Figure 11.7). The seniors' education level is generally improved and is expected to improve even further.

The new Chinese seniors are more open to digital technologies. The Cyberspace Administration of China states that the 'Internet keeps spreading into the middle-aged and aged groups' [1].

Education level of the elderly on the rise

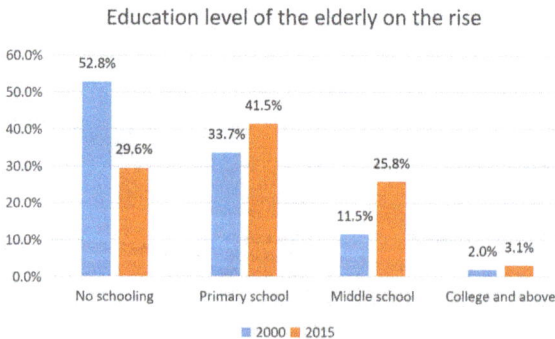

Figure 11.7   *Education level of the elderly on the rise [1]*

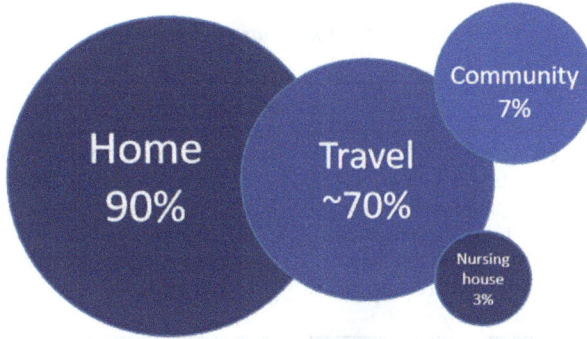

Figure 11.8   Four modes of elderly care and their percentage in China [1]

11.3.2.5   Impacts of epidemics such as COVID-19

The research concludes three major ways people live the retired life and one trend is adopted by the majority (Figure 11.8) [1]. Shanghai government first created the concept of '9073', 'where 90% of the elderly spend their life at home, 7% at community care centres and 3% in institutions' [1].

The Ministry of Civil Affairs has issued a guideline in February 2020 to strictly limit the movement of elderly living in institutions [30]. Although 'very few cases of COVID-19 were reported' in Chinese institutions 'thanks to the effective execution', 100% of the institutions are facing unprecedented ordeals [1]. The situations of these institutions are shown in Table 11.7.

However, despite the relatively terrible situations of the institutions for elderly living, there does exist a trend that institution-based care will possibly be an important pillar according to the reports from FORWARD Research Institute [27]. Table 11.8 presents the possible reasons.

Although we cannot deny the possible trend of institution-based care, there are still a large number of elderly who prefer or have to spend their lives at home. While COVID-19 temporarily suspended Chinese 'to-door elderly care services', the pandemic cannot reverse the trend [1]. 'After the social distancing is lifted', there will be a huge market potential for to-door services in elderly care in the near future [1]. As more professional caregivers instead of family members participate in

Table 11.7   Situations of institutions for elderly living

Financial data	Took a 20% loss in revenue and 30% increase in operational costs, compared to the same period last year, according to the Ministry of Civil Affairs [31].
Objective causes	COVID-19 made it more difficult and even impossible to come back to nursing homes which raised a need for home care [1]. There are 250 million senior citizens in China and 7.6 million beds in various institutions [31]. There thus exists a supply-demand imbalance.

Table 11.8   Reasons for the choice of institution-based care

Reasons	Results
More families come into 'a 4-2-1 structure (4 grandparents, 2 parents and 1 child)' [1]. There exist 'private companies offering big-data-enabling, cloud-based, information-integrated systems for such institutions' [1]. More feasible solutions are expected to emerge sooner or later [1].	Traditional home-based elderly care is facing severe challenges [1]. The supply-demand imbalance (shown in Table 11.4) and the problems discovered through COVID-19 will be solved then.

home-based care through digital technology, more intelligent solutions with to-door elderly care services will emerge in China in the era after COVID-19 [1].

11.3.3   Existing digital technology in aged care in China

Whether it is because of the market trend or government promotion, more and more digital technologies in aged care are emerging in China. Several examples are presented in Table 11.9.

In the meantime, existing digital technology in health and aged care has attracted significant investment in China because of 'its potential to bring revolutionary changes to the medical system' [8]. In 2014, $20 million was invested in 'QuYi's APP "to the hospital"' by the High Light Capital; $170 million was invested in 'Ding Xiangyuan (the online medical network) and Guahao (Registered network)' by Tencent; 'Temasek's affiliated company Pavilion Capital invested $500 million in Spring Rain Doctors' (an application that can link users to over '5,000 doctors in China's leading hospitals, and users can consult doctors by paying a nominal fee of up to 25 yuan and generally receive a professional consultation within minutes') [8].

11.3.4   Development prospect

The problem of providing for the aged is changing from a family problem to a social problem. In response to the severe situation of the ageing society, and to effectively connect the demand for the aged and the supply of the aged, digital technologies are carried out to reform on the supply side to meet the actual needs of the aged.

There is no doubt that advanced digital technologies improve the quality of elderly care services significantly. The services provided by technologies could also be conducive to the independent living of the elderly [22]. Currently, multiple efforts are underway. In the meantime, some suggestions can be given to further improve it. Table 11.10 gives a summary of the roles of digital technologies, current efforts and suggestions to digital technologies in aged care in China.

Digital technology in aged care in China will be an important force in the future elderly care industry whether from the top design, rigid demand or scientific and practical convenience. There is a lot of opportunities despite challenge in the current stage of the development of the digital aged care environment in China. It is

Table 11.9 *Examples of digital technologies in aged care in China*

Company	Products	Purpose
Lan-chuang Network Technology Corp	A set of devices with a setup box, a webcam paired with a TV set and a Siri-like voice assistant 'Xiaoyi' [32]	Allow customers to access telemedicine, an SOS system and for-pay services that include housekeeping and meal deliveries [32]
	A small robot (2 yuan per day) [32]	Ring up a medical centre in response to verbal calls for help
	A smart care system (220,000 elderly clients signed up in 16 cities in August 2019) [32]	Attract more users and make money from providers of offline services [32]
	A smartphone for seniors (with China Mobile Ltd 0941.HK) [32]	
Elsevier	'Elderly Care China', an online platform [33]	Deliver nursing education to address the growing demand for quality geriatric care management services in China [33]; more focused on the cultivation and aid of geriatric care professionals in China
	Later: extend across a mobile platform and other point terminals [33]	
	The above online platform at launch (online version)	Focus on 'nursing education content centred on geriatric management around daily care, preventive care, mental health issues and neurological diseases', which will be gradually expanded later [33]
	The above online platform (running) (content refreshing regularly)	Refreshing content to help China's aged care professionals keep updated with the latest developments [33]
	The above online platform (current)	Bridge the gap between too many old people and relatively too few aged care nurses, which can help 'equip China's nursing professionals with quality, comprehensive and practical skills to meet the requirements of China's elderly care management' [33]

(Continues)

Table 11.9 Continued

Company	Products	Purpose
Hitachi	An 'Internet + Community Home-based care Service Platform' and a 'Smart health service platform for the elderly' focusing on home-based aged care (with Pinghu Municipal Government) [34]	Launched according to the market research that began in 2014; work out the local needs based on the local actual situation and the specific requirements of the elderly [34]; provide IT solutions for pension institutions [34];
	the above platform: solve practical problems for the local government, including:	
	1. monitoring the operation of care centres;	
	2. supervising the daily operation of elderly care service institutions;	
	3. a scientific assessment of the abilities and needs of the elderly, followed by the provision of precise services, while monitoring the time and quality of home visits;	
	4. 24-hr care for the lonely, lost, empty nest and other special elderly [34]	
	An 'indoor positioning system' technology used in the above platforms	Determine the position of the elderly in their home through sensors, so as to master their activities in detail, and the information can be shared with relatives living in other places, elderly care service centres and other relevant parties [34]
	Jointly build the elderly care operation system with the above platform as the core with the local government [34]	Ensure that the platforms can meet the needs of the elderly in a more detailed and thoughtful manner [34]
	Plan to set up nursing stations or sign contracts with nearby hospitals	Realize the combination of medical care and nursing care, so as to provide professional institutional services and meet the convenience of home-based services [34]
Sinopha-rm Fuxin Elderly Care Corp	A smart elderly care big data platform	Link multiple nursing service institutions and can quickly obtain the age, address, health status, nursing level and other data and information of the elderly [35]
	Professional overall operation and intelligent transformation	For more than 1 000 elderly care institutions and community elderly care service centre in Hunan and Anhui provinces [35]

Table 11.10 *Summary of generalized roles of digital technologies and suggestions*

Generalized roles	Help elderly care services to improve accuracy and efficiency. After analyzing the data collected, they may also assist elderly care institutions by finding out the demands of their customers, thus making the right decisions. In developed countries: help 'improve existing systems of healthcare' [8]. In developing countries: play a more crucial role – acting as the main channel 'to introduce training, resources and services that might otherwise remain non-existent or out of reach for the vast majority of the population' [8]
Current efforts	Local industry associations: set up industry technical standards, which will bring the possibility of platforms' opening up between each other and thus promote the rapid popularization of digital technology for elderly care [36].
Suggestions	Digital technologies should be entirely involved in smart cities to resolve Information Isolated Island issues. All the data from the medical system, the elderly care system and other systems should be connected in an efficient way to support a smart elderly care system using digital technology. Considering the limited mHealth for aged health literature in China, in order 'to ensure patients have access to the best possible resources, rigorous researches are required to help produce high-quality and evidence-based mHealth programs' [8]. 'Greater cooperation among network operators, equipment manufacturers and healthcare professionals' should be encouraged to 'innovate and speed up the growth of the mHealth market' and improve the adoption of digital technology in aged care [8]. 'The technical standards for the elderly care services should be formulated as soon as possible' to avoid the chaotic development of the aged smart home care and prevent the incompatibility due to product heterogeneity [22]. 'The existing public and private smart home for elderly care platforms should be combined' to 'optimize resource allocation and management and avoid the waste of public resources' [22]. Enterprises related to 'smart home care services should implement' a customer-oriented tactic [22].

significant to understand the role of digital technology, and clarify these opportunities and challenges to promote the development of China's smart aged care.

11.4   Case study of Haiyang Group

11.4.1   Description of business

11.4.1.1   Description of the venture

Shanghai Haiyang Internet Elderly Services Co., LTD. (hereinafter referred to as 'Haiyang'), founded in 2004, provides the whole pension industry chain services including life services, life care, nursing homes, nursing homes and so on. It is the leading comprehensive provider of pension services in China. At present, Haiyang elderly service has covered 28 cities in ten provinces, including Shanghai, Zhejiang and Jiangsu. There are more than three million elderly platforms, more than 50 000 end-users, and more than 320 employees in the call centre.

11.4.1.2 Product(s) and/or service(s)

The main product is Continuing Care Home-based Community (CCHC), a smart pension model. CCHC consists of many products that will be discussed in Section 4.3.1. CCHC's smart pension platform is the integration and innovative development of new technologies, new business forms and new models in the pension industry. CCHC focuses on developing a service platform and researching the key technologies to support the platform services and industrial development.

11.4.2 Description of industry

11.4.2.1 Type of industry

China is facing the pension status of ageing, senility, low birth rate, ageing before getting rich, empty nesters and so on. Taking care of the elderly has become an important issue in today's society in China. The industry is a service-based industry, trying to enable the elderly to live a better life as well as make old people's children feel at ease. Currently, digital technologies are entering the industry and improving it tremendously.

11.4.2.2 Future outlook and tends of industry

As discussed in Section 11.3, the industry has good prospects (reasons are listed in Table 11.11).

11.4.2.3 Analysis of competitors

At present, there are many providers of various aged service systems in the market, such as Shecuntong, Northwest Star of Chinese Academy of Sciences, and Yixun, but most of these suppliers are only system providers and professional software service providers.

Table 11.11   Reasons for the good prospects of aged care industry

Reasons	Plans and promotions of the government
	Wide acceptance by the elderly
	'Silver economy' prosperity
	Large scale of the mobile medical industry
	'New Chinese seniors' who are more educated and open to digital technologies
	Impacts of epidemics such as COVID-19

Table 11.12   Shortcomings of the traditional manual process of work order processing

Shortcomings	Cannot effectively track and understand the whole process of work order
	Human error and time delay, resulting in the decline of service efficiency
	Manual management cannot carry out quantitative statistics, which is not conducive to query, report and performance assessment

Regarding work order processing, the traditional process has shortcomings (Table 11.12).

11.4.3   Technology

11.4.3.1   Description of technology
Haiyang has launched several products in aged care using digital technologies (Table 11.13).

11.4.3.2   Technology comparison
Several technology comparisons between Haiyang and its competitors together with Haiyang's superiorities are shown in Table 11.14.

11.4.4   Description of market

11.4.4.1   Market segment
Haiyang's products are facing the elderly care service market. The target customers are mainly people aged 65 and older in China, who we call 'the elderly'. Sometimes, the children of the elderly purchase the product and arrange the corresponding living conditions for the elderly.

11.4.4.2   Promotion
Thanks to the long-time engagement of Haiyang in elderly service field, most of Haiyang's business is spread by word of mouth. In addition, with the further expansion of Haiyang's business to the community, the service staff of Haiyang is the best mobile advertisement.

As discussed in Section 11.4.3.2, Haiyang cooperates with the government. The government helps to promote Haiyang's elderly care services, which can make Haiyang's products become trustworthy to the elderly.

11.4.4.3   Product or service
Using digital technologies, Haiyang Group has launched many aged care services. Many of them are presented in the form of a visible product such as a digital

Table 11.13   Digital technology products of Haiyang Group

Products	Details and roles
Seven Internet service systems (emergency rescue system, active care system, home care system, medical rehabilitation system, health service system, two cards and two machines system); **Three cloud service platforms** (smart pension service platform, smart life service platform and emergency relief platform).	1. use digital technologies such as the advanced Internet technology, cloud computing, big data technology and wearable technology equipment; 2. realize the connectivity between different subjects; 3. children or guardians can view relevant information of the elderly in real time through the digital information service platform.
Automation of work order management, using workflow technology; **Multi-point tour path planning technology** applying to the formulation of service personnel's travel routes (When service personnel receive multiple work orders at different locations, they need to use navigation for path planning.)	1. reduce human error and delay, improve the efficiency of work order processing and finally improve the benefits of enterprises; 2. automatically identify the optimal path for service personnel to go through each service point and return to the company, which saves the time of service personnel and improves their work efficiency.
A systematic elderly care service complex, using cloud computing, Internet of Things, mobile Internet and other technologies.	1. realize the link between personal terminals and smart homes; 2. realize human–computer interaction.
Applications for the elderly such as remote health monitoring, emergency assistance, home security and learning and education; **Sensors to monitor** the behaviour data such as breathing, blood pressure, heart rate and living environment data such as gas leak, suspected human or animal invasion outside; **One-button alarm** all day long, calling for medical aid workers or their children (the '95002' platform and the user side will alarm at the same time; the platform will timely follow up the situation of device users).	1. 'within reach' service guarantee for the old; 2. meet the personalized and diversified needs of the elderly; 3. the elderly: no need to carry out any active operation, just normal life and rest in the room; 4. promote the innovative development of the pension industry through the cross-border integration and coordination of the pension industry and new technology; 5. avoid the embarrassment that the device alarms but no one will handle the situation of device users.

Table 11.14   Technology comparison

Haiyang	Competitor	Advantage
A comprehensive pension service platform, covering three models: institutional pension, community pension and home pension at the same time.	Only single service providers	Haiyang's comprehensive platform ensures the excellent integration of information and better service for the elderly.
Introduces context information such as location information and real-time working status through technology	Traditional: weakness (Table 11.2)	It effectively tracks each link of the service and manages the service more efficiently.
Haiyang has been engaged in the elderly service field for more than 10 years and has accumulated **a large number of users**.		1. enable Haiyang to become one of the leaders in the industry; 2. solid customer group: protects Haiyang from the competitors.
Brand advantage		1. drive its development;
An elderly service hotline, '95002', officially launched in 31 provinces across the country. The hotline is a part of Haiyang's comprehensive digital system.		2. seven years since the application in 2013, during which a large number of users have been accumulated. 3. make people trust Haiyang more.
A long-term cooperation with the government		1. make aged service information all available;
Many of its projects are purchased by the government. When the government is promoting elderly services, the product of Haiyang serves as an official platform.		2. enable interconnected sharing of data from aged care institutions, community-based or home-based care, comprehensive old-age allowance and long-term care insurance;
Encourage the government, enterprises and institutions in the pension industry to actively join the service platform, then the platform can rely on the sea of civil administration data		3. serve for industry management; 4. improve work efficiency; 5. help the government make decisions.

Table 11.15   Summary of companies' digital products and their specific roles in aged care in China

Companies' products	Specific roles
Lanchuang Network Technology Corp: smart home care devices and systems	1. give the elderly the convenience to stay at home and access the services remotely; 2. 'ring up a medical centre in response to verbal calls for help' to make sure that someone notices the old people is ill [32].
Elsevier: online platform 'Elderly Care China' (in continuous innovation)	1. provide better and more updated nursing education for aged care; 2. bridge the gap between too many old people and relatively too few aged care nurses; 3. 'equip China's nursing professionals with quality, comprehensive and practical skills' to hit the spots of elderly care [33].
Hitachi: two home-based care service platforms with an 'indoor positioning system' technology	1. monitor the operation of care centres and elderly care institutions; 2. a scientific assessment of the specific abilities and needs of the elderly, providing precise and tailored services; 3. monitor the time and quality of caretakers' home visits; 4. provide 24-hr care for the special elderly; 5. master the old people's activities, and share the information with relevant people and parties [34].
Sinopharm Fuxin Elderly Care Corp: a smart elderly care big data platform	1. link multiple nursing service institutions with high efficiency; 2. enable multiple institutions to obtain the required data and information of the elderly in detail immediately [35]

visualization platform; however, they are essentially services. They serve to take better care of the elderly in China.

11.5   Discussion

Research has shown that there is an increasing need for aged care in China. The government and the industry have noticed the trend and released policies to promote the development of aged care in China and the digital technologies used in aged care. According to the market analysis, more aged people are becoming to accept the usage of digital technologies and smart home care services, which ensures the technologies in aged care can take their due responsibilities to fully serve the elderly. In the meantime, the Chinese 'silver economy' is prospering because of the increasing number of aged people with higher income. Furthermore, the continuous trend of home-based elderly care guarantees the continuous important role of technologies.

Various digital technologies are emerging to improve the aged care industry (Table 11.15).

Although digital technology has already been playing an important role in China's aged care, more efforts are still needed to further advance its development. First, the elderly should be more educated and popularized on how to make better use of digital technologies. Second, all the data from different systems should be connected efficiently to support the smart elderly care system. Third, best possible resources should be accessible to patients by launching mHealth programs with high quality. Fourth, relevant parties should cooperate to improve the adoption of digital technology in aged care. Fifth, standards should be formulated for elderly care services to prevent disorderly development. Finally, the elderly care industry should combine public and private platforms to make full use of resources.

11.6 Study limitations

This chapter is highly dependent on the keywords that were chosen and the databases selected. To minimize this, we conducted a background and exploratory study prior to our review to ensure selection bias was avoided as much as possible. In addition, because the topic embraced complexity and sought to discuss all the contents related to digital technology in aged care in China, the search was quite broad. However, we could still only cover a limited number of papers, published mostly after 2018 to ensure timeliness.

In addition, the selection of articles may have been affected by the use of limited keywords and data sources. To address this issue, we tried different combinations of keywords to search in different databases. We also searched the reference lists of the selected articles to find any relevant articles that matched the objectives of this review.

11.7 Conclusion

This chapter has provided an overview of the role of digital technologies and services for aged care in China. Various data and existing technologies in aged care industry have been analyzed. The case study of Haiyang Group has shown how a pension company takes advantage of digital technologies. It will help readers to better understand the importance of digital health services for healthy ageing.

Nowadays, digital technologies have been playing an unrivalled and powerful role in today's aged care in China. The acceptance and the popularity of technology usage are also increasing, which enables the digital technologies to innovate and better improve the aged care industry. The government and the industry are working together in this direction.

In the future, with the emerging and improvement of more digital technologies (e.g., AI, AR/VR, drones and robots) in aged care industry, the role of technology will become even more indispensable. For example, when more advanced digital technology smart home systems and telepresence robots will enable nurses to care for the elderly from remote locations. This technology is discussed in more detail in the Chapter 16 of this book. More research is needed to establish the effectiveness of such technologies in aged care.

Acknowledgement

This research was partially supported by Shanghai Haiyang Internet Elderly Services Co., LTD.

References

[1]   Daxue Consulting. *COVID-19 impact on elderly care in China* [online]. 2020. Available from https://daxueconsulting.com/covid-19-impact-on-elderly-care-in-china/ [Accessed Dec 2020].

[2]   Wang Z. *'The central committee of the communist party of china (CPC) has issued an open letter to all communist party members of the communist youth league on controlling china's population growth'*. Yearbook of China's Reform and Opening up in the New Era; 1980. pp. 798–9.

[3]   The CPC Central Committee and the State Council. *Decision on implementing the universal two-child policy reform and improving the management of family planning services* [online]. 2015. Available from http://www.gov.cn/gongbao/content/2016/content_5033853.htm [Accessed Dec 2020].

[4]   IBRD.IDA. *Options for aged care in China: building an efficient and sustainable aged care system (English)* [online]. 2018. Available from https://www.shihang.org/zh/news/press-release/2018/12/13/world-bank-report-offers-options-for-elderly-care-in-china [Accessed Dec 2020].

[5]   The CPC Central Committee and the State Council. *The state plan for active response to population ageing* [online]. 2019. Available from http://www.gov.cn/zhengce/2019-11/23/content_5454778.htm [Accessed Dec 2020].

[6]   National Health and Family Planning Commission Family Division. *China Family Development Report (2015)*. Beijing: China Population Publishing House; 2015. pp. 1–165.

[7]   iiMedia Research. *2019 China silver economy consumer market research report* [online]. 2019. Available from https://www.iimedia.cn/c400/64579.html [Accessed Dec 2020].

[8]   Sun J., Guo Y., Wang X., Zeng Q. 'mHealth for aging China: opportunities and challenges'. *Aging and Disease*. 2016, vol. 7(1), pp. 53–67.

[9]   Cipresso P., Serino S., Villani D., *et al.* 'Is your phone so smart to affect your state? An exploratory study based on psychophysiological measures'. *Neurocomputing*. 2012, vol. 84, pp. 23–30.

[10] Sun X., Yan W., Zhou H., *et al.* 'Internet use and need for digital health technology among the elderly: a cross-sectional survey in China'. *BMC Public Health*. 2020, vol. 20(1),1386.

[11] Salovaara A., Lehmuskallio A., Hedman L., Valkonen P., Näsänen J., *et al.* 'Information technologies and transitions in the lives of 55–65-year-olds: the

case of colliding life interests'. *International Journal of Human-Computer Studies*. 2010, vol. 68(11), pp. 803–21.

[12] Moher D., Liberati A., Tetzlaff J., Altman D.G., PRISMA Group. 'Preferred reporting items for systematic reviews and meta-analyses: the PRISMA statement'. *Annals of Internal Medicine*. 2009, vol. 151(4), pp. 264–9.

[13] General office of the State Council of China. *Suggestions on promoting the development of elderly care services* [online]. 2019. Available from http://www.gov.cn/zhengce/content/2019-04/16/content_5383270.htm [Accessed Dec 2020].

[14] Ministry of Civil Affairs of China. *Suggestions on further expanding the supply of elderly care services and promoting the consumption of elderly care services* [online]. 2019. Available from http://www.cncaprc.gov.cn/zcfg/190500.jhtml [Accessed Dec 2020].

[15] Ministry of Civil Affairs of China. *Measures for the management of pension institutions* [online]. 2020. Available from http://www.cncaprc.gov.cn/zcfg/191564.jhtml [Accessed Dec 2020].

[16] Health commission of the Autonomous Region, Development and Reform Commission. *Notice on the implementation measures for the construction of the elderly health service system in the autonomous region* [online]. 2020. Available from http://www.cncaprc.gov.cn/zcfg/191200.jhtml [Accessed Dec 2020].

[17] Ministry of Industry and Information Technology and China Disabled Persons Federation (CDPF). *Guidelines on promoting information accessibility* [online]. 2020. Available from http://www.gov.cn/zhengce/zhengceku/2020-09/23/content_5546271.htm [Accessed Dec 2020].

[18] General office of the State Council of China. *Notice on the implementation plan to effectively solve the difficulties of the elderly in using intelligent technology* [online]. 2020. Available from http://www.gov.cn/zhengce/content/2020-11/24/content_5563804.htm [Accessed Dec 2020].

[19] Department of Ageing Health. *Notice on carrying out the 'wisdom to help the elderly' campaign* [online]. 2020. Available from http://www.nhc.gov.cn/lljks/pqt/202012/3e8b6ac9653f4d2193ba09cba8ea8116.shtml [Accessed Dec 2020].

[20] General office of the National Health Commission. *Notice on further promoting the pilot work of 'internet + nursing services'* [online]. 2020. Available from http://www.gov.cn/zhengce/zhengceku/2020-12/16/content_5569982.htm [Accessed Dec 2020].

[21] Ministry of Civil Affairs, Development and Reform Commission, Ministry of Education. *Implementation plan of encouraging private capital to participate in the development of elderly care service industry* [online]. 2015. Available from http://www.cncaprc.gov.cn/zcfg/73852.jhtml [Accessed Dec 2020].

[22] Zhang Q., Li M., Wu Y. 'Smart home for elderly care: development and challenges in China'. *BMC Geriatrics*. 2020, vol. 20(1),318.

[23] Zhang Q., Li L., Ji G. 'Challenges and solutions to the coordinated development of smart home for elderly care in Qingdao'. Outstanding Research

Compilation of Human Resources and Social Security Department of Shandong Province, China; 2018.

[24]   Silverstein M., Cong Z., Li S. 'Intergenerational transfers and living arrangements of older people in rural China: consequences for psychological well-being'. *The Journals of Gerontology Series B: Psychological Sciences and Social Sciences*. 2006, vol. 61(5), pp. S256–66.

[25]   Suryadevara N.K., Mukhopadhyay S.C. 'Wireless sensor network based home monitoring system for wellness determination of elderly'. *IEEE Sensors Journal*. 2012, vol. 12(12), pp. 1965–72.

[26]   Meng Q., Hong Z., Li Z., *et al*. 'Opportunities and challenges for Chinese elderly care industry in smart environment based on occupants' needs and preferences'. *Frontiers in Psychology*. 2020, vol. 11,1029.

[27]   FORWARD Business Information Co., Ltd. *Report of prospects and investment strategy planning on China pension industry (2020-2025)* [online]. 2019. Available from https://bg.qianzhan.com/trends/detail/506/191231-a98bd81d.html [Accessed Dec 2020].

[28]   FORWARD Business Information Co., Ltd. *Analysis on the future development Trend of China's mobile medical industry with a market size of over 50 billion yuan in 2020* [online]. 2018. Available from https://www.qianzhan.com/analyst/detail/220/181206-f7ba5244.html [Accessed Dec 2020].

[29]   China Scientific Research Center on Ageing. *Data released from the fourth sample survey on the living conditions of China's urban and rural elderly population* [online]. 2019. Available from http://www.crca.cn/sjfw/2019-11-21/1564.html [Accessed Dec 2020].

[30]   Ministry of Civil Affairs. *Deployment of 'one old and one small' service agencies for epidemic prevention and control* [online]. 2020. Available from http://www.mca.gov.cn/article/xw/mzyw/202002/20200200025018.shtml [Accessed Dec 2020].

[31]   Ministry of Civil Affairs. *Guidelines on timely adjustment and improvement of COVID-19 prevention and control strategies for orderly restoration of old-age care institutions* [online]. 2020. Available from http://www.mca.gov.cn/article/xw/tzgg/202004/20200400026691.shtml [Accessed Dec 2020].

[32]   Lanchuang Continuous Innovation. *Smart elderly care and home-based care for aged* [online]. 2019. Available from http://www.ilanchuang.com/ [Accessed Dec 2020].

[33]   Elsevier. *Our solutions* [online]. 2020. Available from http://www.elsevier-china.com/ [Accessed Dec 2020].

[34]   Hitachi, Ltd. *Hitachi works with Pinghu municipal government to build an 'Internet plus smart elderly care service platform* [online]. 2018. Available from https://social-innovation.hitachi/zh-cn/case_studies/pinghu/?WT.mc_id=20CnCnCh-keyword -search [Accessed Dec 2020].

[35]   China National Committee on Ageing. *The momentum of the health care and old-age care industry has been speeded up* [online]. 2020. Available from http://www.cncaprc.gov.cn/llsy/191812.jhtml [Accessed Dec 2020].

[36]   Peine A. 'Understanding the dynamics of technological configurations: a conceptual framework and the case of smart homes'. *Technological Forecasting and Social Change*. 2009, vol. 76(3), pp. 396–409.

Part III

Digital Tools for Healthy Ageing

Chapter 12

Using powered exoskeletons for rehabilitation in healthy ageing – a societal perspective

J. Artur Serrano[1], Eduard Fosch-Villaronga[2], and Roger A. Søraa[1]

This chapter explores how powered exoskeletons may be used in rehabilitation for older adults. It argues that combining characteristics of social robots with state-of-the-art exoskeletons, to create a social exoskeleton, will promote a disruptive innovation in the use of this technology for care. In order to implement technology into existing societal infrastructures, careful attention has to be given to the potential impacts. This chapter draws attention to these in the light of the concept of Responsible Research and Innovation (RRI). Seven specific sociotechnical considerations for technologists, regarding namely accessibility, economy, inclusivity, environment, culture, law, and ethics, are discussed.

Keywords

Exoskeletons, Rehabilitation, Healthy Aging, Social Robots, Gerontechnology

12.1 Introduction

A powered exoskeleton uses robot technology that integrates sensing, control, information, and computer science to provide a wearable mechanical device, mainly targeted to provide power assistance and rehabilitation to older adults and patients with lower limb motor dysfunctions [1].

Powered exoskeletons have recently been given increased attention in the scientific literature, with over 2 600 entries in PubMed (Figure 12.1) and over 34 000 in Google Scholar, in the last 10 years.

[1]Department of Neuromedicine and Movement Science, NTNU/Norwegian University of Science and Technology, Trondheim, Norway
[2]eLaw Center for Law and Digital Technologies, Leiden University, Leiden, The Netherlands

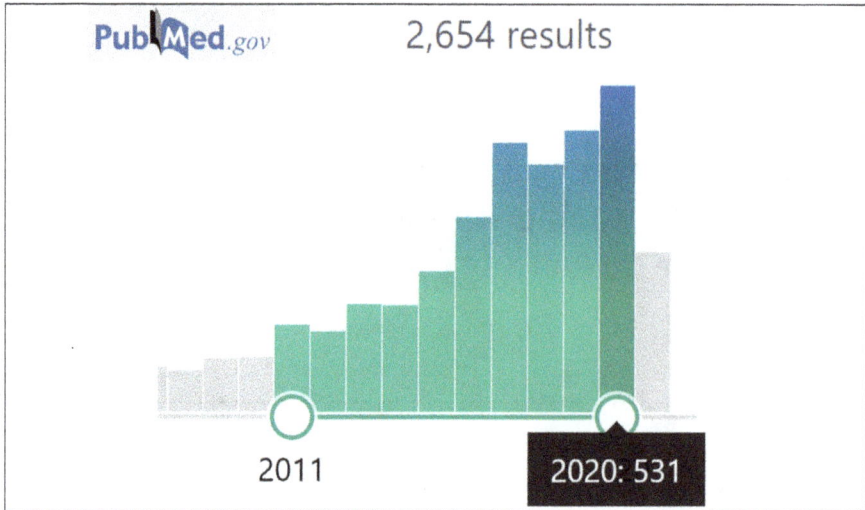

Figure 12.1   Search results in PubMed for the term "exoskeleton"

The common denominator for the interest in use of a powered exoskeleton is the desire to overcome limitations and improve physical ability. Perhaps the most investigated type is the lower limb exoskeleton, which has the potential to increase a person's capacity of bearing weight, either their own body weight or with additional load. This capacity has immediate application to any activity where the person is asked to lift and carry weight, which can be cargo, weapons used in combat, or patients in care facilities. But the use of exoskeletons is not just about increasing natural abilities but also to overcome limitations caused by disease, accidents, or genetics. Much research and technology development have been dedicated to the use of lower limb exoskeletons in patients with spinal cord injury [2, 3]. Because of their potential in this specific area, we will use it as a case study.

Although the advances in mechatronics technology, including hardware, such as sensors and actuators, and software, such as movement analysis algorithms, have been impressive, we claim that there is still a lack of development on the human–robot Interaction (HRI) component. This limits additional functionalities such as user feedback and negotiated training, that is, adjusting of the training level, intensity, or diversity in a negotiated way between the user and the robotic platform.

A patient with a spinal cord injury, may be bound to a wheelchair for life, but an exoskeleton may be able to help the person stand up and create a walking motion. Scientific studies report different results on the actual medical benefits of exoskeletons, calling for more research both on their usefulness from a physical perspective and on the societal aspects [4].

An important aspect of this technology is related to their impact on social interaction. Being able to stand, have a conversation with friends or colleagues, and saying goodbye with a hug while both standing as equals, can be a real social benefit for a patient and reduce stigma. Although a person may have lost the ability to walk, an exoskeleton can partly offer that possibility back. Regaining the ability to walk independently may transform the lifestyle of a patient in many positive ways. However, the potential offered by exoskeletons is far from achieved in the current state of the technology. We claim that, as in most technologies that interface with humans, the capability of powered exoskeletons of aiding a patient in their activities of daily living is dependent on a close interaction between the device and its user. Fosch-Villaronga and Özcan [5] have called attention to the fact that this particular kind of interaction has scarcely been covered in the HRI literature. In this chapter, holistic interaction features associated with social robots will be investigated as a possible addition to the current solutions offered by existing powered exoskeletons.

Moreover, exoskeletons can help people of all ages. Passive walking aids, such as clutches and walkers, may be replaced or supported by the use exoskeletons, as a way to help frail people to continue to walk a while longer independently. These capabilities are constantly being developed as lighter and smaller exoskeletons are offered to the users, as will be presented in the next section.

12.2 Powered exoskeletons and their function – a summary of current technologies

Using a powered exoskeleton in rehabilitation therapy may not only provide better outcomes to the patient but also reduce the use of human resources. Back injuries are some of the most common ailments to affect workers. Exoskeletons are not meant to replace physiotherapists, quite the opposite. They are tools meant to augment existing rehabilitation programs and reduce the injury rate of practitioners in the field [6].

While it is true that exoskeletons still have strong limitations before they are ready to be widely adopted as an integrating part of rehabilitation programs, the already existing products and prototypes can serve as an example as to the impact this technology will most likely have in the future.

In a general classification according to the application of powered exoskeletons in rehabilitation, these robotic platforms can be divided into two categories *treadmill-based robotic systems* and *overground robotic wearable exoskeletons*. In the former category, the system comprises an exoskeleton that is used to provide assistance to leg movement [3] and a body weight support system required to adjust the weight applied onto the legs and also ensure safety and help with balance (Figure 12.2). These include Lokomat [7], ALEX [8], and LOPES [9]. In the latter category, the system helps the patient in training the overground gait (Figure 12.3). These include: Indego [10], Exowalk [11], Ekso [12], and HAL (Hybrid Assistive Limb) [13]. Cyberdyne, the producer of HAL, claims it is able to detect a patient's intention to move through measurement of bio-electrical signals captured at the skin level. The brain is then able to learn the way to send the appropriate signals for walking. HAL then recognizes what sort of motions the wearer wants to perform. Hereafter are presented some relevant commercial and academic-related robotic platforms already in use in rehabilitation therapy.

Commercial platforms, such as Lokomat, produced by Hocoma, have been used in a number of studies with the focus on producing effective gait training [7]. A robot-assisted

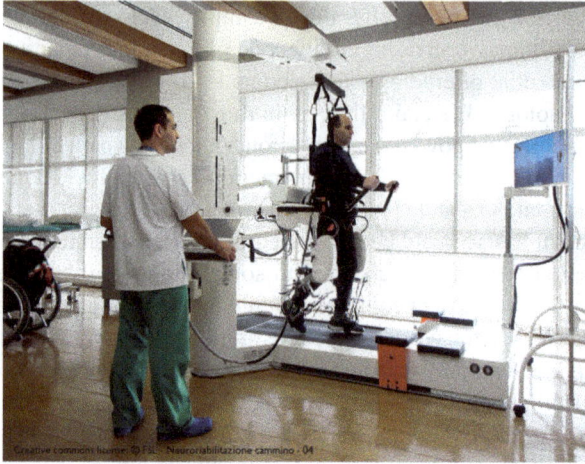

Figure 12.2   The Lokomat treadmill-based robotic system

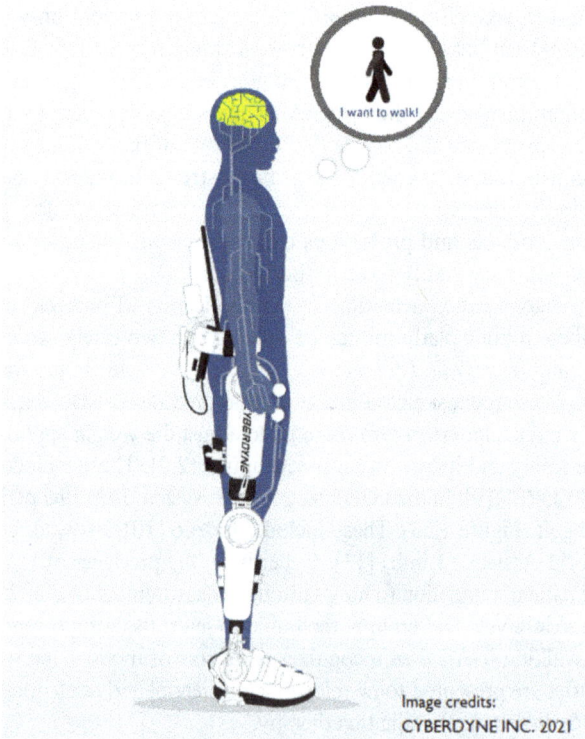

Figure 12.3   Overground exoskeleton – HAL® robot

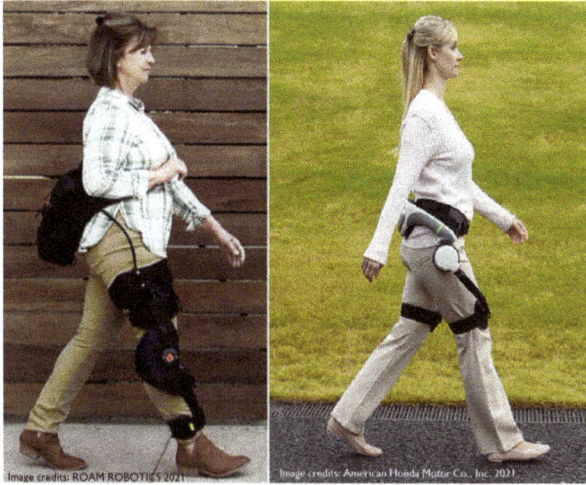

Figure 12.4   Lightweight-powered exoskeletons

therapy may help enable effective and intensive training and ensure optimal exploitation of neuroplasticity and recovery potential [14]. From academia, the Project March at the Delft University of Technology, is developing an innovative and versatile exoskeleton that can be used to let people with a spinal cord injury stand up and walk again [15]. Industry is also involved in research by partnering up with researchers to show evidence on technology effects in clinical use. As an example, the study reported in [11] is a randomized controlled trial to assess the effects of electromechanical-assisted gait training with the commercial platform Exowalk on walking ability of chronic stroke patients. Exowalk is an exoskeletal walk-robotic device developed for any patients with gait difficulty to do gait training by providing a proper walking pattern.

In recent years, the weight of powered exoskeletons has been steadily decreasing, partially due to the developments in battery technology. Some commercial exoskeletons, such as the Indego Personal, have weights below 15 kg (33 lb). Moreover, producers have started to offer a larger diversity in the size of the exoskeleton, from a full lower limb device to more focused designs, with considerably lower weights. Examples of minimalistic exoskeletons with weights as low as 2.7 kg (6 lb) are given in Figure 12.4. Roam Robotics Ascend® (Figure 12.4, left side) is a lightweight power actuated pneumatic orthosis designed to support movement at the knee level [16]. The Honda Walking Assist Device® (Figure 12.4, right side) is a wearable robotic device with actuators placed at the hip joint assist flexion and extension movements allowing it to be used for gait training [17].

12.3   A symbiosis between powered exoskeletons and social robots

Studies have shown that exoskeletons can be used safely in gait training when applied in a clinical environment [18]. However, there is still a lack of research prompting a need for knowledge in certain key areas, including their use outside of a clinical setting [19], even as there is the suggestion that they could offer a great deal of independence in a variety of everyday settings [20].

Attempting to integrate elements of Artificial Intelligence (AI), such an expert component and learning ability, with an exoskeleton, could help exoskeletons to be used outside of the rehabilitation clinic and eventually be part of a more continuous rehabilitation routine during the activities of daily living. Other robotic technological innovations, such as assisted force-feedback for balance and movement, image gait analysis, etc., could also be a valuable addition to an exoskeleton.

12.3.1   Can a social enhanced exoskeleton help in healthy aging?

Being able to move freely is at the core of human life. When a person becomes immobile, there is a domino of negative effects: decline in health, decrease of social interactions, and rise of depression. Exoskeletons aim to rehabilitate patients who are wheelchair-bound in order to restore their mobility to some degree of normal gait functioning and eventually regaining their walking ability. By producing an AI-enabled exoskeleton, integrating a user-interface with social capabilities, such as speech interaction, to allow a motivating, reliable, and safe human–robot communication, and able to supervise, train, coach, and learn together with its user, would have a potential for inducing faster recovery. This device would integrate the following two main technological components: an exoskeleton and an AI system. These two components have synergic functions, and both receive inputs and give feedback to the patient, respectively, at the motoric and speech levels. The integration of socially assistive capabilities into exoskeletons would allow to create a disruptive innovation path on the way rehabilitation procedures are conducted today.

Aging-related conditions such as stroke require increased care resources. In fact, stroke-related care requires more bed days in hospitals and rehabilitation facilities than any other somatic illness [21]. This problem is set to increase significantly with an aging population. There is, therefore, an urgent need to develop evidence-based and clinically novel approaches to personalized ischemic stroke assessment and rehabilitation. Spinal cord injuries often affect older adults [22]. For this section of the population, a spinal cord injury greatly increases both morbidity and mortality [23]. Such injuries affect not only the motor function but also the digestive system, urinary tract, lungs, sex life, etc. The patient usually becomes dependent on a wheelchair in everyday life and mostly will be dependent on additional help to cope throughout the day. A wheelchair-bound life can also cause secondary complications such as pressure sores, hypertension, and osteoporosis, which can affect the patient's quality of life and mood [24].

12.3.2 From a rehabilitation device to a companion

To achieve positive outcomes, however, such device would need to be seen by the patient, not only as a rehabilitation equipment but also as a companion and motivator assistant, an intelligent wearable robot to help in the rehabilitation program.

An expert system would establish the necessary knowledge to support and train the rehabilitation training of the patients. Moreover, the system could learn from the experience with its user, measuring progress, evaluating the best working motivational strategies, suggesting further exercises, and promoting gait improvement.

Perspectives for improved quality of life are exciting. However, the interdisciplinary nature of this research field demands the cooperation of experts from different fields or areas of knowledge, including, but not limited to movement science, physiotherapy, robot technology, computing science, Science and Technology Studies (STS), human cognition, and Human–Machine Interaction, including the subfield of HRI, ethics, and legal aspects.

The symbiosis between powered exoskeletons and social robots, a *social exoskeleton*, opens a new strategy into technology-based physiotherapy and robotic physical rehabilitation. The synergy between these areas is found in the realm of the interdisciplinary field "Welfare Technologies," in the EU context, or "Assistive Technologies" in the UK/US/AU and Asian countries context.

Typically named healthcare robots, care robots, or carebots, these robots are service robots that perform useful tasks for humans by processing information acquired through various sensors, in the context of healthcare. Care robots support impaired individuals, extend the work of doctors in medical interventions, help in patient care and rehabilitation activities, and also support individuals in prevention programs. These robots are part of a larger group of technologies, which promote better welfare. Technologies supporting aging, such as care and well-being technologies, give people the opportunity to better cope with health and strengthen their life through innovation and the application of new technologies to be happier. These technologies make the welfare system better equipped to meet society's future challenges, including demographic trends toward an aging society, technological isolation, and lack of resources. In other words, these technologies contribute directly toward improvement in the quality of life of humans (ISO 13482:2014).

From the six areas of innovation generally related to this healthcare domain, including robotics for medical intervention, supporting professional care, preventive therapies and diagnosis, assistive technology, and rehabilitation treatment, this chapter focuses on assistive and rehabilitation technology. In concrete, we focus on the integration of different care and well-being technologies to promote independent and autonomous living. Indeed, the inclusion of these technologies at home support people's self-reliance, personal monitorization, and enhanced knowledge about one's health status, encourage social contact with caregivers, friends, and loved ones.

12.3.3 *Assessing social exoskeletons using Robot Impact Assessment (ROBIA)*

When technologies are developed to use within the care field, it is of the utmost importance to guarantee that issues related to privacy, safety, liability, autonomy and human dignity are covered. A sociotechnical method called ROBIA [25] helps roboticists to identify, analyze, and mitigate the legal and ethical risks associated with robot technology. The primary goal of ROBIA is to provide a legal assessment of a robot, in this case an exoskeleton, and to provide positive feedback to the creation process of such robots at any point in time i.e., idea, concept, prototype, pre-launch, launch, and post-launch.

A ROBIA includes the following steps: (1) Establish the context (context of use, including workers, technological ecosystem), (2) Describe robot type and characteristics (embodiment, HRI, autonomy, sensors, and functionalities, integrated technology), (3) Identify the relevant legal framework (existing binding legislation, standard setting, agencies recommendations), and (4) Identify associated risks.

12.4 RRI and societal considerations for exoskeletons' implementation

Implementing technology into existing societal infrastructures and practices of technology, care and health do not happen in a vacuum [26, 27]. Rather, it has implications and impacts on a wider societal scale. The importance to draw particular attention to these broader consequences can be seen through the concept of Responsible Research & Innovation (RRI) advocated by the European Union's Framework Programmes, which is an overarching concept that captures crucial aspects concerning what researchers can do to ensure that research and innovation have desirable outcomes [28]. The European Commission defines RRI as "an approach that anticipates and assesses potential implications and societal expectations concerning research and innovation, intending to foster the design of inclusive and sustainable research and innovation" [29].

However, it is often the case that such good intentions struggle to translate into specific, practical, and widely adopted actions [26, 29]. Building on previous research on wearable robots and the self, wearable robots and the other, and wearable robots in society conducted under the H2020 Cost Action 16116 on Wearable Robots [30], we pay particular attention to the latter. We have identified seven specific societal considerations for designers, developers, and deployers of exoskeletons to heed. These seven considerations can help to think about how to implement exoskeletons to foster inclusion and access and are mindful of the ulterior consequences these devices have to society by being respectful to the broader ecosystem where different societal stakeholders intersect.

12.4.1   Accessibility considerations

A disability may constitute a potential vulnerability for persons with reduced mobility. However, other contextual factors, such as access to a high level of care and social support, have also a determinant impact on their lives. The presence or absence of these factors may contribute to or avoid creating "cascading vulnerabilities" [30, 31].

In this respect, facilitating good mobility options for people with lack of mobility due to injuries is crucial for an inclusive society. The wheelchair, passive or motorized, and specially adapted cars are assistive devices now used by persons with complete spinal cord injuries that require from ramps and door openers. How can patients who are wheelchair-bound restore degrees of gait functioning and regaining walking abilities and how can technological innovations help people with movement impairments regain autonomy over their daily lives without such societal help? This is going to translate in similar conditions for exoskeleton users, who may need other accessibility requirements, for example, charging stations or even terrains. Public accessibility is not meant to be "at the expense" of gained accessibility from other users [31], but in complement to those [30]. Exoskeletons can be used – and have already given good results with evidence reported in numerous scientific studies – to give access to areas and activities previously with major (dis)ability barriers, for example, can exoskeletons help users to ski?

When it comes to accessibility, we should consider all members of society. That is why some researchers proposed using a life-based design approach to promote access to this technology to all society members, including children [32]. Of course, this entails many design challenges (e.g., outgrowth, learning a new skill instead of restoring a lost function) and questions market viability and implementation challenges. However, ensuring access to health-enhancing technology is essential to provide healthcare to all society members responsibly. For instance, for children, the stakes are incredibly high, especially if used at a critical phase of a child's development, as it holds out the possibility of improving the quality of life and can improve the long-term health prospects.

12.4.2   Economic considerations

Exoskeletons are as of writing an expensive, advanced piece of technological equipment, far beyond the cost level of ordinary citizens – with prices starting from $5,000, but high-end models such as HAL costing 10–20 times more. Training, maintenance, and other costs in addition quickly make owning and operating an exoskeleton something that requires state or other financial support to be made available for its end-users. In order to provide healthcare technologies, economists have to, however, weigh the costs against other investments. For example, research points to positive outcomes in patients with spinal cord injury when using exoskeletons [10], which is difficult to make calculable.

12.4.3   Inclusivity considerations

Developers usually develop exoskeletons relying on the one-size-fits-all approach, generally offering a minor adjustment to fit the person. However, this design approach does not make justice to end-users, which come with many different criteria, including height, weight, and in rehabilitation, health condition [33]. When the inclusion criteria for whom the technology's intended user is rigid, the exclusion criteria are necessarily just as strict. In this respect, by integrating a much deeper understanding of how exoskeletons users are, including gender, age, and other sensible characteristics, exoskeleton technology holds the potential for being more inclusive [33].

12.4.4   Environmental considerations

Technology requires building materials, and it is needed to evaluate environmental costs of the integrated solution to explore sustainability variables, for example, electricity consumption, battery life cycle, and re-usability of existing materials. Health concerns and environmental concerns are both strengthened when working in liaison, for not negatively impacting one when focusing on the other. Environmental considerations are important throughout the UN's Sustainable Development Goals, as is "good health and wellbeing" (SDG3), and "reduced inequalities" (SDG10). Sustainable and environmental considerations are entwined with health and equality, and general awareness of these global goals and implementing them into sociotechnical systems can thus have cascading effects.

12.4.5   Cultural considerations

With any visible major technological artefact, there is a domestication process of making it work–not only in a practical way of making it usable but also symbolically, to make it generate well-being for its users, as well as making it easy to domesticate on a cognitive level by making learning and training feasible and good processes for the users.

As we have mentioned, technology is not created in a vacuum but is also dependant on a wide variety of social actors to implement and use it well. Caregivers, technology providers, logistics, materials, resellers, policymakers, as well as the actual end-users, are all crucial in together using technologies and putting them to use in daily life [Ref. 34, 35].

12.4.6   Legal considerations

Although many regulatory instruments apply to robots, emerging technologies tend to fall into an "institutional void" [36]. Given this multiplicity of instruments, it can be challenging to understand, both during development and deployment, which regulations apply and how they apply to a precise technology [29]. For exoskeletons, experts usually highlight the overall lack of clarity on the legal frameworks governing exoskeleton use, especially about the relationship between private standards and medical device regulation. It is also unclear whether an exoskeleton is classified as a medical device [37]. Multiple nonbinding resolutions governing the use of robots and AI are making their way into the European institution panorama, confusing further what legal obligations developers should respect [29]. A significant development in this area is the evolution of the understanding of the concept of safety, which traditionally was reserved for physical safety, but that now the community and policymakers start to acknowledge the different dimensions of safety, including physical, psychological, and societal safety, will be probably important.

12.4.7   Ethical considerations

Ensuring that technology actually benefits the user in an ethically responsible way requires technology to be created in an ethically responsible way. Any research and innovation must have a proactive approach to user-engagement implementing responsible dimensions.

For the European Union, to help innovate responsibly and contribute to ensuring a desirable future for humanity translates into the RRI approach [38]. The RRI approach provides a suitable framework to guide all the social actors involved in research and innovation (R&I) processes toward this aim. From the lens of RRI, the principles of anticipation, reflection, inclusion, responsiveness, and transparency typically guide R&I processes [39].

A recurrent notable ethical concern is whether exoskeleton normalization may make users appear less than human. This feeling appears both in rehabilitation contexts, where the stigmatization of the disability would be more evident caused to the use of the device and factories where workers using exoskeletons could be considered hybrid machine-optimized bodies employed for increased efficiency reasons, resonating existing discourses on the dehumanization of work and the workers' possible exploitation [37].

12.5   Conclusion

What is the cultural impact of living with such a technology as a social exoskeleton? In looking at impact, we utilize the concept of domestication theory, from STS to critically examine how technology is used on a practical, symbolic, and cognitive level by its users, who co-produce technology in the process of adapting it to their everyday lives.

The problem of limited mobility is exacerbated when a person is far from large metropolitan centers, which can offer home delivery of goods, transportation to and from services and healthcare, activities, and social events.

Reduced mobility impacts especially older adults, which is worsened considering the fact that their relatives may live in distant places. One of the primary needs in a sustainable implementation of healthcare robot technologies and solutions is defining their use through regulatory initiatives. However, the area of research relating to the use of AI and robotic platforms in healthcare is so new that is scarcely regulated. To provide a thorough analysis of concrete legal and regulatory issues in relation to cyber-physical systems in healthcare settings and devise specific-domain and robot-type sensitive policy recommendations for healthcare is novel in comparison to the general recommendations for robot governance that have been released so far (Robolaw Project 2014, RockEU 2016, Resolution 2015/2103 (INL) 2017, AI Now Report 2017, Intel Report 2017).

We have argued that the current level of development of rehabilitation-oriented powered exoskeletons have not yet addressed the need of an aging population. The integration in these technologies of social characteristics already common in care robots, may provoke a disruptive innovation. However, implementing robotic care technologies brings implications and impacts on society that must be carefully analyzed. Together with a suggested assessment method called ROBIA, we have built on the concept of RRI in line with the European Commission, to introduce seven societal considerations that may help designers, developers, and deployers to think and plan the path for the future of social exoskeletons.

12.5.1 Acknowledgments

We would like to thank CoRobotics for the hospitality in Pontedera, Italy during the execution of this work, and to its CEO Manuele Bonaccorsi and its Chief Research Officer Filippo Cavallo, Professor at the BioRobotics Institute, Scuola Superiore Sant'Anna in Pisa, Italy, for the important discussions.

12.5.2 Disclosure statement

There are no conflicts of interest to declare.

12.5.3 Funding

This work was supported by the EU Horizon 2020 Programme Marie Skłodowska-Curie Research and Innovation Staff Exchange (MSCA-RISE) under the project "LIFEBOTS Exchange" Grant agreement ID: 824047.

References

[1]   Shi D., Zhang W., Zhang W., Ding X. 'A review on lower limb rehabilitation exoskeleton robots'. *Chinese Journal of Mechanical Engineering*. 2019, vol. 32(1), p. 74.

[2]   Baunsgaard C., Nissen U., Brust A., *et al.* 'Exoskeleton gait training after spinal cord injury: an exploratory study on secondary health conditions'. *Journal of Rehabilitation Medicine*. 2018, vol. 50(9), pp. 806–13.

[3]   Gorgey A.S., Sumrell R., Goetz L.L. 'Exoskeletal assisted rehabilitation after spinal cord injury'. *Atlas of Orthoses and Assistive Devices*. 2019, pp. 440–7.

[4]   Esquenazi A., Talaty M. 'Robotics for lower limb rehabilitation'. *Physical Medicine and Rehabilitation Clinics of North America*. 2019, vol. 30(2), pp. 385–97.

[5]   Fosch-Villaronga E., Özcan B. 'The progressive intertwinement between design, human needs and the regulation of care technology: the case of

lower-limb exoskeletons'. *International Journal of Social Robotics*. 2020, vol. 12(4), pp. 959–72.

[6] Marinov B. 'Why wearable exoskeleton technology?' *Exoskeleton Report*. 2017.

[7] Nam K.Y., Kim H.J., Kwon B.S., Park J.-W., Lee H.J., Yoo A. 'Robot-assisted gait training (Lokomat) improves walking function and activity in people with spinal cord injury: a systematic review'. *Journal of Neuroengineering and Rehabilitation*. 2017, vol. 14(1), p. 24.

[8] Banala S.K., Kim S.H., Agrawal S.K., Scholz J.P. 'Robot assisted gait training with active leg exoskeleton (ALEX)'. *IEEE Transactions on Neural Systems and Rehabilitation Engineering : A Publication of the IEEE Engineering in Medicine and Biology Society*. 2009, vol. 17(1), pp. 2–8.

[9] van Asseldonk E.H., van der Kooij H. 'Robot-aided gait training with LOPES'. Neurorehabilitation Technology; 2012. pp. 379–96.

[10] Tefertiller C., Hays K., Jones J., *et al.* 'Initial outcomes from a multicenter study utilizing the Indego powered exoskeleton in spinal cord injury'. *Topics in Spinal Cord Injury Rehabilitation*. 2018, vol. 24(1), pp. 78–85.

[11] Kwon B.S., Nam Y.G., Lee H.J., Jo E.H., Lee J.W. 'Effects of electromechanical assisted gait training with Exowalk® on walking ability of chronic stroke patients: a randomized controlled trial'. *Annals of Physical and Rehabilitation Medicine*. 2018, vol. 61, p. e35.

[12] Lajeunesse V., Vincent C., Routhier F., Careau E., Michaud F. 'Exoskeletons' design and usefulness evidence according to a systematic review of lower limb exoskeletons used for functional mobility by people with spinal cord injury'. *Disability and Rehabilitation. Assistive Technology*. 2016, vol. 11(7), pp. 535–47.

[13] HAL [Hybrid Assistive Limb]. *Cyborg-type robot [online]*. 2021. Available from https://www.cyberdyne.jp/english/products/HAL/.

[14] Lokomat. *Relearning to walk from the beginning [online]*. 2021. Available from https://www.hocoma.com/solutions/lokomat-2/.

[15] Project March. 2021. Available from https://www.projectmarch.nl/ [Accessed 15 Jun 2021].

[16] Ascend. *Roam robotics, CA, United States [online]*. 2021. Available from https://www.roamrobotics.com/health/.

[17] Koseki K., Yozu A., Takano H., *et al.* 'Gait training using the Honda walking assist Device® for individuals with Transfemoral amputation: a report of two cases'. *Journal of Back and Musculoskeletal Rehabilitation*. 2020, vol. 33(2), pp. 339–44.

[18] Louie D.R., Eng J.J. 'Powered robotic exoskeletons in post-stroke rehabilitation of gait: a scoping review'. *Journal of NeuroEngineering and Rehabilitation*. 2016, vol. 13(1), p. 53.

[19] Chen G., Chan C.K., Guo Z., Yu H. 'A review of lower extremity assistive robotic exoskeletons in rehabilitation therapy'. *Critical Reviews in Biomedical Engineering*. 2013, vol. 41(4-5), pp. 343–63.

[20] Gorgey A., Sumrell R., Goetz L. *Exoskeletal Assisted Rehabilitation After Spinal Cord Injury. Atlas of Orthoses and Assistive Devices, 5e*. Canada: Elsevier; 2018. pp. 440–7.

[21] Glader E. V. 'Stroke care in Sweden'. Umeå University Medical Dissertations. ISBN 91-7305-426-7; 2003.

[22] Toda M., Nakatani E., Omae K., Fukushima M., Chin T. 'Age-specific characterization of spinal cord injuries over a 19-year period at a Japanese rehabilitation center'. *PloS one*. 2018, vol. 13(3), p. e0195120.

[23] Fassett D.R., Harrop J.S., Maltenfort M., *et al*. 'Mortality rates in geriatric patients with spinal cord injuries'. *Journal of Neurosurgery. Spine*. 2007, vol. 7(3), pp. 277–81.

[24] Federici S., Meloni F., Bracalenti M. *Gait Rehabilitation with Exoskeletons. Handbook of Human Motion. Chapter: 80*. Berlin: Springer; 2016.

[25] Fosch-Villaronga E. *Robot Impact Assessment: Robots, Healthcare, and The Law*. 1st edition. London: Routledge; 2019. p. 18.

[26] Bijker W.E., Hughes T.P., Pinch T.J. (eds.). *The Social Construction of Technological Systems: New Directions in The Sociology and History of Technology*. Cambridge, MA: MIT Press; 1987.

[27] Forlizzi J. 'How robotic products become social products: an ethnographic study of cleaning in the home'. 2007 2nd ACM/IEEE International Conference on Human-Robot interaction; 2007. pp. 129–36.

[28] Stahl B.C., McBride N., Wakunuma K., Flick C. 'The empathic care robot: a prototype of responsible research and innovation'. *Technological Forecasting and Social Change*. 2014, vol. 84(11), pp. 74–85.

[29] European Commission. *Responsible research & innovation [online]*. 2019. Available from https://ec.europa.eu/programmes/horizon2020/en/h2020-section/responsible-research-innovation.

[30] Kapeller A., Felzmann H., Fosch-Villaronga E., Hughes A.-M. 'A taxonomy of ethical, legal and social implications of wearable robots: an expert perspective'. *Science and engineering ethics*. 2020, vol. 26, pp. 3229–47.

[31] Luna F. 'Identifying and evaluating layers of vulnerability – a way forward'. *Developing World Bioethics*. 2019, vol. 19(2), pp. 86–95.

[32] Fosch-Villaronga E., Čartolovni A., Pierce R.L. 'Promoting inclusiveness in exoskeleton robotics: addressing challenges for pediatric access'. *Paladyn, Journal of Behavioral Robotics*. 2020, vol. 11(1), pp. 327–39.

[33] Søraa R.A., Fosch-Villaronga E. 'Exoskeletons for all: the interplay between exoskeletons, inclusion, gender, and intersectionality'. *Paladyn, Journal of Behavioral Robotics*. 2020, vol. 11(1), pp. 217–27.

[34] Søraa R.A., Nyvoll P., Tøndel G., Fosch-Villaronga E., Serrano J.A. 'The social dimension of domesticating technology: interactions between older adults, caregivers, and robots in the home'. *Technological Forecasting and Social Change*. 2021, vol. 167(1), 120678.

[35] Søraa R.A., Fostervold M.E. 'Social domestication of service robots: the secret lives of automated guided vehicles (AGVs) at a Norwegian Hospital'. *International Journal of Human-Computer Studies*. 2021, vol. 152(2), 102627.

[36]   Hajer M. 'Policy without polity? Policy analysis and the institutional void'. *Policy Sciences*. 2003, vol. 36(2), pp. 175–95.

[37]   Fosch-Villaronga E., Özcan B. 'The progressive intertwinement between design, human needs and the regulation of care technology: the case of lower-limb exoskeletons'. *International Journal of Social Robotics*. 2020, vol. 12(4), pp. 959–72.

[38]   European Commission. *Options for strengthening responsible research & innovation [online]*. 2012. Available from https://ec.europa.eu/research/science-society/document_library/pdf_06/options-for-strengthening_en.pdf.

[39]   Aymerich-Franch L., Fosch-Villaronga E. 'A Self-Guiding tool to conduct research with embodiment technologies responsibly'. *Frontiers in Robotics and AI*. 2020, vol. 7, p. 22.

Chapter 13

SENSE-GARDEN – A concept and technology for care and well-being in dementia treatment

J. Artur Serrano[1]

13.1 Introduction

This chapter describes the original SENSE-GARDEN concept and its supporting technology. In addition, it gives an updated reporting on the current implementations in real care settings. The chapter has a technical perspective but gives insights into both the clinical and the sociological perspectives. For the validation of the SENSE-GARDEN the test sites have conducted a clinical study designed as a multisite before-after controlled trial.

The SENSE-GARDEN is an innovative and disruptive method for dementia treatment, using an immersive environment supported by digital technology, and aimed at creating sensory stimuli to practice reminiscence in individually designed sessions with the person living with dementia (PwD) and a caregiver. The concept was presented to the European Union Programme Active and Assisted Living (AAL) in 2016 and partially implemented during the SENSE-GARDEN project [1], funded under this programme. The work on that project started in June 2017 and was concluded in November 2019. The project team, including caregivers, care managers, and researchers, elected as the essence of the project "Emotions reconnect us," a sentence creating a consensus around the SENSE-GARDEN concept. Since the project has ended, the SENSE-GARDEN concept has been continuously implemented through a series of innitiatives involving the previous project partners and new actors.

The SENSE-GARDEN method aims at creating awareness in PwD by providing stimuli to the different senses, such as sight, touch, hearing, balance and smell, and ultimately leading to a re-connection with the reality around. The SENSE-GARDEN spaces consist in self-contained physical rooms equipped with digital technology to create an immersive environment and are installed in care facilities. The SENSE-GARDEN space integrates digital technologies and biographical media to produce reminiscence effects in the PwD. The media displayed in the SENSE-GARDEN space is personalised to create targeted therapy sessions for the PwD.

[1]Department of Neuromedicine and Movement Science, NTNU/Norwegian University of Science and Technology, Trondheim, Norway

Digital playlists tailored to each specific visitor's life experience are played in the space in order to promote reminisce and interaction with a caregiver. The playlists are composed based on knowledge relating to each visitor, which includes photos, videos and music. The photos and videos may be taken by the family or by the visitor in earlier days and can also be general media with public access but relevant in some way to the PwD. Scents and ambient lights related to the media being displayed complement the experience by giving a further sense of immersion and helping to create the feeling of safety and comfort necessary for a successful session. The SENSE-GARDEN uses, catalyses, establishes, and expands emotional connection, using life stories to uncover, recover, and recreate a more truthful sense of self or identity. One that is not based on what one owns, such as factual memories, as commonly done, but what one is, and that can be called the emotional capacity. A capacity of connection, of relating to people, to situations, to emotionally charged visual, olfactory and auditory stimuli, as proposed by, and already being practiced in the SENSE-GARDEN.

13.1.1   The concept

The professional caregiver (Peter) and the PwD (Maria) arrive at the entrance of the SENSE-GARDEN room, a specially designed space for reminiscence, promoting a feeling of safety (Figure 13.1). Peter scans Maria's bracelet on the RFID[a] reader placed outside on the door. The system recognises Maria and loads her Art of Life Memory Album (ALMA)[5], a life related collection of photos, films, landscapes, music, scents, and games that are collected based on what was told by Maria's family about her past experiences. The necessary information to compose the Maria's ALMA had been previously collected by using a questionnaire presented to the family of the PwD. This is called the ALMA questionnaire, focusing on life events, preferences' and emotional aspects relating to PwD. Media is collected from private items provided by the family and publicly accessible items identified in connection to the information in the ALMA questionnaire. These media are therefore relevant for her. The green light placed above the door turns to red to indicate that the SENSE-GARDEN session has started. This is the beginning of the SENSE-GARDEN live session. Peter and Maria walk through the entrance of the SENSE-GARDEN, whilst a specific soundscape and landscape are played, a scent dispersed, and a mood light creating the ambiance. Peter then selects a SENSE-GARDEN activity on the control tablet. Peter can now choose between "Play Video," which starts a video automatically chosen for Maria, or he can select "New Video," which is then manually chosen by him from the available ALMA selection for Maria. This procedure can be done any number of times for any of the activities in the SENSE-GARDEN. When Peter and Maria are finished and exit the SENSE-GARDEN, Peter scans the bracelet again. This automatically ends the SENSE-GARDEN live session.

[a]Radio-frequency identification (RFID) uses electromagnetic fields to automatically identify and track tags attached to objects (Wikipedia 2021). The tag, in the case of SENSE-GARDEN, is attached to the user's bracelet.

As seen in this scenario, relatives will have a key role in the initial adaptation of the space by providing information regarding the past of the user. After such initial setting, the SENSE-GARDEN will automatically adjust the contents to the individual user. During a session, the PwD enters the SENSE-GARDEN room accompanied by a caregiver. Together they interact with the various activities and stimuli offered by the space. These include browsing through family photographs on an interactive touchscreen or looking at preferred scenery projected onto a large wall with accompanying scents and soundscapes. An app installed in a small tablet is used by the caregiver to control the session and register feedback from the PwD in response to the media contents used in the session.

As originally written in the text of the proposal of the SENSE-GARDEN, people with dementia progressively disconnect from the world as a result of the condition; they experience loss of function, especially memory, eventually affecting their verbal communication. Language loss is a major factor for disconnecting from close ones such as family and friends. This progress is exacerbated by the lack of external stimuli, which can happen due to reduced activity and apathy in general. This is especially the case when the person enters an unfamiliar environment such as a care or nursing home. After some weeks in the new and alien place, it is common that the person reduces the interaction with others and turns increasingly inwards.

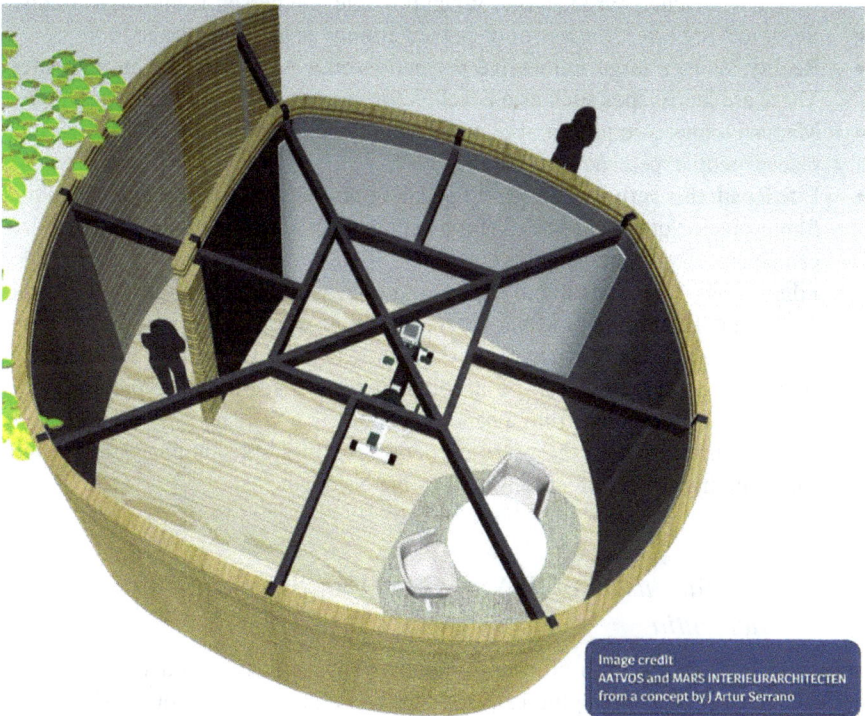

Image credit
AATVOS and MARS INTERIEURARCHITECTEN
from a concept by J Artur Serrano

Figure 13.1   The SENSE-GARDEN space – architectural concept

In an attempt to circumvent these unwanted effects, the SENSE-GARDEN method was proposed as an alternative. SENSE-GARDENs are immersive and digital spaces filled with familiar music, videos, and photos from known places and with known people. Pictures and videos are combined with music – maybe a large image of mountains together with singing birds. Smells – the odor of a pine forest – dispersed with a scent delivery system. This provides an immersive space automatically adjusted to each visitor, creating a connection to the more preserved areas of the memory and activating deeply emotional reminiscences.

During a SENSE-GARDEN visit, the PwD, together with a caregiver, takes a journey to the past and simultaneously in a space that feels safe and familiar. Activities in the SENSE-GARDEN are designed to preserve and stimulate cognitive capacity and also maintain or improve physical condition.

An activity in SENSE-GARDEN consists of a sequence of media contents that have been chosen for a specific PwD. Each activity has a defined focus and target. The following activities can be experienced in a visit to the SENSE-GARDEN. A visit can include all the activities, or a subset of activities can be chosen for that visit:

- Move to Improve: this activity consists of a very simple interactive game adjusted to the level of functioning of the user. For example, a digital interactive projection for picking apples. The game can be played from a sitting position, from a wheelchair for example. When possible, the person is invited to stand.
- Scent to Memories: the use of dispersed aromas as a reminiscence tool.
- Reality Wall: a large immersive projection on a wall to create an ambience. These are landscapes such as a beach, a forest, the ocean, mountaintops, etc.
- Memory Lane: a sequence of pictures from the past of the person. May include places, people, pets, activities, job, etc.
- Life Road: this activity consists of pedaling on a stationary bike connected to a film projected on a wall screen (for a person who is not able to pedal, a handset can be used for the same effect).
- Films of My Life: assisting to clips of old films with the aim of triggering reminiscence ("The Sound of Music", "Wizard of Oz", "Gone with the Wind", etc.)
- Music Touches Me: the use of music with which the person has an emotional connection. The music can be accompanied by a sequence of pictures, or a video such as a concert from a band or a choir.
- Sounds Surround Me: the use of soundscapes in a surrounding sound setup. Birds singing, sound of wind, waves in the ocean, etc.

13.1.2   *Primary users of SENSE-GARDEN: persons living with dementia*

Dementia is a syndrome (a group of related symptoms) associated with an ongoing decline of brain functioning [2]. Both cognitive decline symptoms, which may include memory loss and difficulties with thinking, problem-solving, or language [3], and reduction of behavioral abilities [4] are normally present in various degrees of severity. Dementia ranges in severity from the mildest stage, when it is just beginning to affect a person's functioning, to the most severe stage, when the person must depend completely on others for basic activities of daily living [4]. The SENSE-GARDEN method has been designed for PwD in stage 2 (moderate) or stage 3 (severe) according to the Clinical Dementia Rating (CDR) Scale [5]. However, the extension of its use to give access to other user groups, such as persons suffering from addictions, loneliness, depression, and other mental health diagnoses, is already underway.

Dementia can be caused by a variety of diseases, which conduce to the following recognized types of dementia. "Alzheimer disease is the most common form of dementia and may contribute to 60–70% of cases. Other major forms include vascular dementia, dementia with Lewy bodies, and a group of diseases that contribute to frontotemporal dementia. The boundaries between different forms of dementia are indistinct and mixed forms often coexist" [6]. Estimates of the various dementia types vary greatly, and mixed-type cases are very common (almost half of all cases). There are also cases where it is unclear the distinction between dementia types, as symptoms may overlap.

Dementia is really a condition of the mind that is caused by a disease of the brain [7]. It is important to note that age-specific incidence of dementia (analyzed over three decades) is declining in high-income countries [8]. According to the current version of the Diagnostic and Statistical Manual of Mental Disorders (DSM-V) [9], the term dementia is replaced by "major neurocognitive disorder" (major NCD). However, dementia is still recognized in both the scientific community and in clinical practice as an acceptable alternative term. The DSM-V lists the following, which may be affected in NCD: complex attention, executive function, learning and memory, language, perceptual motor function, and social cognition.

Dementia has currently no cure. However, our study results indicate that SENSE-GARDEN may help in reducing disease progression, improving quality of life, and have a positive effect on the emotional state. Meaningful activities, such as the ones provided in the SENSE-GARDEN, can play an important role in this process [10]. Such activities promote a reconnection to the person's identity through a walkthrough over events, places, and situations with a positive emotional charge. The SENSE-GARDEN space can provide the PwD with feelings of safety and belonging.

13.2 History of SENSE-GARDEN

The initial idea of SENSE-GARDEN began to take shape during the author's stay at the city of Tromsø, in Northern Norway. At that time, the municipality had implemented a new approach for dementia treatment with the creation of outside gardens with winding paths with various plants that could be walked and experienced using various senses like sight, smell, and touch. The idea was interesting but proved of difficult implementation due to high use of human resources for maintenance aggravated during the winter months and with limited use during such colder periods, which are long in that region with several months of snow.

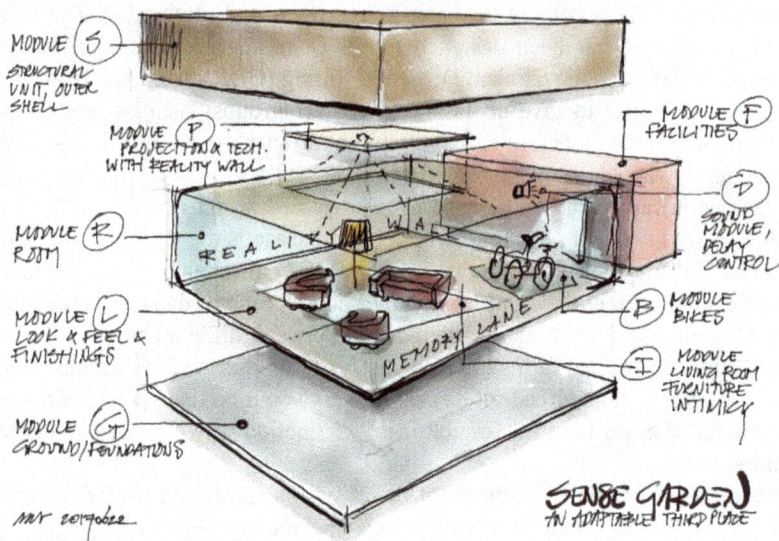

Figure 13.2   The first sketch of the SENSE-GARDEN concept produced by Aat Vos during a design session with J Artur Serrano in June 2017

A second part of the puzzle was gathered during a working period as a care helper in a local care home. In a specific situation, the author realized that memory could be stimulated in PwD by relating to events that were particularly meaningful to them and with strong emotional content. The specific situation related to mentioning scientific names of flowers to a resident who had been a gardener. This person had not spoken for over three months. He had stopped any verbal communication a few weeks after he had been admitted to the care home. Unexpectedly, when listening to the names of flowers, he began to repeat some of them. The author was surprised as he had been told of the muteness of this person.

The idea continued to develop during a series of meetings with care homes' administrators, nurses, and gerontologists, this time in the Netherlands. The concept envisioned by the author was to simulate an experience of walking outside, but in a context that was familiar to the person, so that the sensorial stimuli were targeted to arouse memories of specific moments that were meaningful in the person's life. The concept included joining activities with meaningful media contents, for example, cycling in a known forest path, singing along to the preferred music, looking at family photos, or even combining senses by looking at musical videos, or seeing pictures of baking cakes while smelling the aroma of vanilla. This idea

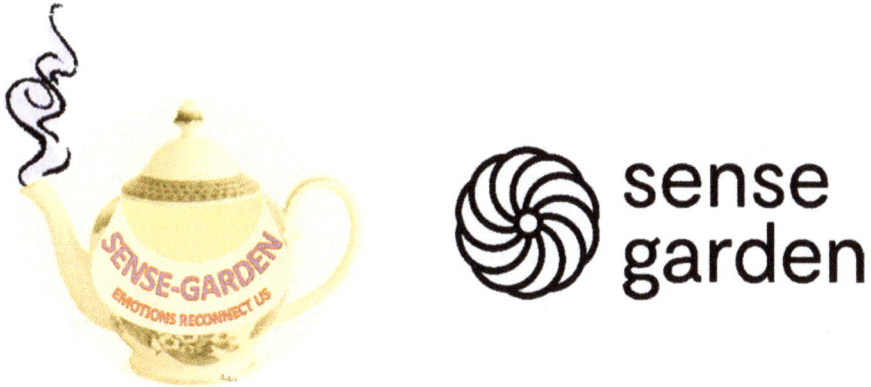

Figure 13.3   The initial logo of SENSE-GARDEN (left) and the new logo (right)

transformed into reality with the awarding of the EU grant to fund the SENSE-GARDEN project.[b]

At the initial stages of the project, a design session was set up at the site in Hamont-Achel (Belgium) to discuss possible architectures of the physical space that would, in the future, accommodate the various activities defined for the SENSE-GARDEN (Figure 13.2).

Together with the development of the system, it was important to develop a brand. The initial logo, informally developed by the author, depicted a teapot symbolizing the combination of senses: the smell and taste of the tea, together with the feeling of warmth conveyed by the vapor going up from the pot (Figure 13.3). The new logo, on the right side of the figure, tries to get a simpler visual effect with a combination of several elements of the letter "S," from "sense," displayed in a circle symbolizing a flower.

13.3   Design and development of SENSE-GARDEN technology and method

This section gives a total perspective of the process of creating the SENSE-GARDEN technology and method following a timeline from the early stages of design to the final produced technology: the SENSE-GARDEN rooms and SENSE-GARDEN system.

The project integrated a multidisciplinary team, including elements from a wide range of professional activities such as caregiving, medical aid, technology, law, architecture, business, research, etc. This wide range of competencies provided a

---

[b]SENSE-GARDEN project (AAL/Call2016/054-b/2017) www.sense-garden.eu.

F/ NF	#	Description	Purport (why we do this, why is it important to the users and/or research)	Prior ity	Read iness	Follow-up comments
f	UR14	Life road. Starting and stopping pedaling will start and stop the video motion, respectively.	This will improve the sense of immersion.	c	d	"What about correlating the speed and walking or cycling with the speed the images run with" (Professional caregiver)
f	UR19	The system will automatically adapt in response to the emotional status of the PwD. For example, the system will automatically change a piece of music upon recognising that the PwD is agitated.	It is important to understand the needs of the PwD and adhere to these needs. Having a system which can automatically adapt to these needs will be beneficial.	f	w	This is a part of the advanced AI module to be considered in the future. "Maybe in the future the system will recognise the emotional status of the user, by itself, and play accordingly" (IT manager)
f	UR20	The guide will be able to adjust levels of sensory stimulation. For example, the guide may only choose to use SurroundMe during the SENSE-GARDEN session.	Several user representatives raised the issue of overstimulation. Having the choice of using as many or as few SG components at once will help to avoid negative side effects of under or overstimulation.	c	d	"Never use too many stimuli once. The effect of overstimulation will be the opposite of what we expect." (Professional caregiver)
f	UR22	Introduce smiley ratings per activity	This way we can know what the PwD likes to do in the SENSE-GARDEN. How much time they use in activity and which ones they choose by themselves	c	d	Two ways of collecting the data: automatic based on the time spent on the activity. The manual one is input by the caregiver when the PwD can decide waht is the activity they want to do next. (IT specialist)
nf	UR10	Visual memory markers should be integrated into the Liferoad content.	It is important to create a sense of story/coherence across the sessions. This may also aid memory improvement.	f	w	"Walking or cycling with a clear aim, purpose and marks (stops where the story can be developed), in order to stimulate interest and a sense of coherence." (Informal caregiver)
nf	UR11	The PwD has a means of stopping the SENSE-GARDEN session immediately if they wish to do so	It is important to give the PwD a sense of autonomy/control over the sessions	c	d	"Use 'Stop' keywords or other modality for the user to be in control and to stop the experience when he or she wants to. Maybe you can use Alexa for it "Alexa, stop this now." (Informal caregiver)

Table caption

Priority					
c	Compulsory	n	Negotiable	f	Future work

Readiness		
d	Done	w	Whish list

Figure 13.4   An excerpt of the SENSE-GARDEN user requirements list

wide range of perspectives on what should be achieved, what may be achieved, and how to achieve it. This rich mixture of perspectives created its own path in the development of the project. This process can be analyzed through a sociotechnical network approach [11]. The result was the creation of four innovative spaces in Norway, Belgium, Portugal, and Romania that implemented the original concept and idea of technology.

13.3.1   User-centered design process

The process of developing the SENSE-GARDEN technology followed a User-Centered Design (UCD) process with the involvement of end users, including PwD and carers. Both care professionals and family carers contributed to the design process.

UCD followed an iterative approach consisting of three phases where users were involved from the start and during the full project life cycle. In this approach, the users were progressively more involved, thus minimizing the risk of failure in the introduction of the technology. Evaluation sessions have been conducted in all the four sites.

The first phase aimed at a first impression of the user experience with nonfunctional low-fidelity prototypes (e.g., mock-ups) and involved small groups of users (from 3 to 5) in care facilities. The focus was on users who are normally engaged and positive in testing new solutions and technologies – referred to as "super-users." That is, users who: are themselves PwD, adopt an intrigued and active attitude toward new technologies targeted to their condition, and are willing to try out and give feedback on the technology and services produced in the project.

The second phase focused on individual users and aimed at a deeper understanding of the users' needs and requirements. At this stage, an Alpha version of the SENSE-GARDEN system was already available for testing with a large part of the functionality included. Methods used included semi-structured interviews and usability testing with the help of use cases. This has been performed in a controlled laboratory environment and not in real settings.

The third phase corresponded to a pre-trial and was then conducted in the real settings, the SENSE-GARDEN rooms. We started with a small number of users for technical feasibility testing (1–2 users per site).

An excerpt of the final user requirements list produced as a result of the UCD process is given in Figure 13.4.

After this process, the trials were initiated in the various test sites. At this stage, a collaborative requirements list supported by a spreadsheet was not ideal for the users in the test sites. For this reason, the Consortium switched to the use of a ticketing system where requirements from users could be issued through email sent directly to the helpdesk system. These emails were automatically transcribed into tickets, which constituted the new adjusted requirements to be resolved by the development team. The nature of these requirements was normally related to improvements in the system functionality and on the user interface.

13.3.2   SENSE-GARDEN system architecture

The foundation of the SENSE-GARDEN system architecture is a data structure defined as a UML Class Model [12]. This model is reproduced below in Figure 13.5. The figure was divided in two parts due to page size limitation. This model represents the structure for the data repository (local cloud) in each organization owning a SENSE-GARDEN. This structure holds all the data (media elements such as images and videos) and metadata (information about the media elements such as place, date, etc.). It also holds all the information regarding the sessions in the SENSE-GARDEN as explained hereafter. All personal data is encrypted and local to the institution. Access is only possible by use of username and password, and accesses are limited by each individual user, defining which caregivers have access to which PwD's data.

The UML model includes all the information regarding the users and their experiences in the visits to the SENSE-GARDEN. Data are resulting of two methods: direct input from the caregivers and automatically collected by the equipment in the SENSE-GARDEN.

The connection between the SENSE-GARDEN User Profile ("User") and the SENSE-GARDEN Content Data Storage ("MediaRepository") is done through the concept of playlists, called "Flows." Each session in the SENSE-GARDEN is called a "LiveSession" and is composed of a series of "Flows."

Any SENSE-GARDEN Session includes a PwD ("Primary user") and a "Caregiver" with the constraint: each caregiver in the SENSE-GARDEN can only

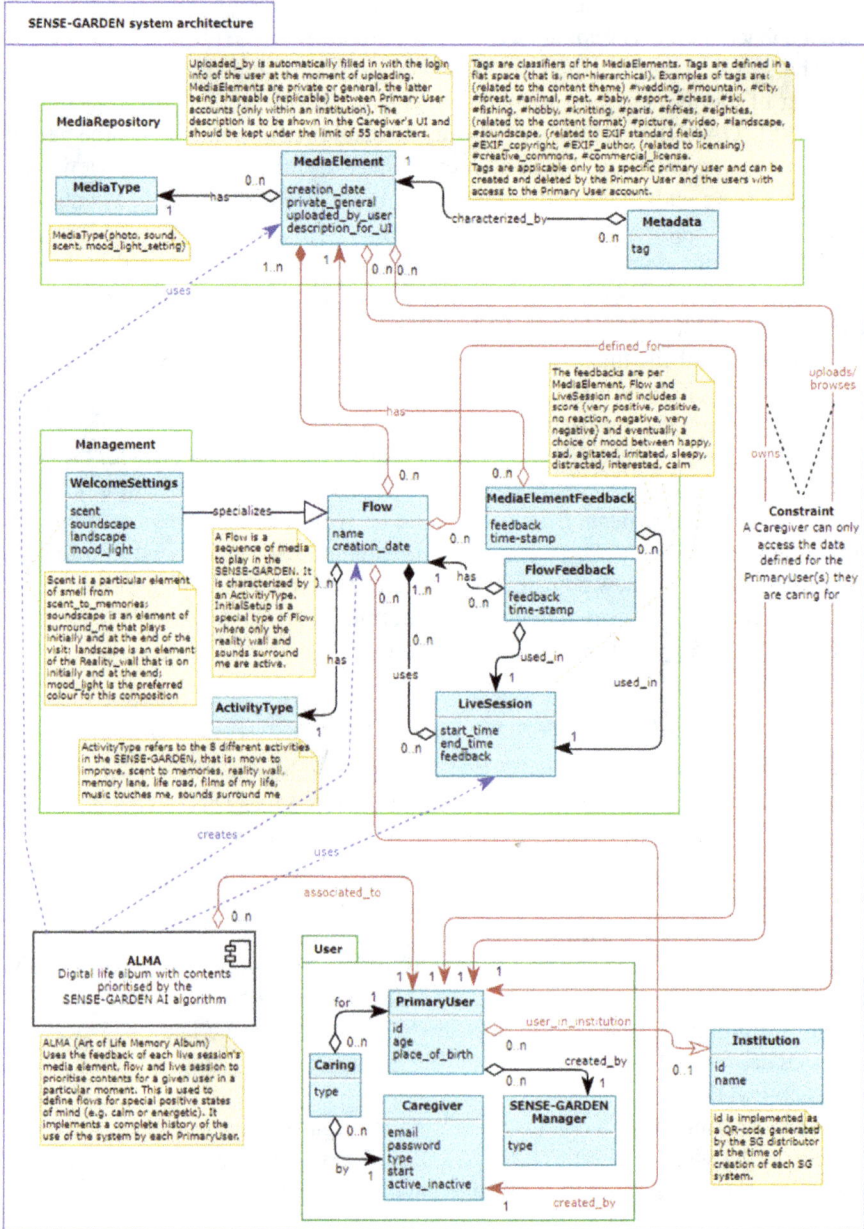

Figure 13.5   The SENSE-GARDEN system architecture

access data owned by PwD they care for ("Caring"). A "LiveSession" has a start time, an end time. Each LiveSession can receive a "feedback" evaluation given by

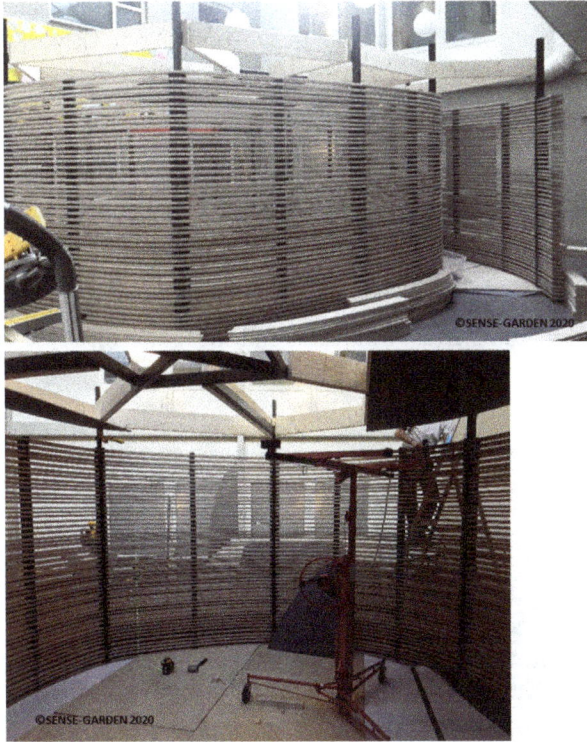

Figure 13.6   The construction of the SENSE-GARDEN room in Odda, Norway

the caregiver through the User Interface in the tablet at the end of each session. To note that each individual session element, a media element used in the live session, such as a video, a music track, or a picture, can also receive a "feedback" evaluation by the caregiver during the session.

13.3.3   Building a SENSE-GARDEN room

The SENSE-GARDEN space takes the form of a physical room usually built inside a dementia care environment, such as a care home, a daily care center, or an hospital. The room provides both a physical and emotional shelter to the user, helping to promote feelings of comfort and safety. Inside this room, personalized music, films, photographs, and dispersed scents, together with soothing lights, are combined to create a fully immersive environment specially tailored to each person's life story, interests, and preferences. The process of creating a SENSE-GARDEN room starts by finding the appropriate space. This can be an open area inside the organization, such as a large hall or common area. The space must be large enough to accommodate the SENSE-GARDEN hut, which measures approximately 25 m^2 (typically 4.5 × 5.5 m). In a simpler setting, it can also be created as an adaptation of an existing empty room that can be prepared to function as a SENSE-GARDEN room.

The example in the pictures (Figure 13.6) shows the construction of a hut using a CNC[c] process, with technical production by Artisan Tech, Oslo, with the creative direction of Aat Vos and Mars Interieurarchitecten, following a concept by J Artur Serrano.

13.3.4   The final technology: a SENSE-GARDEN room and system

The product to be sold is a configurable care and well-being technology for the treatment of persons with moderate to advanced dementia. The SENSE-GARDEN offers an immersive experience that stimulates the senses of the user (smell, sight, audition, and proprioception) in order to create a safe space where reconnection to emotional memory can increase awareness and strengthen the sense of self. Unlike

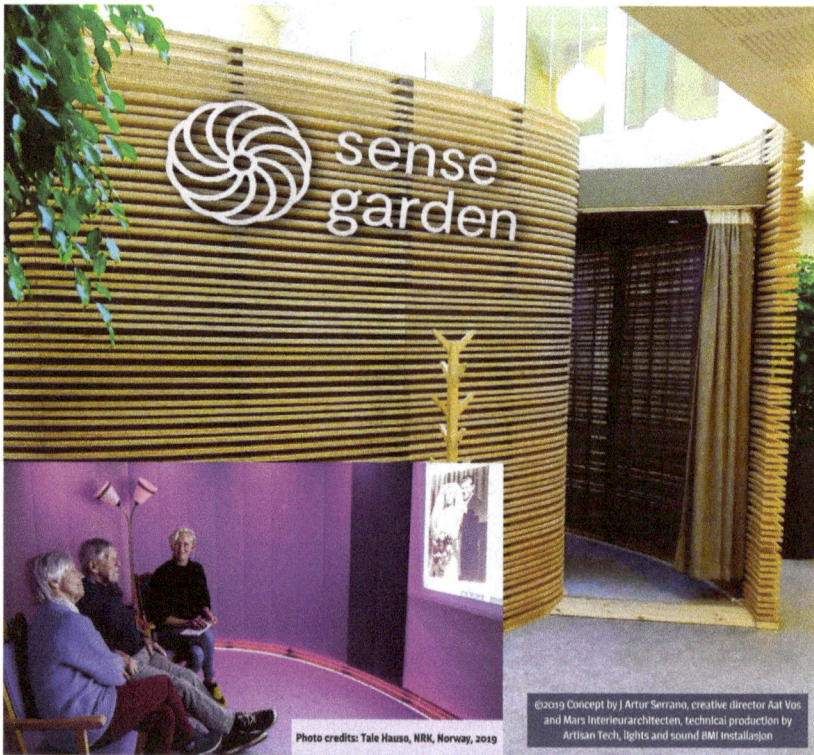

Figure 13.7   *The SENSE-GARDEN in Bokkotunet care home, Odda, Norway*

[c]CNC stands for "computer numerical control," and CNC machining is a subtractive manufacturing process, which typically employs computerized controls and machine tools to remove layers of material from a stock piece – known as the blank or workpiece – and produces a custom-designed part. (Based on definition by Thomas Publishing Company, https://www.thomasnet.com/articles/custom-manufacturing-fabricating/understanding-cnc-machining/, accessed on 02/03/2021.)

current products based on reminiscence or Snoezelen, where the kits are generic and not personalized, the SENSE-GARDEN offers a totally individualized experience based on the events lived by each individual customer.

The target market was, at the start, limited to the four countries in the Consortium (Norway, Belgium, Portugal, and Romania) and is progressively expanding to the neighboring countries, that is, Sweden, Denmark, the Netherlands, and Spain. Two companies in Europe will sell the SENSE-GARDEN with a model of one-time payment of hardware and an annual license fee for software maintenance and general support.

13.4 The existing SENSE-GARDENs

In the course of the SENSE-GARDEN project four rooms were constructed in four countries, which became operational during 2018 and 2019. The SENSE-GARDEN rooms had already received over 700 visits by the end of 2020. All these four rooms are currently in routine operation, although under some restrictions imposed by the regulations associated with the COVID-19 pandemic. Three of these SENSE-GARDENs were constructed inside care homes, while one of them was built inside an hospital facility. Short descriptions of the existing SENSE-GARDENs are given below.

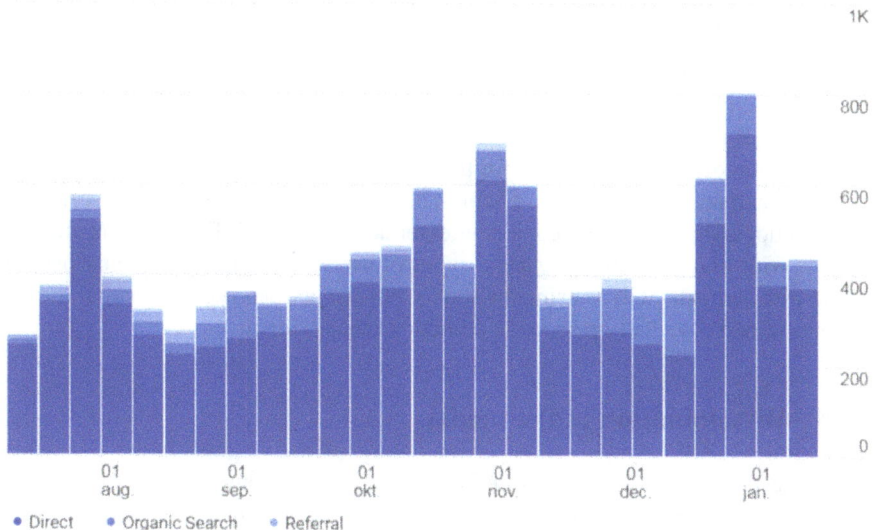

Figure 13.8   *Results of Google analytics regarding visits to the SENSE-GARDEN website during the months of July 2020 to January 2021*

13.4.1   Bokkotunet care home, Odda (Norway)

The care home is located in the centre of Odda, a small city of less than 5 000 inhabitants, located in the Hardanger district. It is owned by the municipality and provides accommodation, daily care, and occupational activities. The room has been built in an inside large hall, as has the shape of a "shell" constructed in wood with interiors covered in wool. In Figure 13.7, the exterior and the interior of the SENSE-GARDEN room are shown.

13.4.2   Aan de Beverdijk care home, Hamont-Achel (Belgium)

Located in a calm country-side area, in the municipality of Hamont-Achel in the Belgian province of Limburg, the carehome is one of the 33 care homes owned by the VULPIA care group. The SENSE-GARDEN room was constructed by renovating a small room inside the facility.

13.4.3   Lar Santa Joana Princesa care home, Lisbon (Portugal)

The SENSE-GARDEN room placed in Lisbon, the capital city of Portugal, has been built inside a care facility located in the centre of this large metropolis. The facility is a part of the patrimony of Lisbon Holy House of Mercy MHIH, a charitable organisation, with public activity responsibility, and overseen by the public Secretary of State for Social Security. The SENSE-GARDEN room features a large round projection wall and, as the other SENSE-GARDENs, adjustable ambient lights, and surround sound to provide an immersive experience to its users.

13.4.4   ELIAS Emergency University Hospital in Bucharest (Romania)

This is the only SENSE-GARDEN built inside an hospital facility. It has been created in a room part of the rehabilitation clinic at the ELIAS Emergency University Hospital in Bucharest.

Inclusion of different contexts for the construction of SENSE-GARDENs, such as private and public managed care homes, hospitals and other types of care-oriented organizations, shows that the scope of intervention of the SENSE-GARDEN method is quite wide and adaptable to various types of users. In the future not only people living with dementia will be using the rooms, but also various types of mental illness diagnoses, and eventually persons in addiction rehabilitation.

13.5   Dissemination in the media

The project has had a large exposure in the media, when comparing to the average exposure of projects in the AAL EU-Programme. This includes 13 presentations at conferences and 12 in mass media including newspapers, official social media, and TV. The project was featured in national broadcasting news agencies in Romania, Belgium, and Norway. During the final months of 2020 and January of 2021, the website of the project had an average of over 500-page hits per week, with the last week in December reaching 800 hits (Figure 13.8).

13.6   Testing the SENSE-GARDEN technology

This chapter is primarily targeting the SENSE-GARDEN technology, and therefore only a brief summary of the more clinically oriented research is presented herein. For detailed information on each of the particular studies, the reader is invited to refer to the published research mentioned in this section. The studies conducted in the scope of the SENSE-GARDEN EU-project were a part of the overall multisite before–after controlled trial executed in the test sites of the project.

The protocol for this trial has been published [13], and various studies, both qualitative and quantitative, have been conducted in the scope of the trial. Below are given the summaries of the obtained results. Part of the quantitative data is under analysis at the moment of publishing of this chapter and, therefore, only preliminary data is available; the complete results are expected to be published in the course the current year (2021).

Users involved in the trial included the primary users: persons with intermediate to advanced dementia, 55 years of age and above; formal secondary users: care staff; informal secondary users: mostly family but also neighbors and friends; and tertiary users: care home managers and insurance companies.

Total number of users involved:

> Primary: 27 completed the study (in addition to this number were several drop-outs due to death)
> Secondary formal: 11
> Secondary informal: between 20 and 25.

The mean age of primary users was 81.44 years. The participants were 16 females and 11 males. Twenty participants had moderate dementia, and seven had severe dementia according to the CDR Scale.

In the following sections, a summary of the results obtained in the studies is given. The impact will be analyzed in two dimensions: qualitative and quantitative.

13.6.1   Qualitative impact studies

A study on the user perspectives toward the SENSE-GARDEN concept explored the initial responses from user groups across Belgium, Norway, Portugal, and Romania. Through exploring these responses, subsequent development of the SENSE-GARDEN could be shaped to meet the desires and needs of the users. Additionally, it was important to identify any potential concerns that the users may have had. Six themes were generated from thematic analysis of the interview transcripts. These included: benefits for all, focus on the individual, past and present, emotional stimulation, shared experiences, and challenges to consider [14].

A second qualitative study explored the experiences of care staff in all the test sites, in their use of SENSE-GARDEN. Reflexive thematic analysis of the interviews was used to generate themes and their respective subthemes. A paper on this study has been submitted for publication [15].

The third and last qualitative study explored the experiences of PwD and their caregivers within the SENSE-GARDEN from a transactional perspective with the aim to explore how narrative identity and interpersonal relationships are shaped by the use of technology. Three themes were generated from reflective thematic analysis: openness, learning, and connecting. The first theme, openness, reflects the way in which SENSE-GARDEN encouraged individuals (not only participants with dementia) to become more open in their communication with one another, particularly with regards to expressing emotions and discussing personal subjects. The second theme, learning, addresses the way in which SENSE-GARDEN can provide knowledge on (a) optimizing care through the use of personalized environments and individual focus on the resident, (b) understanding the PwD, and (c) learning more about the unique life story of the resident, even for family members. The third theme, connecting, encapsulates how connections are made between individuals while using SENSE-GARDEN together. This connection can happen through: (a) "care" reporting on how facilitated sessions enhanced the caregiver-resident relationship and the overall SENSE-GARDEN experience, (b) "technology" reporting on how the technology used in SENSE-GARDEN prompted conversation and connected participants to their own sense of identity, (c) "space" reporting on how participants considered the SENSE-GARDEN space to help them feel safe and connected, and (d) "memories" reporting on how participants connected through reminiscing about memories that were triggered and shared during the sessions, and how these memories remained intact after the sessions [16].

13.6.2   *Quantitative impact studies*

For the acquisition of quantitative data during the trials, we have used the following scales: BPSD: behavioral and psychological symptoms of dementia; CMAI: Cohen–Mansfield Agitation Inventory; BANS-S: Bedford Alzheimer Nursing Scale–Severity; QUALID: Quality of Life in Late Stage Dementia scale; CSDD: Cornell Scale for Depression in Dementia; OERS: Observed Emotion Rating Scale; OME: Observational Measurement of Engagement; VNVIS-CR: Verbal and Nonverbal Interaction Scale; Mini-Cog: 3-min instrument to screen for cognitive impairment in older adults; FAST: Functional Assessment Staging Tool; GDS: Global Deterioration Scale; ICF: International Classification of Functioning, Disability and Health; WHODAS 2.0: World Health Organization Disability Assessment Schedule 2.0; FRT: Functional Reach Test; ZBI: Zarit Burden Interview; Brief-COPE: abbreviated version of the Coping Orientation to Problems Experienced inventory, a self-report questionnaire [13].

These scales have been transferred into spreadsheets, producing over 1 000 lines of data. Publication of the results is currently under preparation [17, 18].

13.6.3 Ethical concerns

The SENSE-GARDEN trial was conducted across Norway, Portugal, Belgium, and Romania. The ethical acceptance procedures followed national guidelines; these included: In Norway, the regulating body is the Regional Committee for Medical and Health Research Ethics to which an application was submitted and approved. In Belgium and Portugal, no ethical guidelines are defined for dementia care interventions, and only signed informed consent is required from participants. In Romania, ethical approval is issued by a commission established at the hospital where the trial is conducted. To note that in the case a participant is not able to give informed consent, as was the case with several persons with dementia in the trial, the consent was given by proxy, normally a family member.

Additional information of the safety issues around the SENSE-GARDEN intervention can be found in the publication by Ciobanu *et al.* [19].

13.7 SENSE-GARDEN resources

The main source of updated information on SENSE-GARDEN is its website www.sense-garden.eu. The site includes information about the currently implemented SENSE-GARDENs, the process on how to order a SENSE-GARDEN, the published dissemination materials, and the activities of the SENSE-GARDEN Association.

The data produced during the SENSE-GARDEN studies are openly available in Zenodo.

The terminology used in the SENSE-GARDEN method can be found at the "SENSE-GARDEN Glossary of terms" in https://sites.google.com/view/sense-garden-glossary-of-terms/home.

13.8 The future SENSE-GARDENs

The tailoring and personalization in the SENSE-GARDEN method distinguishes it from other multisensory interventions [20]. Future developments in the SENSE-GARDEN will bring Artificial Intelligence (AI) algorithms and emotions-based analysis. AI will be used to identify a user's affective state. Sensors can automatically detect the affect of the user [21], and AI algorithms may be used to tailor the user experience based on this data. The use of state-of-the art automatic affect detection methods in combination with adaptive Human-Computer Interaction (HCI) components will be the novel and disruptive addition to the SENSE-GARDEN technology. This has the potential of enabling the system to adapt itself automatically to the user's needs and preferences. Once the system detects a user's affect, it will combine this information with other information it can gather from the situation, for example, what media was the person interacting with, and what it knows about the individual, for example, what activities the person enjoys, what music do they like, in order to adjust the experience to the user.

Using the information collected by the AI engine, the system will then be able to offer the user relevant activities and dynamically refine the user's profile (ALMA). The ALMA digital patient profile will then become a living digital document, constantly being updated with more targeted media to the current state of development of the disease. The ALMA will be a mirror of the condition of the PwD at every moment. New visits to the SENSE-GARDEN will improve the accuracy of the ALMA. This will be used to automatically adjust the contents of the SENSE-GARDEN sessions and at the same time give professional caregivers and family an updated picture of the progression of the disease for each PwD.

The produced SENSE-GARDEN system achieved a technology readiness level TRL7 (system prototype demonstration in operational environment) with a full trial executed across the test sites. The current steps in the SENSE-GARDEN strategy consist in offering a SENSE-GARDEN as a commercial product, which means achieving a TRL9 (actual system proven in operational environment). To note that all the four SENSE-GARDEN spaces constructed during the original project are in continuous operation, and the responsible institutions have allocated resources that guarantee their sustainability.

Two directions are envisaged that will happen in parallel: a commercial way and a further development of research aspects mainly in the AI area. A commercial front is being planned in Norway led by Prof. J. Artur Serrano.

13.9   Conclusion

The chapter presented the concepts underlying the technological innovation called SENSE-GARDEN method.

Findings from the studies conducted in four SENSE-GARDEN installations have shown that for the person with dementia (PwD) the SENSE-GARDEN helps preserving identity and self-awareness. Through exposure to different stimuli to the senses, totally related to the person's life story it is possible to create individualised experiences to trigger emotional connection and promote a reconnection with past and present. Through meaningful activities, the SENSE-GARDEN experience can catalyse the interpersonal relationships amongst people living with dementia and their caregivers. For the caregivers, both staff and family members, SENSE-GARDEN helps to deeply connect with the person with dementia despite the daily challenges that the condition presents.

The above findings suggest that the SENSE-GARDEN therapy has positive outcomes for both the persons with dementia and their caregivers. The reconnection with life experiences facilitated in the SENSE-GARDEN has proven to be very valuable to care staff in providing detailed knowledge about the PwD. There were also cases that new knowledge has shed more light on the life story of the person for family caregivers: "The experience itself has probably caused me to open my eyes to small things that I have not noticed before. Things I had no idea meant anything to him" [16].

A strong international network of institutions from several countries has been created and is in constant expansion. The network includes the four countries involved in the studies, that is, Norway, Portugal, Romania, and Belgium, which feature one SENSE-GARDEN each, with plans for several extensions with new SENSE-GARDENs being added. In addition to these countries, several institutions and organizations from Canada, Switzerland, and the Netherlands have been supporting efforts in the new developments related to the SENSE-GARDEN concept.

13.10 Acknowledgments

The author would like to thank all the participants in the SENSE-GARDEN project, especially to the professionals working at the test sites involved in the conduction of the studies, led by Dr. Rita Valadas, in Portugal, with the local coordination of Dr. Sigrid Eitrheim, Norway, Nurse Marleen Custers, Belgium, and the clinical team in Romania lead by Prof. Dr. Mihai Berteanu, which includes Dr. Ileana Ciobanu, Dr. Andreea Marin, and Dr. Rozeta Draghici; the technology development team led by Iulian Anghelache; Ronny Broekx who was both collaborating in the technology improvement and leading the marketing strategy; the researchers responsible for the data collection and reporting, led by Dr. Gemma Goodall, with the collaboration of Dr. Lara André; the expert guidance of Dr. Christophe Van Dijken, MD, Specialist in Gerontology and Geriatrics in the concept definition phase, and of Prof. Katrin Losleben in the understanding of soundscapes; and finally all the involved PwD and their families.

13.11 Disclosure statement

There are no conflicts of interest to declare.

13.12 Funding

This work was supported by AAL under Grant AAL/Call2016/054-b/2017, co-funded by the European Commission and National Funding Agencies of Norway, Belgium, Romania, and Portugal.

References

[1] SENSE-GARDEN. 2018. Available from http://www.sense-garden.eu/.

[2] NHS. *About dementia – dementia guide* [online]. 2020. Available from https://www.nhs.uk/conditions/dementia/about/ [Accessed 06 July 2021].

[3] Alzheimer's Society. *What is dementia?* [online] Factsheet 400LP. Alzheimer's Society; 2017. Available from https://www.alzheimers.org.uk/sites/default/files/pdf/what_is_dementia.pdf [Accessed 15 Jun 2021].

[4]   US National Institute on Aging. *Alzheimer's disease fact sheet* [online]. 2021. Available from https://www.nia.nih.gov/health/alzheimers-disease-fact-sheet.

[5]   Hughes C.P., Berg L., Danziger W.L., Coben L.A., Martin R.L. 'A new clinical scale for the staging of dementia'. *The British Journal of Psychiatry : The Journal of Mental Science.* 1982, vol. 140, pp. 566–72.

[6]   Qiu C., De Ronchi D., Fratiglioni L. 'The epidemiology of the dementias: an update'. *Current Opinion in Psychiatry.* 2007, vol. 20(4), pp. 380–5.

[7]   Dolan D. *A conversation about frontotemporal degeneration (FTD): transcription from the alzheimer's podcast 2011* [online]. 2011. Available from https://dementiasherpa.com/episode86/.

[8]   Satizabal C.L., Beiser A.S., Chouraki V., Chêne G., Dufouil C., Seshadri S. 'Incidence of dementia over three decades in the Framingham heart study'. *New England Journal of Medicine.* 2016, vol. 374(6), pp. 523–32.

[9]   American Psychiatric Association. *Diagnostic and Statistical Manual of Mental Disorders (Dsm-5®).* Philadelphia: American Psychiatric Pub; 2013.

[10]   Goodall G., Taraldsen K., Serrano J.A. 'The use of technology in creating individualized, meaningful activities for people living with dementia: a systematic review'. *Dementia.* 2021, vol. 20(4), pp. 1442–69.

[11]   Sørgaard J., Berteanu M., Serrano J.A. 'Reconnecting with past and present – personalizing sensory stimulated reminiscence through immersive technologies – developing a multidisciplinary perspective on the SENSE-GARDEN room'. *Proceedings of the 4th International Conference on Information and Communication Technologies for Ageing Well and e-Health.* 2018, vol. 1, pp. 234–40.

[12]   Fowler M. *UML Distilled: A Brief Guide to the Standard Object Modeling Language.* Third Edition. Addison-Wesley Professional. ISBN: 9780321193681; 2003.

[13]   Goodall G., Ciobanu I., Taraldsen K., *et al.* 'The use of virtual and immersive technology in creating personalized multisensory spaces for people living with dementia (SENSE-GARDEN): protocol for a multisite before-after trial'. *JMIR Research Protocols.* 2019, vol. 8(9),e14096.

[14]   Goodall G., Ciobanu I., Broekx R., *et al.* 'The role of adaptive immersive technology in creating personalised environments for emotional connection and preservation of identity in dementia care - Insights from user perspectives towards SENSE-GARDEN'. *International Journal on Advances in Life Sciences.* 2019, vol. 2, pp. 13–22.

[15]   Goodall G., Taraldsen K., Granbo R., Serrano J.A. 'Towards personalized dementia care through meaningful activities supported by technology: a multisite qualitative study with care professionals'. *Submitted for publication.* 2021, vol. 111.

[16]   Goodall G., Andrea L., Taraldsen K., Serrano J.A. 'Supporting identity and relationships amongst people with dementia through the use of technology: a qualitative interview study'. *International Journal of Qualitative Studies on Health and Well-being.* 2020, vol. 16(1), pp. 1–26.

[17] Ciobanu I., Marin A.G., Zamfir M.-V. 'Case series of an ICT-based multi-modal intervention program for persons with major neurocognitive disorders: the SENSE-GARDEN project'. *Submitted for publication.* 2021.

[18] Serrano J.A., Andre L., Goodall G. 'Results from the SENSE-GARDEN multisite before-after controlled trial'. *Manuscript in preparation.* 2021.

[19] Ciobanu I., Marin A.G., Draghici R., *et al.* 'Safety aspects in developing new technologies for reminiscence therapy: insights from the SENSE-GARDEN project'. *Romanian Journal of Gerontology and Geriatrics.* 2019, vol. 8(1-2), pp. 3–8.

[20] Marin A., Ciobanu I., Serrano A., Berteanu M. 'The emotional response as outcome in reminiscence therapy'. ELAPSYT1 First International Conference on Emotions, Language Processing and Psycholinguistic Testing; Bucharest, Romania, 12–15 October; 2017. pp. 31–32.

[21] Schmidt P., Reiss A., Dürichen R., Laerhoven K.V. 'Wearable-Based affect Recognition-A review'. *Sensors.* 2019, vol. 19(19),4079.

Chapter 14

Challenges and opportunities in the adoption of IoT for the elderly's health and well-being: a systematic review

Dr Golam Sorwar[1] and Md. Rakibul Hoque[2]

Abstract

With the advent of medical science and treatment, the aging population is increasing each year globally. Supporting regular care for the aging population at a large scale is a matter of great expense and labor-intensive. Without using new technologies, it might be a challenge for most countries, if not all, to support elderlies' needs with limited resources. To address this challenge, technologies like wearable's and smart homes, powered by the Internet of Things (IoT), are now being employed to offer innovative ways to enable the elderly population to an independent living and improve health and well-being. While IoT is meant to ease the life and care of elderlies, the adoption of IoT-based devices is reported very low. Therefore, new studies should be conducted periodically to gain updated knowledge in terms of use cases and efficiency. Consequently, the authors have conducted an integrative review of the existing literature reviews on the use of IoT for older people. Twenty-six review studies were reviewed as the sources of secondary data. Broadly, three themes were identified: (1) Use Cases, (2) Adoption Barriers, and (3) Future Research Directions. The review identified that the use cases of IoT solutions fall into different categories such as physiological monitoring, emergency detection, safety monitoring, social interaction, and cognitive assistance at various levels. On the other hand, the most frequently reported barriers were privacy, security, cost, perceived usefulness, and interoperability. The most common future research directions were suggested about the inclusion of users' perspectives and use of artificial intelligence in future research. The authors conclude that a lack of formal clinical studies and contradictions in existing study findings are frequently reported. Hence, the authors suggest gathering more empirical evidence as a strong basis for a large-scale adoption of IoTs by the older population.

[1]Faculty of Science and Engineering, Southern Cross University, Lismore, Australia
[2]Department of Management Information Systems, University of Dhaka, Dhaka, Bangladesh

14.1 Introduction

The use of technology like the Internet of Things (IoT) is gaining popularity in many areas of human life, especially in the daily lives of elderlies, to make their lives convenient. While the elderly population worldwide has been increased in the last two decades due to the advancement in medical science and treatment [1], their high longevity has become a concerning matter because of the challenges of ensuring age-friendly environments for them [2, 3]. The number of people aging above 60 globally is more than the number of children below 5 years old. Today, people are expected to live beyond the age of 60 more than before. According to WHO, the older population worldwide is expected to reach nearly 22 per cent in 2050 from 12 per cent in 2015 [4]. WHO has also predicted that 80 per cent of elderlies globally will be living in the least developing and developed countries. Consequently, elderlies' families will need cost-effective solutions to assist them in their own homes and nursing homes [3]. They will require to adopt newer technologies to help the elderly population age in place with safety and convenience instead of relying on the old care homes' model.

Despite the increase in longevity, better healthcare, and more economic safety than their previous generation, today's elderlies encounter more physical and mental health challenges, including various types of cognitive and social health issues [5]. Therefore, newer technologies are being continuously used to improve their declining physical and mental capacity and support their independent livings, healthcare, safety, and comfort. The development and application of newer technologies can be part of a sustainable commitment facilitating the healthy aging of elderly people. Additionally, it will be difficult for most countries to support elderlies, which is a labor-intensive task, with limited resources without the use of assistive technologies [6]. To address this, technology like IoT is now employed to contribute innovative ways to develop integrated health systems, enable independent living, and support the well-being and healthy life of the elderly population [7].

IoT refers to interoperable networks consisting of different objects or things integrated with sensors and software to communicate data with each other [8]. For elderlies, IoT is mainly used for developing technologies like wearables and smart homes, which are often interrelated. Wearables are IoT systems that users wear to monitor their physical activities and health status [9]. On the other hand, smart homes are powered by IoT that enables users to control their home environments, such as temperature and lighting, remotely using mobile applications or even by users' voice commands. In recent times, IoT-based wearable and smart homes have increased to provide better elderly healthcare, safety, and simplicity [10, 11]. As elderlies prefer to remain and live independently, IoT-based smart home technologies are considered potential solutions in their home settings [12].

While IoT is meant to ease the life and care of elderlies, the adoption of IoT-based devices is low yet [13]. Therefore, despite many existing review studies, new studies should be conducted periodically to gain updated knowledge in terms of use cases and efficiency. According to the authors' best knowledge, no recent studies have conducted a systematic literature review of the existing reviews on IoT applications for the elderly population. Therefore, this chapter aims to fulfill this gap by reviewing the recent reviews. Review of reviews is often conducted in Information Systems (IS) to establish an evidence-based overview by synthesizing review studies [14]. This study will contribute as an overall future direction to increase the adoption of these technologies by elderlies and identify specific related issues and evidence.

In total, 26 review studies were reviewed as the sources of secondary data. Subsequently, three common themes are identified from the review studies: (1) Use Cases, (2) Adoption Barriers, and (3) Future Research Directions. Discussion of each theme is divided into two categories, i.e., wearable and smart home. The following sections present the methodology and the findings according to themes derived from secondary data synthesis.

14.2 Methodology

Conducting the literature review, the authors have followed an Integrative Review Method [15, 16] involving the thematic synthesis of secondary data to summarize the findings. The authors searched journal articles published in the last 5 years (2016–2020). The journal databases, namely PubMed, Google Scholar, MEDLINE, Elsevier, and EBSCO were searched using specific keywords: ("review") AND ("IoT" OR "Internet of Things" OR "Wearable" OR "Smart Home") AND ("elderly" OR "old" OR "senior" OR "aged").

In total, 398 studies were initially found from the database search. However, only 26 articles were reviewed as the sources of secondary data. These 26 articles were included for full-text review only when the authors agreed to review based on specific inclusion and exclusion criteria [17]. The authors only included the review studies for review related to IoT applications for elderlies and conducted in English. The authors excluded the studies related to assistive technology that were not related to Smart homes and wearables. Also, the review studies that did not primarily focus on elderlies were excluded.

14.3 Use cases of IoT

When employing IoT-based sensors, supporting seniors' independent livings using a low-cost remote monitoring system is mostly focused. The use cases are categorized into two broad categories, as presented below.

14.3.1 Use cases of wearables

By reviewing 327 journal articles, Baig *et al.* [17] conducted a systematic study indicating that IoT-integrated wearable is mostly used to detect falls and daily life activities [17]. The systematic review by Chen *et al.* [18] reported another use case of IoT, which uses wearable devices for gait analysis (assessing gait degradation and fall risks) for measuring fall risks and monitoring falls for the elderly [18]. The IoT-integrated sensors can generate data about the kinetic information of muscle activities in the gait area. Table 14.1 shows selected review studies on IoT and their use cases. When Malwade *et al.* [19] reviewed the studies on wearable technologies for aging people's healthcare, they found that IoT-based wearable devices, when used in coordination with mobile monitoring system, can enhance the quality of life of the elderly population by remotely monitoring their sleeping patterns, chronic diseases, and frailty [19].

Similarly, a recent reflective review by Tun, Madanian, and Mirza [9] focused on using IoT-based wearables for elderlies [9]. Overall, they identified 11 areas of application of wearables. Some important areas are monitoring chronic diseases, emergency conditions, human activity recognition, mental health, movement disorder, fall prevention and detection, monitoring users' vital signs, and accessing healthcare services. Apart from finding the areas of use cases, they also have categorized the data collected by IoT into five broad classes: biomechanical and physiological measures, physical mobility, blood profile, electro-cardiogram, and vital signs.

Moreover, Gordon's systematic review study shows wearables like smartwatches; smart bands are mainly used for fall detection and prevention [6]. He found that wearables can provide between 80 per cent and 100 per cent accuracy in fall detection. Besides, wearables are also used as a useful reminder for medication adherence. Another use case of wearables is to assess tremors or handshaking and neurological disorders such as dementia and Parkinson's Disease. Likewise, wearables are found convenient and beneficial in longitudinal health status monitoring. Wang *et al.* [21] reported that advanced wearables like smart clothing are used for elderly care, such as fall detection, health monitoring, and activity recognition [21].

A review study by Leirós-Rodríguez, García-Soidán, and Romo-Pérez [22] reported wearable accelerometers for assessing the balance of elderly to prevent falls [22]. Qi *et al.* [23] mentioned the use of IoT-based wearables for physical activity recognition (e.g., sleeping or resting) and health monitoring (e.g., functions of lung and heart) [23]. In a recent study, Zhong and Rau [26] reported the cost-benefit of using wearable for gait analysis for elderlies [26]. Based on 34 studies, Husebo *et al.* [24] reported that IoT-based devices are useful for targeted clinical applications such as monitoring dementia conditions and treatment response [24]. On the other hand, Rovini, Maremmani, and Cavallo [25] specifically reviewed the use cases of wearable devices to identify and monitor tremors, body motion, and motor fluctuations for the elderly with Parkinson's Disease [25].

14.3.2   Use cases of smart homes

Evaluating the impact of the use of smart homes for elderlies, Liu *et al.* [1] synthesized 14 articles in a systematic review [1]. They found smart homes positively impact the mental health of the aging population with chronic diseases with long-term (longer than a year) intervention. However, in the short-term intervention of smart home adoption, no significant impact has been reported. In an earlier systematic review, Liu *et al.* [27] analyzed 43 studies and summarized the use cases of

Table 14.1   Use cases of IoT for elderly people

Article no.	Review on	Articles reviewed	Use Cases, Barriers, and Future Directions
1	Wearables [17]	14	*Use Cases*: • Fall detection • Physical activity *Barriers*: • Low usability/user-friendly • Lack of interoperability • Low reliability of the power and battery • Limiting the users' movement *Future Directions*: • Applying artificial intelligence • Increasing interoperability
2	Wearables [18]	35	*Use Cases*: • Fall detection • Gait analysis *Barriers*: • Higher operating cost • Low wearability *Future Directions*: • Development of more reliable evaluation metrics
3	Wearables [19]	Not mentioned	*Use Cases*: • Sleeping patterns • Chronic diseases • Frailty *Barriers*: • Personalized care *Future Directions*: • Acceptability
4	Wearables [9]	54	*Use Cases*: • Chronic diseases • Emergency conditions • Human activity recognition • Mental health • Movement disorder • Fall prevention and detection • Access to healthcare services • Biomechanical and physiological measures *Future Directions*: • Users' perspective • More clinical point of views • Integrated ecosystem

(Continues)

Table 14.1   Continued

Article no.	Review on	Articles reviewed	Use Cases, Barriers, and Future Directions
5	Wearables [20]	44	*Use Cases*: • Fall detection • Physical activity monitoring *Barriers*: • Trust • Perceived value
6	Wearables [6]	8	*Use Cases*: • Fall detection and prevention • Medication adherence • Monitor neurological disorders *Barriers*: • Cost *Future Directions*: • Formal clinical trials
7	Wearables [21]	12	*Use Cases*: • Fall detection • Health monitoring • Activity recognition *Barriers*: • Cost • Convenience • Privacy *Future Directions*: • Smart clothing • Artificial intelligence
8	Wearables [22]	19	*Use Cases*: • Fall detection • Physical activity monitoring • Health monitoring
9	Wearables [23]	17	*Use Cases*: • Fall detection • Physical activity monitoring *Barriers*: • Cost *Future Directions*: • Scalability • Extensibility • Cost-efficiency
10	Wearables [24]	34	*Use Cases*: • Monitoring dementia
11	Wearables [25]	136	*Use Cases*: • Monitoring tremor • Body motion • Motor fluctuations *Future Directions*: • User interface

(Continues)

Table 14.1   Continued

Article no.	Review on	Articles reviewed	Use Cases, Barriers, and Future Directions
12	Wearables [26]	21	*Use Cases*: • Gait analysis *Future Directions*: • Involving family members, relatives, and caregivers in studies
13	Smart home [1]	14	*Use cases*: • Mental health • Chronic diseases *Barriers*: • Privacy *Future Directions*: • Cost-saving • Safely • Privacy • Data security • Personalized service • Easy accessibility • Interoperability
14	Smart home [27]	48	*Use Cases*: • Physical health • Mental and cognitive health *Barriers*: • Perceived usefulness • Privacy • Technology readiness • Lack of information • Proper repayment scheme • Cost-effectiveness *Future Directions*: • Compare with economic and clinical benefits with alternatives
15	Smart home [28]	31	*Use Cases*: • Independent living • Health monitoring *Barriers*: • Technology readiness • Privacy • Data security • Fear of social isolation *Future Directions*: • Privacy • Safety • Cost-effectiveness

(Continues)

Table 14.1   Continued

Article no.	Review on	Articles reviewed	Use Cases, Barriers, and Future Directions
16	Smart home [29]	16	*Use Cases*: • Daily life • Healthy living • Monitoring safety • Social communication *Barriers*: • Lack of active participation of elderlies in studies *Future Directions*: • Client-centered studies
17	Smart home [30]	13	*Use Cases*: • Health monitoring *Barriers*: • Privacy • Security • Cost • Usefulness *Future Directions*: • Context • Users' perspective
18	Smart home [31]	54	*Use Cases*: • Health monitoring
19	Smart home [32]	5	*Use cases*: • Anomaly detection • Remote home • Health monitoring • Social interaction *Future Directions*: • Users' perspective
20	Smart home [33]	53	*Use Cases*: • Social isolation *Future Directions*: • Data mining • Artificial intelligence

(Continues)

Table 14.1 Continued

Article no.	Review on	Articles reviewed	Use Cases, Barriers, and Future Directions
21	Smart home [34]	42	*Use Cases*: • Operational functions • Distant medical care • Chronic conditions • Socialization *Barriers*: • Security • Usability • Privacy • Reliability • Complexity • Price • Cost of installation and maintenance • Technology resistance • Lack of prior knowledge *Future Directions*: • Users' perspective
22	Smart home [35]	31	*Use Cases*: • Fall detection • Medication reminder • Assessing cognitive functions • Health monitoring • Environmental warning, indoor tracking • Indoor intrusion • Assistive navigation • Personal hygiene • Home cleaning • Social engagement • Planning • Watching TV
23	Smart home [12]	16	*Use Cases*: • Fall detection • Physical activity monitoring *Barriers*: • Privacy • Obtrusiveness • Decreased human touch *Future Directions*: • Reliability

(Continues)

Table 14.1   Continued

Article no.	Review on	Articles reviewed	Use Cases, Barriers, and Future Directions
24	Smart home [36]	33	*Use Cases*: • Physiological monitoring • Emergency detection • Safety monitoring • Social interaction • Cognitive assistance *Barriers*: • Technological readiness • Privacy • Security • Usability • Cost *Future Directions*: • Investigating long-term economic benefits
25	Smart home [37]	15	*Use Cases*: • Health monitoring • Wellness prediction *Future Directions*: • Applying textile technologies • Low power consumption • Artificial intelligence
26	Smart home [3]	8	*Use Cases*: • Fall detection • Physical activity monitoring *Barriers*: • Quality • Cost • Complexity • Privacy • User-centered design

smart homes for elderlies [27]. They found that smart homes, combined with mobile technology, are used for the physical, mental, and cognitive health of aging people. Overall, they found that smart homes are used for health monitoring, safety monitoring, social interaction, cognitive and sensory assistance, and emergency condition identification.

Furthermore, their study reported high evidence of improvement of heart health monitoring using smart homes along with home health-monitoring devices. However, their study has not found any significant evidence that smart homes can prevent the falling of the elderly. They also reported that although smart homes are used for monitoring lung disease, conflicting findings are present regarding the outcome of their use.

A systematic review study by Pal *et al.* [28] concluded that elderlies, in general, show a positive attitude toward smart home use for independent living and health status monitoring [28]. Turjamaa *et al.* [29] conducted an integrative review based on 16 research articles to investigate how smart homes are used to support elderlies [29]. The primary use cases they found support daily life and healthy living, monitoring safety, and social communication. Correspondingly, elderly users also reported that the use of smart homes increased their sense of security and improved their quality of daily life. Prabowo *et al.* [31] found in their systematic review that smart home technology can be used for health monitoring to improve and increase happiness [31]. Likewise, Maresova *et al.* [30] showed that a smart environment is useful for health state monitoring and mobility support [30].

Fernando *et al.* [32] studied five case studies and found that the primary use cases of smart homes by elderlies are anomaly detection, remote home and health monitoring, and social interaction [32]. Campos *et al.* [33] reviewed 53 studies and found that IoT-enabled Ambient Intelligence (AmI) can help in the early detection of social isolation and facilitate the social integration of elderlies through social networking sites [33]. Marikyan, Papagiannidis, and Alamanos systematically reviewed articles on smart homes and found that smart homes can support elderly people in operational functions, accessibility to distant medical care, and monitoring and managing chronic conditions [34]. They also found that smart home adoption helps improve socialization and overcome elderly people's isolation issues.

Kon *et al.* [35] reviewed 31 articles and showed that the major use cases of smart home are: fall detection, medication reminder, assessing cognitive functions, health status monitoring and alerting, environmental warning, indoor tracking, indoor intrusion, assistive navigation, and guidance, personal hygiene, home cleaning, social engagement, planning and reminding, and watching TV [35]. They categorized these use cases into six categories: safety measurement, health, and nutrition monitoring, support physical activity, support personal hygiene and care, facilitate social engagement, and accompany in leisure. Moraitou *et al.* [36], in their systematic review, classified the use of smart homes into five categories: physiological monitoring, emergency detection, safety monitoring, social interaction, and cognitive assistance at various levels [36].

Majumder *et al.* [37] reviewed 15 smart home systems designed for specific purposes, from fall detection to health monitoring to behavior and wellness prediction [37]. Overall, they found that smart home can be integrated with eight components: (1) wearable devices, (2) activity detectors, (3) sleep monitoring devices, (4) environment controlling devices, (5) security devices, (6) energy management devices sensors, (7) home automation devices, and (8) remote service platform.

14.4 Barriers in IoT adoption

14.4.1 Barriers in the adoption of wearables

Addressing the barriers in IoT adoption, presented in Table 14.1, is critical for the elderlies to avail the benefits of using IoT-enabled devices to the greatest extent. Baig *et al.*

[17] highlighted that the most common barriers in IoT solution adoption are low usability/user-friendliness, lack of interoperability, and low reliability of the power and battery [17]. They have also identified the constraint of limiting the users' movement within the monitoring area and the low accuracy of the sensors. However, their study did not highlight the privacy issue. Chen *et al.* [18] synthesized information based on 669 articles and suggested overcoming the barriers such as higher operating cost, low wearability of the device, and challenges in analyzing the data collected from wearable sensors [18]. On the other hand, in their review, Malwade *et al.* [19] mentioned the challenges of continuous and personalized care to the elderlies in their living area, which can be a significant barrier for IoT adoption [19].

Yusif *et al.* [20] have found in their systematic review that privacy is the greatest concern for elderlies when using wearable assistive technologies, followed by two other significant barriers: trust and perceived value [20]. According to Gordon [6], although wearables use cases showed a promising result, mostly for non-communicable diseases, wearables are still a costly alternative to the existing low-cost solutions or devices [6]. In contrast, when considering advanced wearables like smart clothing, Wang *et al.* [21] mentioned that cost, convenience, and privacy are the most significant barriers to adoption [21]. Qi *et al.* [23] mentioned battery life and cost as adoption barriers [23].

14.4.2　*Barriers in the adoption of smart homes*

Liu *et al.* [1] found that privacy is the greatest concern for adopting smart home technology by the elderly [1]. Earlier, Liu *et al.* [27] also found that the elderly's adoption depends on their perceived usefulness and whether smart home technology improves their health [27]. They also found that privacy is a significant barrier, especially the camera setup in smart homes. Moreover, lack of technology readiness and cost-effectiveness might affect the adoption of smart home negatively.

Pal *et al.* [28] found technology readiness, privacy, and data security as the most significant barriers when using smart homes [28]. It is also reported that elderly users fear social isolation if they become increasingly dependent on smart home technology. On the other hand, Turjamaa *et al.* [29] mentioned the lack of active participation of elderlies in designing and developing processes of smart home technology [29]. Such lacking will create a barrier in increasing users' adoption. Maresova *et al.* [30] emphasized that privacy, security, cost, and usefulness are the most critical barriers to adoption if not addressed [30]. Marikyan, Papagiannidis, and Alamanos mentioned in their study that the common barriers in smart home adoption are: security, usability, privacy, reliability, complexity, price, cost of installation and maintenance, technology resistance, and lack of prior knowledge [34].

In another integrative review, Chung *et al.* [12] particularly focused on the ethical issues related to the use of smart homes by elderlies. Subsequently, they identified privacy, obtrusiveness, and decreased human touch as the most significant barriers that can impede smart home adoption [12]. Moraitou *et al.* [36] presented 15 categories of barriers in adopting smart home technologies by elderlies into three types of challenges: (1) technological, (2) psychological, and (3) ethical and economic challenges [36]. They found that interoperability is the greatest technological challenge, whereas privacy, security, and usability as the most common psychological and ethical ones. On the other hand, cost-effectiveness and health benefits are identified as significant economic challenges. Debes *et al.* [3] identified in their review that barriers related to quality, cost, complexity, and privacy are the four most common challenges [3]. They also opined that a transparent privacy policy and user-centered design are essential to increase elderly users' acceptance.

14.5 Future directions of IoTs study

14.5.1 Future directions for wearable studies

Findings from review studies can be a critical foundation for future research direction. When using wearable devices, Baig *et al.* [17] emphasized further research on the scope of using real-time data for applying machine learning and artificial intelligence and increasing interoperability [17]. Chen *et al.* [18] suggested developing more reliable evaluation metrics to make the application of wearable devices more reliable for clinical diagnosis [18]. Malwade *et al.* [19] stressed a further study on the design, implementation, and acceptability of wearable devices by the aging population [19]. On the other hand, Tun, Madanian, and Mirza identified in their review study that most of the studies cover the technological aspects primarily. There is a considerable lack in investigating the users' perspective, which future studies should focus on increasing the adoption. They also suggested future studies from a clinical point of view with clinicians' participation, which is set at a negligible level. They also found a lack of a framework and integrated ecosystem where IoT devices can achieve interoperability at system and service levels to lower the cost and increase efficiency.

Majumder *et al.* [37] provided suggestions for applying textile technologies to develop textile-based sensors, lowering the cost and making the wearables comfortable [37]. Gordon [6] recommended that as the use of wearables is increasing more than ever, future studies should focus on formal clinical trials [6]. He also suggested taking into account the elderly user' acceptance and their perceived usefulness of wearables. Wang *et al.* [21] recommended future studies on smart clothing to find the scope of incorporation of artificial intelligence [21]. Qi *et al.* [23] provided future research direction for scalability, extensibility, cost-efficiency for wearables [23]. Rovini *et al.* [25] recommended improving the user interface in future studies [25]. Zhong and Rau [26] suggested involving family members, relatives, and caregivers in the design and development of wearable for elderly people [26].

14.5.2 Future directions for smart home studies

Liu *et al.* [1] emphasized further study on cost-saving, safety, privacy, data security, personalized service, easy accessibility, interoperability of smart homes [1]. Liu *et al.* [27] identified a lack of studies comparing the economic and clinical benefits of using a smart home with other technological interventions [27]. There is also a lack of theory-based studies for testing the elderly users' intention to use smart homes and a lack of perspective regarding the cost-effectiveness of smart homes in the existing studies. Pal, Triyason, and Funilkul [28] suggested that, in addition to privacy, safety, and cost-effectiveness, future studies need to focus on how smart home technology can provide more social companionship boosting the mental state of elderlies [28]. On the other hand, Turjamaa *et al.* [29] recommended client-centered studies in the future [29].

Maresova *et al.* [30] indicated a significant gap in the existing literature, most of the current studies focus on smart home solutions rather than appropriate consideration of context and users' needs [30]. Fernando *et al.* [32] also stressed that the existing studies had not considered the users' perspective (e.g., too complex to use, privacy-invasive, perceived usefulness), which, if unaddressed, can be a significant barrier to adoption [32]. In future studies, Campos *et al.* [33] suggested using data mining and artificial intelligence to develop a predictive model for early detection of social isolation and notify family members and caregivers earlier. On the other hand, Marikyan *et al.* [34] particularly highlighted the lack of existing research that has been conducted from users' perspectives [34]. They also pointed out an important research gap in the current studies: no studies have tested users' perceived benefits and preference for smart home over wearable devices that do not need full setup and cost much lesser.

Chung *et al.* [12] recommended enhancing the reliability of smart home solutions in future development [12]. Moraitou *et al.* [36] suggested investigating the long-term economic benefits of using smart homes in the future [36]. In contrast, Majumder *et al.* [37] provided future research directions for incorporating predicting algorithms, such as machine learning, deep learning, and artificial intelligence [37]. They also emphasized low power consumption for long-term and seamless use.

14.6 Conclusions

This chapter presents a critical review of the existing review studies to investigate the current status of the development and adoption of IoT-based solutions by the elderly. A synthesis of the secondary data from 26 elderly specific review studies identified three main themes (i.e., Use Cases, Adoption Barriers, and Future Research Directions). The discussion under each theme was divided into two categories, wearables and smart homes. The findings indicate that the most use cases of IoT-led solutions are fall detection and prevention, managing chronic conditions, facilitating social interactions, detecting emergency conditions, remote access to healthcare, mental health support and monitoring, physiological data collection and measurement, assisting in independent living and daily activities. On the other hand, the most frequently reported barriers are privacy, security, cost, perceived usefulness, and interoperability. The third theme then highlights that future research should focus on the users' perspective in designing IoT-based solutions and address the demand for personalized care, which might increase the adoption rate. Furthermore, future studies should find ways of integrating artificial intelligence with IoT-based solutions for health status prediction.

The literature review found a lack of formal clinical studies and inconsistency in some findings, which warrant further empirical evidence for large-scale adoption and gaining reliability. Also, there is a lack of Randomised Control Trial (RCT)-based studies to compare the benefits and results of IoT solutions with the existing alternative solutions. RCT also eliminates researchers' bias from the data to provide fair research outcomes and findings. Finally, regarding reliability, the authors of the study suggest that future studies need to focus on developing methodologies and guidelines for quantifying IoT product's reliability requirements. The authors also suggest newer studies to find the best Quality Appraisal criteria and frameworks [29] to systematically measure and compare the evidence from different studies on IoT solutions for elderlies.

References

[1] Liu P., Li G., Jiang S., *et al.* 'The effect of smart homes on older adults with chronic conditions: a systematic review and meta-analysis'. *Geriatric Nursing.* 2019, vol. 40(5), pp. 522–30.

[2] Leskova I.V., Mazurina N.V., Troshina E.A., Ermakov D.N., Didenko E.A., Adamskaya L.V. 'Social and medical aspects of elderly age: obesity and professional longevity'. *Obesity and Metabolism.* 2017, vol. 14(4), pp. 10–15.

[3] Debes C., Merentitis A., Sukhanov S., Niessen M., Frangiadakis N., Bauer A. 'Monitoring activities of daily living in smart homes: understanding human behavior'. *IEEE Signal Processing Magazine.* 2016, vol. 33(2), pp. 81–94.

[4] WHO. *Ageing and health.* 2018. Available from https://www.who.int/news-room/fact-sheets/detail/ageing-and-health [Accessed 15 Jan 2021].

[5] PC National. *Healthy aging in action. Washington [online].* 2016. Available from https://www.cdc.gov/aging/pdf/healthy-aging-in-action508.pdf [Accessed 15, Jan 2021].

[6] Gordon L.A.N. 'Assessment of smart watches for management of non-communicable diseases in the ageing population: a systematic review'. *Geriatrics.* 2018, vol. 3.E56.

[7] Pal D., Funilkul S., Vanijja V., Papasratorn B. 'Analyzing the elderly users' adoption of smart-home services'. *IEEE Access.* 2018, vol. 6, pp. 51238–52.

[8] Kim T.-Hoon., Ramos C., Mohammed S. *Smart City and IoT.* 76. Amsterdam: Elsevier; 2017. pp. 159–62.

[9] Tun S.Y.Y., Madanian S., Mirza F. 'Internet of things (IoT) applications for elderly care: a reflective review'. *Aging clinical and experimental research.* 2021, vol. 33(4), pp. 1–13.

[10] Pal D., Funilkul S., Charoenkitkarn N., Kanthamanon P. 'Internet-of-things and smart homes for elderly healthcare: an end user perspective'. *IEEE Access.* 2018, vol. 6, pp. 10483–96.

[11]   Choi D., Choi H., Shon D. 'Future changes to smart home based on AAL healthcare service'. *Journal of Asian Architecture and Building Engineering.* 2019, vol. 18(3), pp. 190–9.

[12]   Chung J., Demiris G., Thompson H.J. 'Ethical considerations regarding the use of smart home technologies for older adults: an integrative review'. *Annual Review of Nursing Research.* 2016, vol. 34, pp. 155–81.

[13]   Pal D., Papasratorn B., Chutimaskul W., Funilkul S. 'Embracing the smart-home revolution in Asia by the elderly: an end-user negative perception modeling'. *IEEE Access.* 2019, vol. 7, pp. 38535–49.

[14]   Kardas P., Lewek P., Matyjaszczyk M. 'Determinants of patient adherence: a review of systematic reviews'. *Frontiers in Pharmacology.* 2013, vol. 4, 91.

[15]   O'Doherty D., Dromey M., Lougheed J., Hannigan A., Last J., McGrath D. 'Barriers and solutions to online learning in medical education - an integrative review'. *BMC Medical Education.* 2018, vol. 18(1), 130.

[16]   Fogg C., Griffiths P., Meredith P., Bridges J. 'Hospital outcomes of older people with cognitive impairment: an integrative review'. *International Journal of Geriatric Psychiatry.* 2018, vol. 33(9), pp. 1177–97.

[17]   Baig M.M., Afifi S., GholamHosseini H., Mirza F. 'A systematic review of wearable sensors and IoT-Based monitoring applications for older adults – a focus on ageing population and independent living'. *Journal of Medical Systems.* 2019, vol. 43(8), pp. 1–11.

[18]   Chen S., Lach J., Lo B., Yang G.-Z. 'Toward pervasive gait analysis with wearable sensors: a systematic review'. *IEEE Journal of Biomedical and Health Informatics.* 2016, vol. 20(6), pp. 1521–37.

[19]   Malwade S., Abdul S.S., Uddin M., *et al.* 'Mobile and wearable technologies in healthcare for the ageing population'. *Computer Methods and Programs in Biomedicine.* 2018, vol. 161, pp. 233–7.

[20]   Yusif S., Soar J., Hafeez-Baig A. 'Older people, assistive technologies, and the barriers to adoption: a systematic review'. *International journal of medical informatics.* 2016, vol. 94, pp. 112–6.

[21]   Wang Z., Yang Z., Dong T. 'A review of wearable technologies for elderly care that can accurately track indoor position, recognize physical activities and monitor vital signs in real time'. *Sensors.* 2017, vol. 17(2), p. 341.

[22]   Leirós-Rodríguez R., García-Soidán J.L., Romo-Pérez V. 'Analyzing the use of Accelerometers as a method of early diagnosis of alterations in balance in elderly people: a systematic review'. *Sensors.* 2019, vol. 19(18), p. 3883.

[23]   Qi J., Yang P., Waraich A., Deng Z., Zhao Y., Yang Y. 'Examining sensor-based physical activity recognition and monitoring for healthcare using internet of things: a systematic review'. *Journal of Biomedical Informatics.* 2018, vol. 87, pp. 138–53.

[24]   Husebo B.S., Heintz H.L., Berge L.I., Owoyemi P., Rahman A.T., Vahia I V. 'Sensing technology to monitor behavioral and psychological symptoms and to assess treatment response in people with dementia: a systematic review'. *Frontiers in pharmacology.* 2019, vol. 10(2), pp. 1–13.

[25] Rovini E., Maremmani C., Cavallo F. 'How wearable sensors can support Parkinson's disease diagnosis and treatment: a systematic review'. *Frontiers in Neuroscience*. 2017, vol. 11(10), pp. 1–41.

[26] Zhong R., Rau P.-L.P. 'Are cost-effective technologies feasible to measure gait in older adults? A systematic review of evidence-based literature'. *Archives of Gerontology and Geriatrics*. 2020, vol. 87,103970.

[27] Liu L., Stroulia E., Nikolaidis I., Miguel-Cruz A., Rios Rincon A., Rincon A.R. 'Smart homes and home health monitoring technologies for older adults: a systematic review'. *International Journal of Medical Informatics*. 2016, vol. 91, pp. 44–59.

[28] Pal D., Triyason T., Funikul S. 'Smart homes and quality of life for the elderly: a systematic review'. 2017 IEEE International Symposium on Multimedia (ISM). IEEE; 2017. pp. 413–9.

[29] Turjamaa R., Pehkonen A., Kangasniemi M. 'How smart homes are used to support older people: an integrative review'. *International Journal of Older People Nursing*. 2019, vol. 14(4),e12260.

[30] Maresova P., Krejcar O., Barakovic S., *et al.* 'Health–related ict solutions of smart environments for elderly–systematic review'. *IEEE Access*. 2020, vol. 8, pp. 54574–600.

[31] Prabowo H., Hidayanto A.N., Gaol F.L. 'Smart home component using orange technology for elderly people: a systematic literature'. 2018 Indonesian Association for Pattern Recognition International Conference (INAPR). IEEE; 2018. pp. 166–71.

[32] Fernando N., FTC T., Vasa R., Mouzaki K., Aitken I. Examining digital assisted living: towards a case study of smart homes for the elderly. Proceedings of 24th European Conference on Information Systems (ECIS). AIS; 2016; Atlanta, Ga; 2016. pp. 1–11.

[33] Campos W., Martinez A., Sanchez W., Estrada H., Castro-Sánchez N.A., Mujica D. 'A systematic review of proposals for the social integration of elderly people using ambient intelligence and social networking sites'. *Cognitive Computation*. 2016, vol. 8(3), pp. 529–42.

[34] Marikyan D., Papagiannidis S., Alamanos E. 'A systematic review of the smart home literature: a user perspective'. *Technological Forecasting and Social Change*. 2019, vol. 138(16), pp. 139–54.

[35] Kon B., Lam A., Chan J. 'Evolution of smart homes for the elderly'. Proceedings of the 26th International Conference on World Wide Web Companion; 2017. pp. 1095–101.

[36] Moraitou M., Pateli A., Fotiou S. 'Smart health caring home: a systematic review of smart home care for elders and chronic disease patients'. *Advances in Experimental Medicine and Biology*. 2017, vol. 989, pp. 255–64.

[37] Majumder S., Aghayi E., Noferesti M., *et al.* 'Smart homes for elderly healthcare—recent advances and research challenges'. *Sensors*. 2017, vol. 17(11), p. 2496.

Chapter 15

Designing mobile healthcare applications for elderly users

Alan Yang[1]

Abstract

Individuals over the age of 60, categorized as elderly, pose a unique challenge to mobile health application designers. Effective application design for this demographic recognizes and accounts for the average physical and mental obstacles that impair adoption and continued usage of healthcare applications for an older population. Application designers must also acknowledge the aesthetic and content preferences of the elderly and how they may differ from mobile phone users in other age groups. This chapter will present the challenges associated with designing mobile healthcare applications for the elderly followed by a series of recommendations for developers interested in designing an app for this demographic.

15.1 Introduction

The proportion of elderly individuals throughout the world has steadily increased in the last 50 years. In 1980, roughly 400 million individuals worldwide were considered part of the elderly demographic over sixty. In 2017, this value crossed the one billion mark. Modern predictions estimate that the global population of seniors will increase to two billion by the year 2050 [1]. A series of explanations for this upward trend have been proposed, including higher average quality of life, developments in medical care, and relative geopolitical stability [2]. Regardless of the reason for the increase in the elderly population, individuals in the healthcare field need to account for this increasing proportion of the population regardless of their serviced demographic. Individuals specifically designing healthcare interventions for the sixty or

[1]Computer Information Systems Department, University of Nevada, Reno, NV, USA

older demographic need to be aware of the unique challenges and opportunities they may encounter.

Individuals over sixty have on average a higher chance of encountering moderate to severe health conditions compared to younger people [3]. Medical spending for the elderly accounts for a large proportion of the healthcare infrastructures of most nations [4–6]. To offset these costs, medical applications have been proposed and implemented as a solution to address healthcare problems such as medication adherence, fitness, diet, and more to improve healthcare behaviors and lower the burden on healthcare systems worldwide. Medical applications are being increasingly proposed as potential solutions to problems for the elderly demographic because of their ease of deployment once developed, customizability, and the increasing acceptance and usage of technological devices by elderly populations worldwide [7–9].

A common misconception among application designers is that older demographics are not interested, or unable, to utilize more modern technologies. Modern trends in mobile device usage worldwide run counter to this idea. There are more seniors using technology than ever before in the history of the world, and studies show that elderly individuals considered to be "cognitively healthy" utilize mobile devices as often and as well as individuals in younger demographics [10]. These trends can be explained by the spread of technology worldwide and a higher familiarity with technology for the average individual. As populations continue to age, the proportion of individuals in the elderly demographic that are familiar with computing devices will only continue to increase. Designing applications for the growing elderly demographic is a relevant skill that will benefit both current and future generations [3, 11, 12]. This chapter will explore application design for seniors through two facets, that of academic literature and that of practice. After exploring the existing discussion on this topic, we will derive a series of guidelines for individuals interested in pursuing application design for the elderly within the context of healthcare.

15.2   Technology trends for elderly populations in academic literature

When interpreting how elderly populations use newer technologies, academic literature has adapted general theories on technology usage and adoption to the context of elderly users. Many theories exist as a lens through which to interpret technology adoption and usage, including but not limited to: the technology acceptance model (TAM), the unified theory of the acceptance and usage of technology (UTAUT), the theory of reasoned action, the theory of planned behavior, social cognitive theory, and the innovation diffusion theory [13]. To specify the scope of the discussion, this literature review will focus on the TAM and UTAUT theories.

The TAM posits that five constructs affect an individual's usage of a technology. External variables effect the perceived usefulness and perceived ease of use of a technology. These two constructs then effect an individual's attitude toward the usage of a technology and their intention to use it. Intention to use a technology leads to actual usage [14, 15]. The UTAUT is considered a progression of TAM.

Table 15.1   Construct definitions for TAM and UTAUT

Construct	Definition	TAM	UTAUT
Actual usage	Measured usage of a technology	X	X
Usage intention	How likely an individual is to use a technology	X	X
External variables	Environmental factors that may affect an individual's perception of a technology based upon a usage context.	X	X
Perceived usefulness	The amount of utility an individual believes a technology can bring given effective utilization	X	
Perceived ease of use	The degree of ease a technology can be effectively used based upon individual perception	X	
Attitude towards technology	An individual's perception towards utilizing devices in general to accomplish tasks	X	
Performance expectancy	The extent to which an individual believes utilization of a technology will result in a beneficial outcome		X
Effort expectancy	How easy an individual perceives a system is to use based on the cognitive and physical effort they expect to expend		X
Social influence	The degree to which an individual is affected by the opinions of other people close to them regarding a technology's use		X

Five factors influence usage behavior: performance expectancy, effort expectancy, social influence, and facilitating conditions [16]. Table 15.1 contains a summary of the key constructs and their definitions, the constructs of actual usage, usage intention, and external variables are shared across both theories.

Based on these theoretical models, researchers studying technology usage for the elderly have observed patterns among end users and the factors from these models that influence actual usage. These patterns are presented in this section as a series of observations along with a discussion of the cases supporting them, as reported in the cited literature.

Observation One: Social influence is a consistently strong predictor of attitude toward technology. There is often an assumption that elderly individuals utilizing technology do so in a vacuum with no outside influence influencing their decisions. A similar assumption is that elderly individuals do not care what others have to say and will be resolutely stubborn in attempting to adopt a new technology, despite social pressure to do so. A survey study conducted by Hsiao and Tang in 2015 in which 338 surveys were administered, observed that elderly individuals living near younger family members will be influenced by those individuals' attitudes towards technology, which tend to be positive. Similarly, elderly individuals living near older individuals such as peers in a care facility will also be influenced by those individuals' values. If the individuals constituting the social component of the external construct of the UTAUT model have consistent interaction with the elderly individual seeking to use technology, they have a high probability of influencing the elderly individual's attitude toward that technology [17].

Observation Two: Negative preconceptions of desktop computing devices increase perceived effort expectancy. In a study conducted by Cimperman *et al.* in 2016, elderly individuals were observed to be less likely compared to other demographics to distinguish between mobile computing devices such as cell phones, tablets, and laptops and desktop computing devices. From a survey with 400 participants aged 50 years and above, the study designers observed the phenomena that elderly individuals with negative preconceived notions of technology based upon their experiences with desktop computers will exhibit higher anxiety when presented with systems that require usage of those computing devices, such as a web portal or a software program [18]. This then results in a reluctance to adopt a technology because of the perceived effort involved in learning it. Studies involving tablets and mobile devices have had success in overcoming this mental barrier for elderly individuals [12], as touch and voice controls do not appear as daunting or complex compared to devices with keyboard and mice inputs [19]. These mobile devices are ultimately perceived as neutral or even friendly by the end users [20].

Observation Three: Elderly have fewer preconceived notions regarding technology. Despite the possibility of negative preconceptions regarding desktop computing, elderly individuals on average have the least amount of prior knowledge or assumptions about technology compared to other demographics. In a study conducted by Salim, Ali, and Noah in 2017, an application was developed with the UTAUT framework as the primary evaluation component. The study design was limited in its implementation in that only nine individuals were surveyed, but the factors of performance expectancy, perceived usefulness, and perceived ease of use were observed to have smaller effects on attitude toward a technology prior to usage compared to factors such as social influence [21].

Observation Four: Younger demographics are more willing to adopt and operate new technology compared to the elderly. Additional studies focused on the age of an individual as a potential moderating construct between the constructs defined in TAM and UTAUT have made a series of observations regarding the usage of technology by senior populations. Attitudes towards new technology are an important factor contributing to the use of technology [22]. The interaction between age and positive attitudes towards new technology tends to be negatively related, meaning that as an individual ages, their attitude toward newer technologies is less likely to be positive [23, 24]. This will result in individuals in senior demographics to be less likely to engage with new types of technologies. Older demographics also utilize technology with different goals in mind compared to younger demographics [17]. They are more likely to see devices as having a singular usage, are less eager to adopt newer technologies, and on average express less comfort in learning a newer technology compared to younger individuals [25].

Casual observation by individuals of these traits among their family or other individuals within their social circles has led to the stereotype that elderly individuals are completely unable and unwilling to utilize new technology. While research may appear to support this stereotype, the overwhelming majority of studies find that the elderly are willing and capable of utilizing technologies, but are relatively slower to adopt and use newer technologies compared to younger demographics. Elderly demographics are also influenced by social groups and make the same value calculations as younger individuals, although they tend to place a higher emphasis on the functional utility of a device [26].

These observations have affected the way applications have been developed and studied in academia. There is a conscious effort by application developers to move away from complex designs and displays with too much information richness. Instead, design principles for applications targeted toward the elderly promote ease of use, immediacy of feedback, and simplification of information for the sake of the end user [21, 27, 28].

15.3   Design trends for elderly populations in practice

Mobile applications targeted toward senior demographics focus on accessibility and ease of use. While the extent to which accessibility features are created with the intent to facilitate adoption cannot be verified, healthcare applications targeted toward seniors with interfaces focused on readability and visual feedback tend to be more accessible compared to those with an abundance of text and fewer pictorial depictions [29, 30].

Table 15.2 contains a summary table of sample healthcare applications for seniors. The table is a sample of five applications that had ratings of over 3.0 from a search with the keywords of "healthcare; senior" and "health app; senior" on the Google Play store. Applications that were targeted towards healthcare providers were not included; the applications included in the table were designed to be used by elderly demographics.

While the applications had different goals for their users, the features across them are similar. The applications simplify screen navigation, contain large icons with visual depictions of features, and often include videos or photographs demonstrating users performing targeted activities. For those applications that contain a social component, contact numbers are given less prominence in favor of photographs and names of the individuals represented. Most applications also emphasized their key functionalities, menus have three to four icons directing users to their most used options. Settings menus tended to contain more text, along with other customization features. Main navigation menus and functionality screens possessed large pictorial elements that generated immediate user feedback when selected.

15.4   Suggestions for designers

Designers creating health applications targeted towards seniors need to be cognizant of their application features and presentation if they hope for their programs to be adopted and used for prolonged periods of time. The utility of an application

Table 15.2   Summary of sample healthcare applications for seniors

Name of application	Rating	Purpose	Notable features
MyCentura Health	4.3	Patient portal access	Simplified login screen; icon spread with account and messaging profile persistent across bottom bar
Senior Safety Phone	3.9	Phone interface	Contact list enhancement with names and pictures; large keypad, alarm feature with visible delete button
Daily Senior Fitness	3.4	Exercise guide	Exercise focus areas color coded and represented pictorially; exercises contain supporting diagrams
Mango Health	4.3	Health habit tracker	Opening screen displays key habits, visual indicators throughout: progress bars, sliders, and checklists
Seniors Beginner Workout	3.9	Exercise guide	Videos demonstrating exercise sets along with text descriptions, exercises are listed with photos

needs to be immediate with instant feedback to mark a successful utilization of a feature. The design also needs to be accessible; accessibility can manifest in many forms. In general, visual representations are superior to text, text should be used sparingly, and all interactable elements should be easy to comprehend and select. Accessibility should also lead to friendliness of user interface. Warm color schemes, friendly messages, and other forms of positive reinforcement will help to place users into an optimistic frame of mind during utilization of the application and afterwards. Repeated, encouraging reinforcement of desired health-related tasks can ultimately lead to realization of desired health-outcomes.

Figures 15.1 and 15.2 contain two sample designs for a healthcare application. Figure 15.1 is an example of an application missing key features that would be rewarding for the senior demographic and will be referred to as App One, while Figure 15.2 is an application sample containing senior-considerate features and will be referred to as App Two. The font throughout all of App Two is larger, and icons immediately convey the different features of the application both textually and pictorially. The menu screen also offers a quick way to navigate across the different features. App One's exercise screen is devoid of visuals and contains a long description of the exercise in question. In contrast, the exercise in App Two contains a

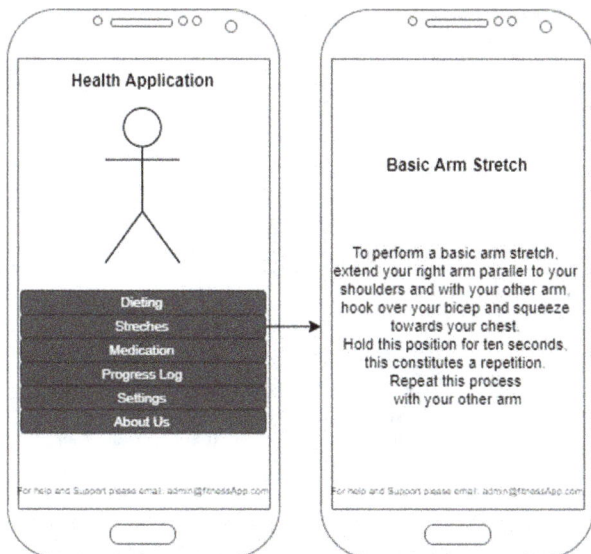

Figure 15.1   An example of application design lacking senior-considerate features

picture to aid in execution of the stretch and the text that is present is broken down and simplified into a series of four steps, rather than being presented without organization. Finally, the contact mechanism for help is a static line of text for App One,

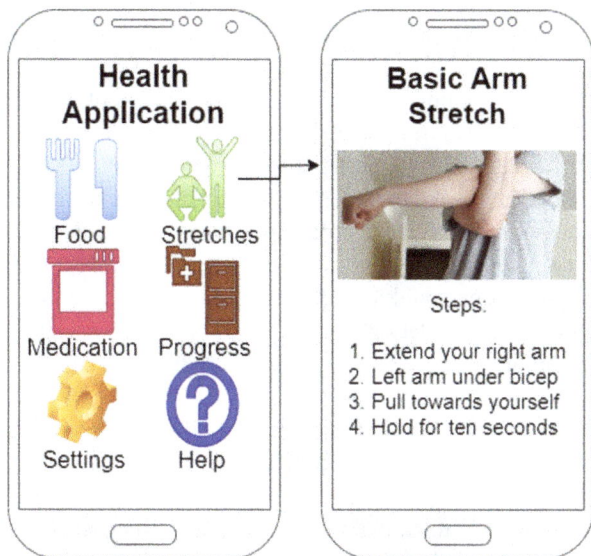

Figure 15.2   An example of application design with senior-considerate features

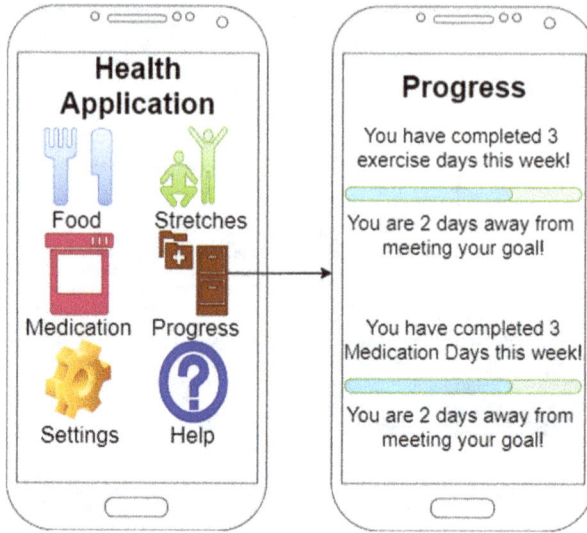

Figure 15.3   An example screen with gamification

requiring a user to go outside of the application and send information to an email address. For App Two, the contact mechanism is directly presented as another icon on the home screen.

An additional functionality that has demonstrated success in adoption of technology and continued usage among elderly demographics is gamification [31]. Gamification is the inclusion of features into a system typically included into recreational environments. These features can include things such as progress bars, achievements, or audio and visual rewards for completing tasks such as cheering or virtual fireworks. Gamification has been used in the context of elderly healthcare to great success in multiple studies [32, 33] and has also been applied more broadly to enact positive behavioral changes across a variety of contexts [9, 34, 35].

Figure 15.3 displays a progress screen for a health application focused on the elderly. A visual progress bar tracks progress as part of a gamified element, encouraging users to complete healthy behaviors to meet goals. More advanced implementations of gamification could include a reward mechanism in the form of visual and audio stimuli upon completion of a goal, virtual incentives such as points and badges with the option to share milestones across social networks, or even financial rewards.

A common feature across mobile apps is the ability to allow users to customize their settings and to give the user autonomy in determining their application experience. The challenge with experience tailoring and customization is that designers wish to give users all the autonomy they can but must also limit the amount of information provided to the user lest they get overwhelmed. Solutions involve a middle ground, providing users the option to customize features but not overwhelming them

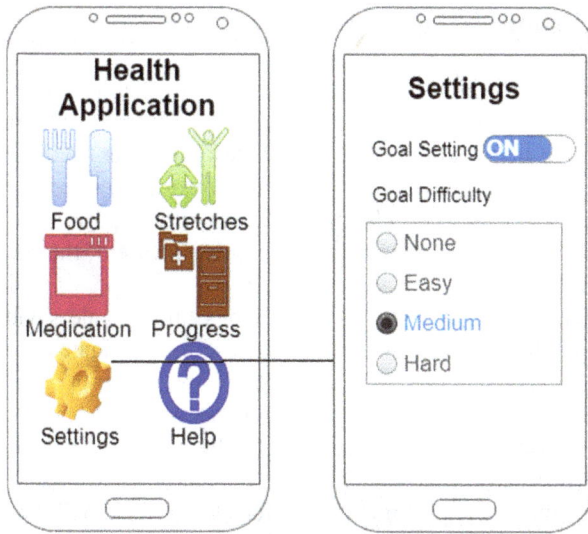

Figure 15.4   An example screen with customization

with information to the point that they become frustrated and give up on the customization features or stop using the application entirely.

Figure 15.4 displays a settings screen for an elderly focused health application. A simple on/off switch enabling goal setting leads to a simple, binary selection. If toggled on, users can select a goal difficulty level from four choices: none, easy, medium, and hard. If users select none, their progress will be tracked but there will be no pressure to meet a weekly goal for healthy behaviors. Easy, medium, and hard settings will correspond to an increasing number of days application users will need to be adherent to healthy behaviors in order to receive rewards implemented through the gamification system.

Along with the considerations discussed, general user design principles still apply. Overt complexity and sparse information will lead to user attrition quickly among the senior demographic. Compared to younger demographics, seniors are more likely to discontinue usage of a technology if they feel that its operation is unclear [30], if they encounter an error, or if they perceive it to have low utility [36]. Designing for seniors may seem like an endeavor filled with obstacles, but opportunities exist for applications that are adopted by the demographic. Seniors have a tendency to use less applications compared to other age groups; but, as a result, the applications that the elderly do use, they use for longer periods of time [10]. Seniors also tend to switch applications less compared to other demographics and demonstrate more app loyalty, so successful adoption of an application by an individual senior on average will result in more overall usage in the six-to-twelve-month range compared to adoption by an individual in another age group [7, 11].

15.5   Conclusion

This chapter explored the possibilities of design for health-related applications focused on senior demographics. By examining how the academic and practitioner disciplines handled the question of designing for seniors, we derived guidelines for design and noted their differences through comparison of two sample applications. We have also identified together the opportunities that exist in designing applications for seniors while remaining aware of the risks and potential downsides.

This chapter explored the usage of applications among seniors with the physical and mental capabilities to operate a mobile device and navigate a mobile application. New developments in this field explore the exciting prospects of implementation of smart assistants for the elderly with a focus on voice feedback [37], along with robotic assistants and more advanced technologies for patients with sever mental illnesses such as dementia [38].

Effective healthcare application design for elderly users will continue to be a relevant topic as average human lifespans continue to increase, and larger proportions of elderly become more and more tech-savvy. By finding ways to design effective applications for seniors, the burden on healthcare infrastructures can be eased and provided healthcare can be supplemented with all the capabilities of the latest information technologies.

References

[1]   Anshu B., Rithu S., World Health Organization. *Ageing. Decade of Healthy Ageing: Baseline Report*. Geneva: World Health Organization; 2020.

[2]   Feng Z. 'Global convergence: aging and long-term care policy challenges in the developing world'. *Journal of Aging & Social Policy*. 2019, vol. 31(4), pp. 291–7.

[3]   Moschis G.P., Lee E., Mathur A. 'Targeting the mature market: opportunities and challenges'. *Journal of Consumer Marketing*. 1997, vol. 14(4), pp. 282–93.

[4]   Jakovljevic M., Timofeyev Y., Ranabhat C.L., *et al.* 'Real GDP growth rates and healthcare spending – comparison between the G7 and the EM7 countries'. *Globalization and Health*. 2020, vol. 16(1),p. 64.

[5]   Cristea M., Noja G.G., Stefea P., Sala A.L. 'The impact of population aging and public health support on EU labor markets'. *International Journal of Environmental Research and Public Health*. 2020, vol. 17(4),p. 1439.

[6]   Dieleman J.L., Cao J., Chapin A., *et al.* 'US health care spending by payer and health condition, 1996-2016'. *JAMA*. 2020, vol. 323(9), pp. 863–84.

[7]   Kim S.-Y., Jung T.-S., Suh E.-H., Hwang H.-S., *et al.* 'Customer segmentation and strategy development based on customer lifetime value: a case study'. *Expert Systems with Applications*. 2006, vol. 31(1), pp. 101–7.

[8]   Camilleri M.A. 'Market segmentation, targeting and positioning'. *Travel Marketing, Tourism Economics and the Airline Product*. Springer; 2018. pp. 69–83.

[9]   Yang A.T., Kaul M., Varshney U. 'Application design to Incentivize medication adherence for chronic care'. 54th Hawaii International Conference on System Sciences; 2020. p. 45.

[10]   Gordon M.L., Gatys L., Guestrin C. 'App usage predicts cognitive ability in older adults'. Proceedings of the 2019 CHI Conference on Human Factors in Computing Systems; 2019. pp. 1–12.

[11]   Rasche P., Wille M., Bröhl C., *et al.* 'Prevalence of health APP use among older adults in Germany: national survey'. *JMIR mHealth and uHealth*. 2018, vol. 6(1),e26.

[12]   Ray P., Li J., Ariani A., Kapadia V. 'Tablet-based well-being check for the elderly: development and evaluation of usability and acceptability'. *JMIR Human Factors*. 2017, vol. 4(2),e12.

[13]   Davis F.D., Bagozzi R.P., Warshaw P.R. 'User acceptance of computer technology: a comparison of two theoretical models'. *Management Science*. 1989, vol. 35(8), pp. 982–1003.

[14]   Lee Y., Kozar K.A., Larsen K.R.T. 'The technology acceptance model: past, present, and future'. *Communications of the Association for Information Systems*. 2003, vol. 12, p. 50.

[15]   King W.R., He J. 'A meta-analysis of the technology acceptance model'. *Information & Management*. 2006, vol. 43(6), pp. 740–55.

[16]   Viswanath V., Michael G.M., Gordon B.D., Fred D.D., *et al.* 'User acceptance of information technology: toward a unified view'. *MIS Quarterly*. 2003, vol. 27(3), pp. 425–78.

[17]   Hsiao C.-H., Tang K.-Y. 'Examining a model of mobile healthcare technology acceptance by the elderly in Taiwan'. *Journal of Global Information Technology Management*. 2015, vol. 18(4), pp. 292–311.

[18]   Cimperman M., Makovec Brenčič M., Trkman P. 'Analyzing older users' home telehealth services acceptance behavior–applying an extended UTAUT model'. *International Journal of Medical Informatics*. 2016, vol. 90, pp. 22–31.

[19]   Muskens L., van Lent R., Vijfvinkel A. 'Never too old to use a tablet: designing tablet applications for the cognitively and physically impaired elderly'. *International Conference on Computers for Handicapped Persons*. Springer; 2014. pp. 391–8.

[20]   Ramprasad C., Tamariz L., Garcia-Barcena J., Nemeth Z., Palacio A. 'The use of tablet technology by older adults in health care settings—Is it effective and satisfying? A systematic review and meta analysis'. *Clinical Gerontologist*. 2019, vol. 42(1), pp. 17–26.

[21]   Salim M.H.M., Ali N.M., Noah S.A.M. 'Mobile application on healthy diet for elderly based on persuasive design'. *International Journal on Advanced Science, Engineering and Information Technology*. 2017, vol. 7, pp. 222–7.

[22] Chen K., Chan A.H.S. 'A review of technology acceptance by older adults'. *Gerontechnology*. 2011, vol. 10(1), pp. 1–12.

[23] Peek S.T.M., Wouters E.J.M., van Hoof J., Luijkx K.G., Boeije H.R., Vrijhoef H.J.M. 'Factors influencing acceptance of technology for aging in place: a systematic review'. *International Journal of Medical Informatics*. 2014, vol. 83(4), pp. 235–48.

[24] Niehaves B., Plattfaut R. 'Internet adoption by the elderly: employing is technology acceptance theories for understanding the age-related digital divide'. *European Journal of Information Systems*. 2014, vol. 23(6), pp. 708–26.

[25] Magsamen-Conrad K., Upadhyaya S., Joa C.Y., Dowd J. 'Bridging the divide: using UTAUT to predict multigenerational tablet adoption practices'. *Computers in Human Behavior*. 2015, vol. 50, pp. 186–96.

[26] Zhang X., Han X., Dang Y., Meng F., Guo X., Lin J. 'User acceptance of mobile health services from users' perspectives: the role of self-efficacy and response-efficacy in technology acceptance'. *Informatics for Health & Social Care*. 2017, vol. 42(2), pp. 194–206.

[27] Seo H.-M. 'The development of user interface usability evaluation of mobile healthcare application for the elderly'. *Journal of Digital Contents Society*. 2018, vol. 19(9), pp. 1759–67.

[28] Akter S., D'Ambra J., Ray P. 'Development and validation of an instrument to measure user perceived service quality of mHealth'. *Information & Management*. 2013, vol. 50(4), pp. 181–95.

[29] Holzinger A., Errath M. 'Mobile computer web-application design in medicine: some research based guidelines'. *Universal Access in the Information Society*. 2007, vol. 6(1), pp. 31–41.

[30] Baharuddin R., Singh D., Razali R. 'Usability dimensions for mobile applications-a review'. *Research Journal of Applied Sciences, Engineering and Technology*. 2013, vol. 5, pp. 2225–31.

[31] Martinho D., Carneiro J., Corchado J.M., Marreiros G., *et al.* 'A systematic review of gamification techniques applied to elderly care'. *Artificial Intelligence Review*. 2020, vol. 53(7), pp. 4863–901.

[32] Talaei-Khoei A., Daniel J. 'How younger elderly realize usefulness of cognitive training video games to maintain their independent living'. *International Journal of Information Management*. 2018, vol. 42(2), pp. 1–12.

[33] de Vette F., Tabak M., Dekker-van Weering M., Vollenbroek-Hutten M. 'Engaging elderly people in telemedicine through gamification'. *JMIR Serious Games*. 2015, vol. 3(2),p. e9.

[34] Korn O. 'Industrial playgrounds: how gamification helps to enrich work for elderly or impaired persons in production'. Proceedings of the 4th ACM SIGCHI symposium on Engineering interactive computing systems; 2012. pp. 313–16.

[35] Stiegler A., Zimmermann G. 'Gamification and accessibility'. International Conference on Human Aspects of IT for the Aged Population. Springer; 2015. pp. 145–54.

[36] Lin T.T.C., Bautista J.R., Core R. 'Seniors and mobiles: a qualitative inquiry of mHealth adoption among Singapore seniors'. *Informatics for health & social care*. 2020, vol. 45(4), pp. 1–14.

[37] Kerr D., Serrano J.Artur., Ray P., *et al.* 'The role of a disruptive digital technology for home-based healthcare of the elderly: telepresence robot'. *Digital Medicine*. 2018, vol. 4, p. 173.

[38] Goodall G., Taraldsen K., Serrano J.A. 'The use of technology in creating individualized, meaningful activities for people living with dementia: a systematic review'. *Dementia*. 2021, vol. 20(4), pp. 1442–69.

Chapter 16

Telepresence robots for healthy ageing

Chongdan Pan[1], Mingzhong Wang[2], and Pradeep Ray[1,3]

Researchers have been investigating the use of robots in the world for elderly in various types of applications, such as communication with relatives and friends at a distance, transportation of medical supplies and equipment across healthcare/aged care facilities, surgical procedures, etc. In China, ground zero of the COVID-19 outbreak, robots are being used in hospitals to deliver food and medication and take patients' temperatures. Drones are deployed to transport supplies, spray disinfectants, and do thermal imaging. This chapter will focus on telepresence robots that have become critically important to perform remote healthcare operations, complying with social distancing measures. The University of New South Wales (UNSW) and University of Sunshine Coast have been partners in the European Union VictoryaHome (VH) project (2014–2016) that involved Australia and EU countries Norway, Sweden, the Netherlands, and Portugal. The project was aimed at better emotional health of the elderly and their security at home. The project identified some major problems, such as the high cost of the robot and its high complexity, making its adoption difficult. This led to the project "Robots for Elderly" as part of the new "Robots for Elderly" project (involving Australia, China, Bangladesh, and EU) in mHealth for Belt and Road (mHBR) Initiative led by the UM-SJTU Joint Institute in China from 2018.

The aim of this study is to design, implement, and test a low-cost telepresence robot for healthcare. The focus has been on implementing a low-cost telepresence robot for healthcare management for the elderly during pandemics like COVID-19.

This project uses an innovative, multi-disciplinary collaboration across disciplines (software, electronics engineering, mechatronics, and public health) involving young university talents from these fields.

[1]Center For Entrepreneurship, University of Michigan Joint Institute (UM), Shanghai Jiao Tong University (SJTU), China
[2]School of Science, Technology and Engineering, University of the Sunshine Coast, Australia
[3]World Health Organization Collaborating Centre on Health, University of New South Wales, Australia

According to preliminary customer feedback, the main functions have already been realized by our robot. The cost is approximately $500, about 20 times less expensive than the Giraff robot used in the VH project.

Many groups all over the world have been trying to develop low-cost robots for various applications. We addressed the needs for the healthcare of elderly, most affected by the COVID-19 and came up with a simple low-cost design of telepresence robot that can be deployed widely in hospitals and aged care establishments. The system is currently in a prototype level and will require an entrepreneur to commercialize it in large scale.

16.1 Introduction

Telepresence robots are robots that provide two-way communication between two persons, which may be widely deployed for general office work, aged care, and healthcare. In the applications in aged care and healthcare, a telepresence robot is generally remotely controlled by caregivers' smart phones or computers to maneuver around the living environment of the target user along with visual and audio communications. With the equipment of mechanical components, telepresence robots can also assist with medication dispensation and other physical supports.

Since COVID-19 is highly contagious, telehealth and mHealth have become very important to protect various types of service providers, particularly health professionals (e.g., doctors and nurses) from close contact with patients and clients. Due to the feature of remote operation, telepresence robots can help with the delivery of medical services while maintaining social distances. They have been widely adopted to fight against the COVID-19 pandemic with applications of telecheckups, telemonitoring, teleconsultation, and teletreatment. During COVID-19, life and death somewhat are tied with the availability of the intensive care unit (ICU), which is unfortunately very scarce regarding the number of patients. Given the acknowledged shortage of intensive care specialists, the alternative is to have one intensive care physician to supervise multiple bedside nurses with real-time and two-way communication support. Telepresence robots, with the aid of physiological and behavioral sensors, enable care providers to remotely observe patients' vital signs and examine medical charts [1]. They can also enable the remote collaboration of a multidisciplinary team without standing beside a patient's bedside [1, 2]. According to feedback from the clinic tests, more than 75 per cent of patients and medical professionals agree that telepresence robots can provide satisfying medical service in ICU.

Moreover, telepresence robots were also deployed in the public area for various tasks, including large-scale temperature monitoring, bathing surfaces with radiation, sanitizing floors, scanning for fevers, spewing anti-microbial gas, and enforcing mask wearing [3–5].

Although there are dozens of different models of telepresence robots available on the market, almost all of them are designed for the general public use without considering the specific needs of the aged population, which is probably the most vulnerable group in pandemics like COVID-19. In fact, only a few of them, such as Giraff [6–8] and Double [9], were trialled with the elder community. Therefore, in this chapter, we analyzed the experiences learnt from these trials to design the FLEXTRA, a FLEXible Telepresence Robot Assembly, to addresses the requirements of flexibility, extensibility, and economy targeting the applications of healthcare in general and with the aged population in specific. The objectives of this chapter include:

- Provide a low-cost mobile telepresence robot to support multimedium communication with elderly people.
- Enable remote healthcare and monitoring of elderly people, such as medicine dispensation.
- Design the telepresence robot with flexibility and extensibility to enable its wide applications in various scenarios, such as COVID-19.

The main strategy has been to exploit recent advances in embedded computing, tablet-based low-cost robot display, and mechatronics dynamics for the robot. Therefore, FLEXTRA is built with off-the-shelf hardware components and open software standards and protocols at the cost of approximately $500, which is only a small fraction of most existing telepresence robots with the same features. It may serve as a basis for many applications of telepresence robots for the elderly, especially in the case of pandemics like COVID-19. In addition, due to its low cost, FLEXTRA will help the wide deployment of telepresence robots for healthcare purposes in developing countries [10].

The chapter is organized as follows. Section 16.2 discusses the specifications and principles of FLEXTRA as well as the methodologies used to design and evaluate FLEXTRA. Section 16.3 presents the results, including the hardware and software implementation of FLEXTRA and relevant evaluations. Sections 16.4 and 16.5 discuss the key features and limitations of FLEXTRA. Section 16.6 concludes our work.

16.2 Research method

16.2.1 Design principles

This project started with the experience of the team in the EU VH[a] project [8]. Hence the initial specification was taken from the robot used in the VH project for which trials were carried out in Australia, Norway, the Netherlands, Portugal, and Sweden. Addressing the issues and experiences with existing telepresence robots, FLEXTRA tries to achieve the following expectations.

---

[a]https://www.youtube.com/watch?v=o2VhThCzFwg

Functionality: The functionality should be similar to Giraff robots, including video communication, remote control, 6-way movement, medication dispensation, and fall detection. Moreover, special considerations should be given to the functionality for the elderly as they usually have different needs and characteristics. For example, the robot should be able to store the pills for a long time when caregivers are away, and the pills should not go bad. It is also common that they need to take different pills at different time. Therefore, the medicine dispenser should be capable of dispensing various combinations of pills each time.

Economy: The cost should be under $1 000 for the required functionality. As the products in the market are above $3 000, it implies that FLEXTRA should focus on the Minimally Viable Product (MVP), and the main challenge is to redesign, simplify the robot, and implement the essential functions at a lower cost.

Stability and usability: As the telepresence robots are controlled remotely via Internet, it becomes important that the quality of control and communication should not be affected by lags or firewalls. The users on both ends should be able to see and hear clearly through the robot, and the remote control should get instant response.

Safety and power: As the robots become part of the living environment of the elderly, safety becomes a critical requirement. The robot structure should be stable to avoid tumbling, and the nominal voltage should be low, e.g., less than 30V. In addition, the robots should have a high-capacity battery so that they do not need frequent charging.

Flexibility and extensibility: Users have varied needs for the robots. Even for the very basic application of video chatting, the elderly may be more familiar with and prefer Skype, Zoom, or others. Therefore, it is important that the robots are extensible and customizable to be tailored with various features and functionality.

16.2.2   Requirements and specifications

Generally, a telepresence robot consists of two component categories, hardware and software, in its implementation. Therefore, a practical approach to design FLEXTRA is to specify the requirements in terms of hardware and software. Based on the principles and expectations shown in the previous section and the experience learned from VH project, we can list the detailed requirements for FLEXTRA as below.

- Hardware

1. The screen, along with its control buttons, should be large enough.
2. The speaker should be loud enough for the elderly.
3. The height of the screen should be suitable for users who might sit in a chair to interact.

Table 16.1   Specifications of FLEXTRA

Item	Unit	Target Value
Speaker loudness	dB	80
Moving speed	m/s	0.2–0.5
Remote control lag	sec.	<0.2
Video lag	sec.	<1
Battery capacity	mAh	20 k
Cost	US dollar	<1 k

4. The medicine dispenser should be located at a suitable height.
5. The medicine dispenser should have large storage.
6. The medicine dispenser should provide dry environment to store the medicine.
7. The moving speed of the chassis should not be too fast or too slow.
8. The battery duration of the robot should last sufficient time.
9. The physical entity of the robot does not contain any sharp edges.
10. The hardware is extensible that new sensors and actuators can be easily added.

• Software

1. The control (both local and remote) of the robot should be easy.
2. Alarm function should be added to remind the elderly to take medicine.
3. The applications are flexible and customizable based on users' preferences.

In addition to the functional requirements listed above, the total cost of the robot should be below $1 000.

Some of these requirements can be quantified as shown in Table 16.1. The target values, except cost and battery capacity, in the table are commonly recommended in the literature for telepresence robots. The 20 000 mAh battery capacity is chosen as a trade-off between the cost and duration.

16.2.3   Design processing using QFD

The design uses Quality Function Deployment (QFD) matrices from the Total Quality Management (TQM) domain [11–13].

The QFD matrices help design systems from relatively vague customer requirements by quantifying them through the QFD process. Its application in FLEXTRA results in a matrix as shown in Figure 16.1, which lists 12 customer requirements and 10 engineering specifications, rates their relationships, and calculates the priority. Each strong relationship counts as 9 points, each moderate relationship counts as 3, and each weak relationship counts as 1. Multiply by the important points of the requirements, we can calculate the weighted average of each specification. The specification with highest weight has the highest priority. As a result, the remote-control

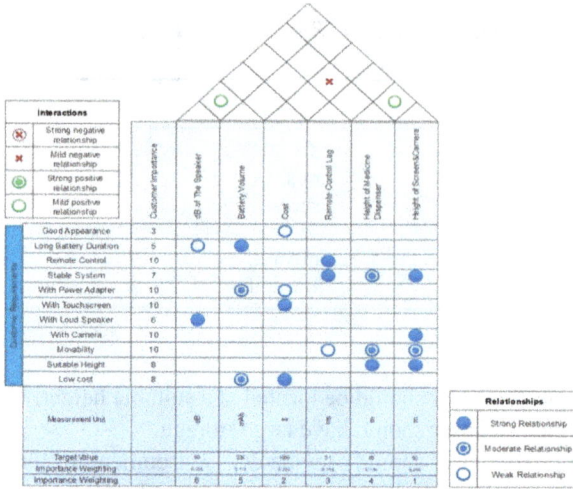

Figure 16.1   QFD table of FLEXTRA project

lag is the most important, and the motor power and the weight follow. The least important is the dB of the speaker.

Once the priorities of the design are decided, one solution needs to be selected from several design choices using Pugh's concept selection method [14].

The FLEXTRA robot consists of multiple components, including Medication Dispenser, Chassis, Controller, Screen, Camera, and the software for video/audio streaming, device management, and control system. Due to the word limit, we demonstrate the selection process with the design of the Medication Dispenser. As other components follow the same process, we only present the outcome of their designs in this chapter.

More than 50 per cent of the older people are living with multiple chronic illnesses [8]. Thus, routine monitoring and assessment of the individual's adherence is crucial to improve their health outcomes. Elderly with multiple chronic conditions face the complex task of medication management that can involve multiple medications of varying doses at different times. Advances in telehealth technologies have resulted in home-based devices for medication management and health monitoring for the elderly. The function of such medication dispensers is to alert the patient when it is the date and time to take their prescribed medication [8]. When the time comes to take the medication, the pill dispenser automatically releases a pre-measured dose for consumption. Some of the features are:

- Provides audible, visible, or vibration alerts
- Dispenser must be locked once medicine is replenished
- Long distance connectivity to track use
- Humidity-resistant and tamper proof
- Dispense only the prescribed amount at the required times.

Selection Criteria	Rating Importance	Weight	Concept 1 (Mixed Pill Manual Sorting)		Concept 2 (Pill Blocks Automatic Sorting)	
			Rating (1-10)	Score	Rating (1-10)	Score
Pill Quantity	Higher is Better	10	4	40	10	100
Ease of Use	Higher is Better	8	4	32	10	80
Manufacturing Cost	Lower is Better	5	8	40	5	25
Manufacturing Complexity	Lower is Better	5	7	35	3	15
Humidity Proof	Higher is Better	15	8	120	5	75
Tamper Proof	Higher is Better	20	8	160	8	160
Dosage Accuracy	Higher is Better	37	8	296	4	148
			Total =	723	Total =	603

Figure 16.2   Concept selection scoreboard

For the medicine dispenser of FLEXTRA, key factors in the design include the budget constraint, the end users, and the safety standards. It means that the design has to operate with few electrical components (motors, servos, etc.), to be simple enough to enable low-cost 3D printing, to be easily handled by the elderly and their caregivers, and to comply with the safety standards (correct dosages, tamper proof, and humidity proof).

Based on the way that the pills would be sorted and delivered to the users, two possible design concepts were proposed:

Mixed pill manual sorting: The daily medication would have to be sorted by the caregiver and the cocktail of medication would have to be put into each slot manually. The dispenser would then rotate at the desired time so that the medication that was in the next slot would fall into a tray and be consumed by the user.

Pill Blocks Automatic Sorting: The dispenser would have blocks in which each block would contain one type of medication, and the system would separate them automatically depending on the demand. The system would dispense into a tray the desired amount of each pill at the designated time. Each block would have its own mechanism to make sure that only a single pill would be released at a time, so that the user would have the correct dosage of medication.

To decide a solution from two optional design concepts, the Mixed Pill Manual Sorting and the Pill Blocks Automatic Sorting, the Pugh method was applied. A scoring matrix was constructed to compare different concepts against the requirements (price, user, and safety), thus ensuring the best decision. Figure 16.2 provides the matrix for comparison between the two concepts.

We can see from the criteria and the weights that the safety aspects of the target medicine dispenser outweigh the usability and cost. Therefore, the Mixed Pill Manual Sorting concept was chosen for FLEXTRA as it has a higher score in the comparison.

The chosen concept leads to the final design of the medical dispenser which consists of five main sections as shown in Figure 16.3.

- The stepper motor, gears, and bearing (orange and red) are responsible for the movement of the dispenser base.
- The support beam (silver) is connected to our chassis, and it supports the gearbox, bottom dispenser base, and the pill tray that are all fixed to it.

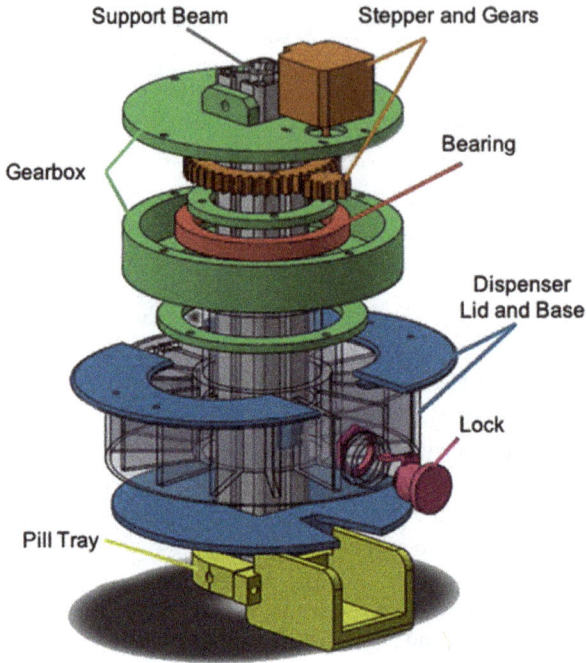

Figure 16.3   3-D view of the medicine dispenser

- The gearbox (green) houses the moving parts, so they are safely away from the users, as well as keeps the dispenser suspended and rotating freely with the bearing.
- The dispenser lid and base (blue and transparent) house the pill boxes and keep them humidity proof. The lock (pink) locks the dispenser lid in place so that once the pill boxes are inside the dispenser. They are tamper proof.
- The pill tray (yellow) receives the pill boxes once they drop from the dispenser, making it easy for the user to administer the drugs.

All the necessary components can either be bought (bearing, stepper motor, and lock) or 3D printed (gearbox, gears, dispenser, and pill tray) to meet our engineering specifications and requirements.

16.2.4   Evaluation methodology

The evaluation of FLEXTRA consists of two parts: the operational functionality of FLEXTRA and its application in real scenarios.

For the operational functionality, there are three major criteria to evaluate the quality of the product: the chassis movement, the medicine dispenser, and the remote video communication. For other engineering specifications such as the loudness of the speaker, the volume of the battery, the height of the screen, and the screen resolution, they can be directly measured or validated by reading the manual for each component used. The detailed operational experiments can be found in the Results section.

Due to the resource limit, we have not done on-site evaluations to verify the capability and suitability of FLEXTRA in the elderly care environment and in the case of pandemics. Instead, we use the paper-based simulation to verify that the functionality of FLEXTRA can achieve the operational requirements in four common operation scenarios of telepresence robots in COVID-19. The detailed requirements of these scenarios and the procedures of operating FLEXTRA to satisfy these can be found in the Results section.

16.3 Results

16.3.1 FLEXTRA

The prototype of the FLEXTRA robot costs only around $500 which is significantly lower than existing products with similar features. Moreover, FLEXTRA utilizes open architecture with open standards, making it easily expandable and scalable. Figure 16.4 shows its appearance with all hardware components assembled.

The interaction of relevant components in practical use is illustrated in Figure 16.5. The robot, which is deployed on the care receiver's side, consists of a pad for the multimedia user interface for the care receiver, the medicine dispenser, and the chassis for moving the robot around. Both medicine dispenser and the chassis are managed by a Raspberry Pi computer installed in the chassis. A caregiver can connect with the robot from any device with a browser, such as a PC or smartphone. Once connected, the control UI is displayed to allow the management of the movement of the chassis and the dispensation of the medicine dispenser. The control commands are issued to the Raspberry Pi computer. Meanwhile, the multimedia interactions, such as video/audio call and remote vision of the environment, are communicated via the pad.

The design and implementation of the medicine dispenser has been explained in the previous section. The other components follow the same design principles and procedures. Therefore, we only present the implementation of the key components in the rest of this section.

16.3.1.1 Chassis implementation

The chassis is the home of wheels and motors that enable the mobility of the robots. Considering the end users of FLEXTRA, the chassis needs to

- be stable enough to support a one-meter-long aluminum rod with a bunch of components installed on it,
- have the required mobility such that it can move freely in narrow places at home,
- have enough space to host electrical components and batteries, and cover them well so that there is no risk of exposing them to hurt the elders.

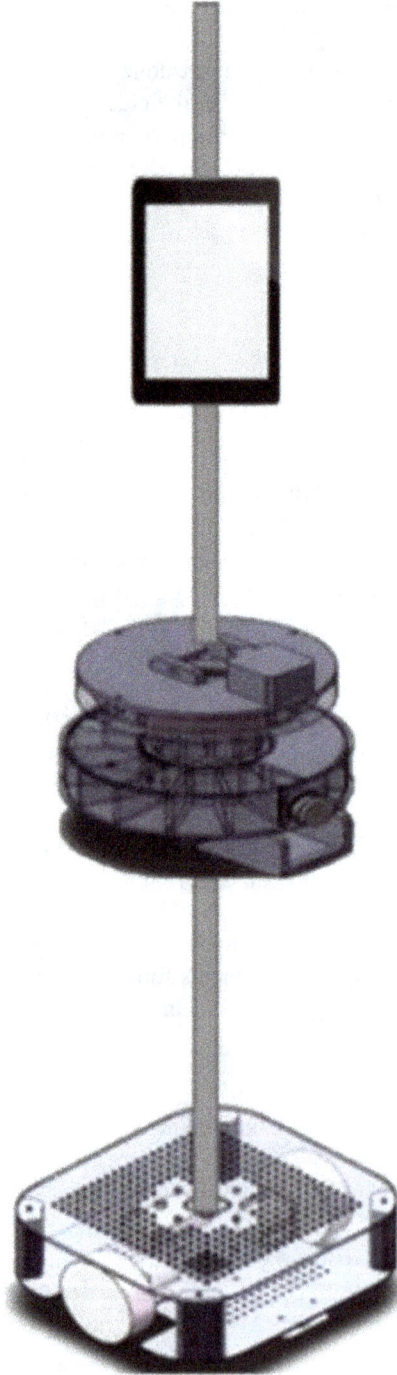

Figure 16.4   FLEXTRA overview

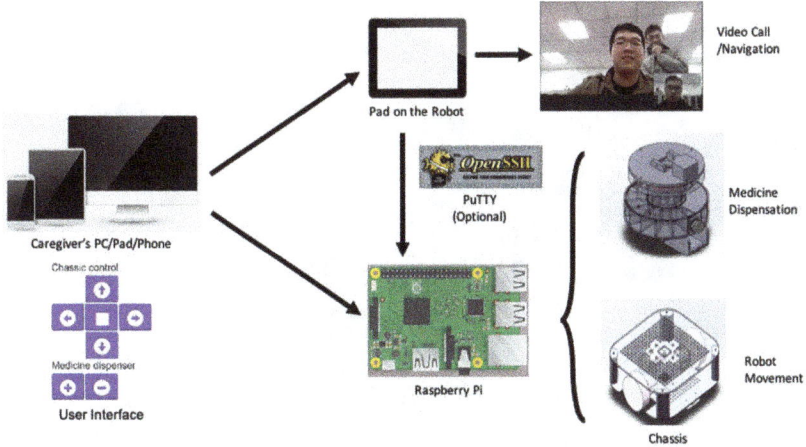

Figure 16.5   Interactions between FLEXTRA components

We use the universal balls at the front and the back, so that the weight center of the robot will not change during turning process. The driving wheels are directly connected to the motors. The batteries are also hosted inside the chassis to supply power to the robots. In the center, a square hole is prepared for the aluminum rod, so that the connection between chassis and upper components are stable (Figure 16.6).

16.3.1.2   Controller, screen, camera, and other actuators and sensors

A big screen is required as the human–computer interaction interface for the elderly as they usually require extra aids in reading. With such a screen, the elderly can communicate with the caregivers visually and freely.

A camera with wide-angle lens and zooming support is also a necessary feature. As such a camera can help caregivers to capture broader scope of the surrounding

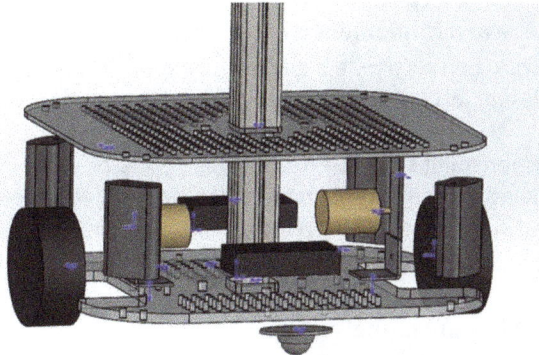

Figure 16.6   Exploded view for chassis design

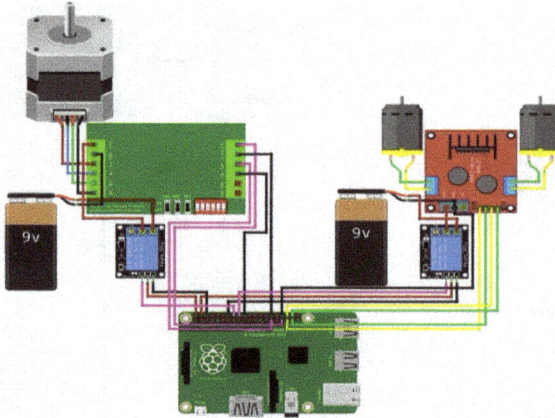

Figure 16.7   Circuit design of the control system

environment or to inspect some spots of interests with greater details, it becomes much easier to control and move the robots.

Actuators and sensors are the add-ons to extend the functionality of the robots. There are no specific add-ons included in the FLEXTRA, but it is important to guarantee the extensibility.

Therefore, FLEXTRA utilizes Raspberry Pi, a low-cost yet powerful and versatile single-board computer, as the controller to connect all hardware components. With the support of Linux operating systems and general-purpose input-output (GPIO) connectors, Raspberry Pi has great extensibility and has won great popularity in embedded computing and robotic communities. The use of Raspberry Pi will benefit the future of FLEXTRA as innovative functionality can be transferred from the open-source community.

Figure 16.7 illustrates the circuit design and the connection of different hardware components.

16.3.1.3   Software implementation

From the software perspective, the engineering specifications and custom requirements of our design lead to the implementation of three major components:

1.   The video streaming system.
2.   Device management system to remotely manage the Raspberry Pi and the pad.
3.   The control system that allows remote control of the robot.

16.3.1.3.1   Video streaming system

To support video communication with the elderly and provide visual guide for the remote control of the robot, a video streaming system is required to exchange real-time information between users. We decided to use a Windows tablet on which the

Chassis switch

Medical dispensor switch

Chassis control

Medicine dispenser

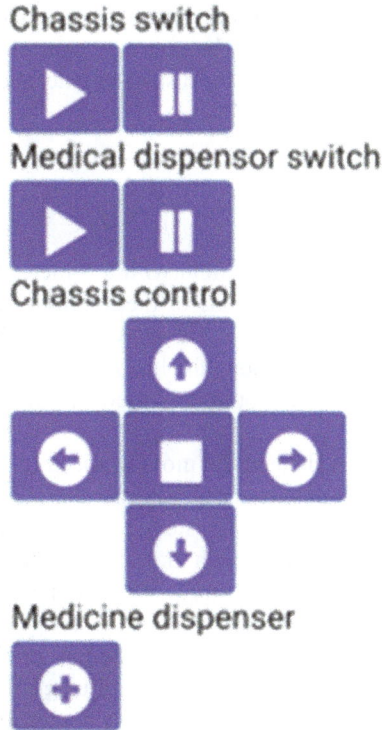

Figure 16.8   User interface of the control system

video communication system is already implemented. With this tablet, users can choose whatever video chatting tools they prefer, such as Skype, Zoom, or WeChat, to use.

16.3.1.3.2   Device management system

As ordinary computers, users need to perform housekeeping jobs (installation, uninstallation, add/delete users, etc.) on the Raspberry Pi and the pad in the FLEXTRA. It is common that caregivers need to do these by remotely logging into the devices. We decide to use TeamViewer, a mature software for remote device control, to realize this function. The inclusion of TeamViewer aligns well with our custom requirement and engineer specifications because it supports multiple platforms and offers stable remote controls. Moreover, TeamViewer offers a private communication channel guarded by the 256-bit AES encryption scheme.

16.3.1.3.3   Control system

To remotely control the movements of robots, we developed a web-based remote-control system running in the Raspberry Pi. Figure 16.8 shows its graphic user interface that is intuitive to use.

The chassis can be remotely controlled to move up and down, turn left and right, and stop. The medicine dispenser can be remotely controlled to move the stepper motor clockwise (+) to open 1 step of the dispenser gate, and counter-clockwise (−) to close 1 step of the gate.

16.3.2   Functionality test

16.3.2.1   Chassis movement

In this experiment, we set up a clear field with a 5-meter line with measurement marks. The robot was placed at one side of the field right on one end of the line. A tester sat at the other side of the field but away from the line end. The robot was remotely controlled to go forward along the line for 5 m, and then turn to the tester. The user that controlled the robot could only view the situation in the field via the camera of FLEXTRA.

In this experiment, we validated the moving speed of the robot and the video streaming specification. The test result shows that the moving speed of the robot is 0.4 m/s, the lag for remote control system is 0.1 s while the user can see the situation around the robot clearly through the camera. The robot can move straight and turn easily following the user's instructions, thus succeeding in moving to the destination.

However, when the robot was asked to speed up or slow down, it wobbled because its gravity center was high. So, we adjusted the layout of the robot chassis after the experiment to lower the gravity center. In the experiment after the adjustment, we experienced no more wobbling issue. A side effect of the adjustment is that the chassis is close to the floor, reducing the pass-through ability of the robot on rough surfaces. Nevertheless, as FLEXTRA is designed to work in hospitals or at home where the ground is generally smooth, we consider this is acceptable.

16.3.2.2   Medicine dispenser

The experiment was initially set up with 10 rounds. In each round, we filled in the medicine dispenser with pills. Then we rotated the dispenser 14 times and saw if the pills could be correctly dispensed. The number of failures was recorded. In each round, pills with different weights were applied.

In this experiment, we validated the functionality of the medicine dispenser, as is required by the engineering specification. The experiment result shows that the medicine dispenser failed 10 times while delivering 100 blocks of pills. The result is unacceptable since its inaccuracy is two times higher than our engineering specification. To increase the accuracy, we decided to add a 3D-printed gear box between the stepped motor and bearing. The gear box increases the time for dispensing but makes it more stable. We repeated the experiment after installing the gear box. The result shows the failure is lower than 1 when delivering 100 blocks. After running the experiments with the gear box repeatedly, the failure rate for the dispenser remains stable at about 0.3%.

16.3.2.3 Remote video communication

In this experiment, we compared FLEXTRA with a stable video communication tool that served as a reference. We turned on the video utility of the robot and the reference tool at the same time. Then a third person recorded the video conference using a camera. By analyzing the time delay between the streaming of these two approaches, we could get the delay of the video utility of the robot.

In this experiment, we validated the engineering specification for the video communication lag. The result shows that the video lag is about 0.8 s, which is lower than our target value 1 s. In this experiment, we also tested the endurance of the battery. The results show that the pad can keep running video communication for more than 6 hours, and the robot can keep moving for 2 hours. The experiment shows the robot meets all our specification for remote video communication.

16.3.4 Suitability for pandemics like COVID-19

Robots for healthcare are built for different purposes, such as medical diagnoses, medical procedures, patient care, and drug stores. However, we focus on the applications that help human fight against COVID-19.

In this section, we demonstrate that FLEXTRA with appropriate attachments can be deployed in four different use scenarios in fighting against COVID-19. For each scenario, we use a flowchart to illustrate the operational procedure and an architecture diagram to demonstrate the robot's control structure.

In the following diagrams, bold text represents existing components of a telepresence robot and their functions, and italic text represents additional hardware sensors/actuators required and their functions.

16.3.4.1 Remote temperature measurement

As fever is a key symptom of COVID-19, temperature measurement becomes a simple but effective approach for the detection of sick persons. Temperature measurement facilities are widely deployed at various venues, such as buildings, stores, and airports. Due to the contagiousness of COVID-19, such facilities require to measure temperatures remotely. With the equipment of temperature sensors, FLEXTRA can achieve this task easily. In addition, the pad on FLEXTRA enables remote video communication or visual guidance to the passengers. Moreover, as FLEXTRA can be remotely controlled to move around, FLEXTRA can be dynamically deployed to the spots in need and be used as a gatekeeper to allow only people with normal temperature to pass. This is illustrated in Figures 16.9 and 16.10.

16.3.4.2 Remote consultation and reception for medical service

The remote consultation robots can effectively avoid potential infection of health workers as they remove the need of close contact with patients who are potential virus carriers. Doctors can update their schedules and send instructions to the robots which provide an easy-to-use user interface for patient interaction. With

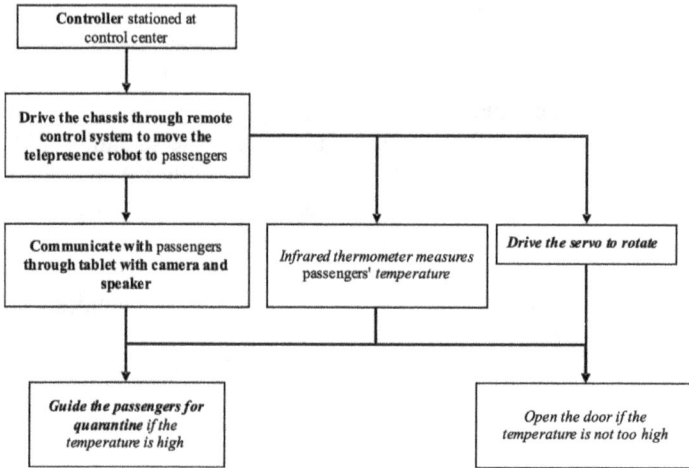

Figure 16.9   Flowchart for remote temperature measurement scenario

relevant sensors and actuators equipped, the FLEXTRA can also support basic medical tests and treatments for patients, such as measuring the temperature. Doctor and patients can also communicate by video calls to make remote diagnosis (see Figures 16.11 and 16.12).

16.3.4.3   Contactless delivery of food and medicines
FLEXTRA supports contactless delivery of food or medicine in hospital wards. In comparison with human delivery, robots are a more cost-effective solution as it does not need protection measures required by human. The medicine dispenser

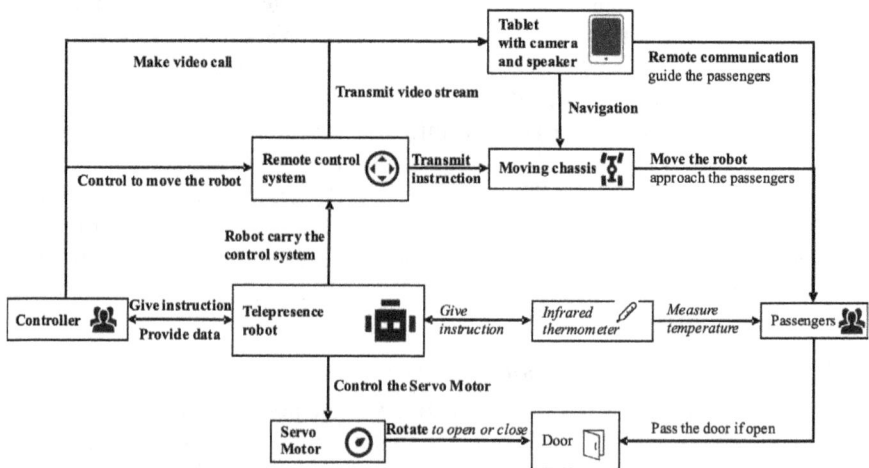

Figure 16.10   Architecture diagram for remote temperature measuring scenario

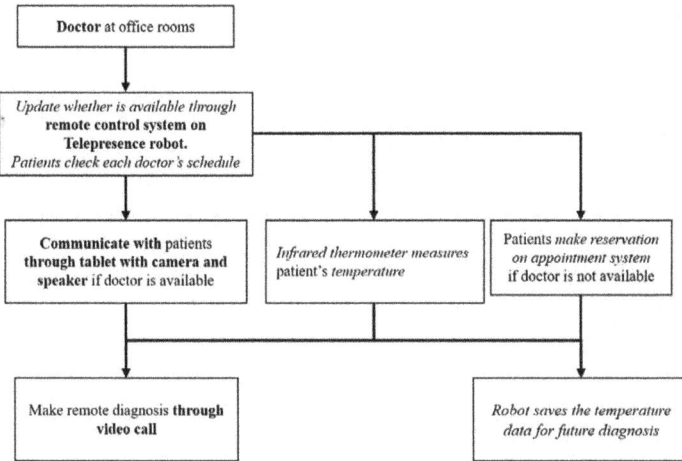

Figure 16.11   Flowchart for remote consultation and reception scenario

of FLEXTRA can be used to dispense food as well. The video call and remote-control system can help doctors to provide guidance and communication with patients. The robot can also measure patient's temperature while delivering food or medicine as shown in Figures 16.13 and 16.14.

16.3.4.4   Disinfect rooms and remove germs

With relevant sensors and actuators equipped, FLEXTRA can be remotely controlled to disinfect rooms and remove germs with chemist spray and ultraviolet light.

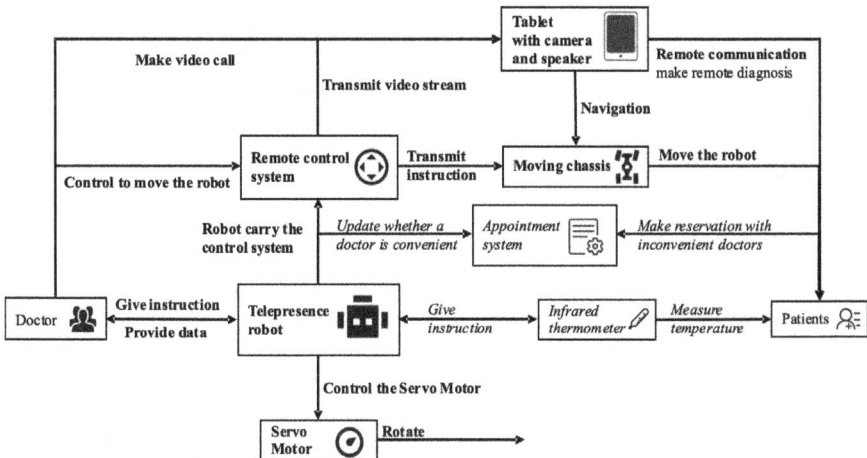

Figure 16.12   Architecture diagram for remote consultation and reception scenario

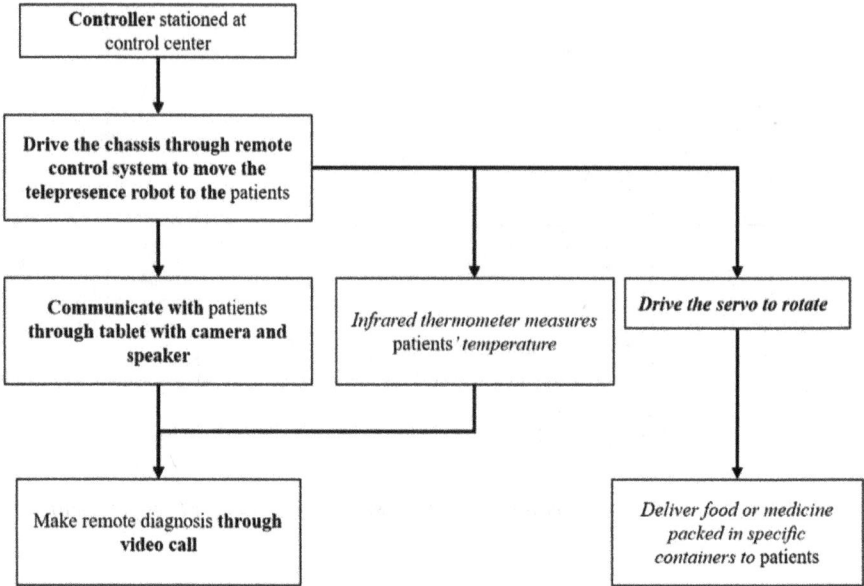

Figure 16.13   Flowchart for contactless delivery scenario

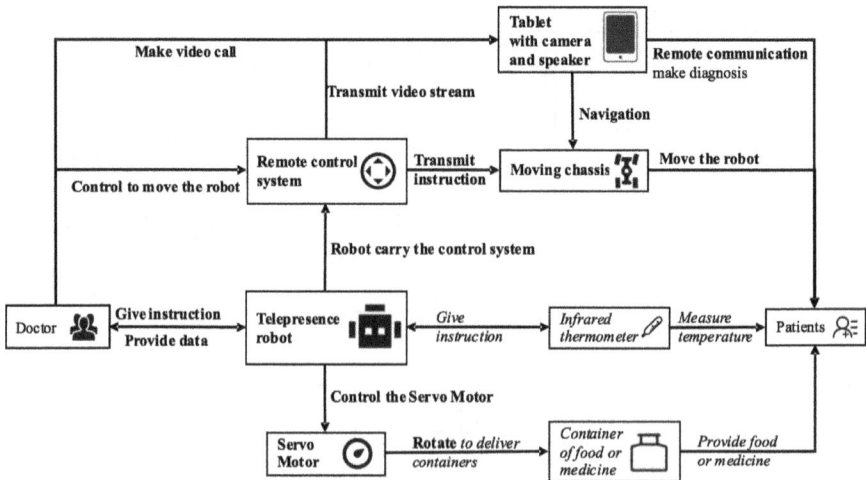

Figure 16.14   Architecture diagram for contactless delivery scenario

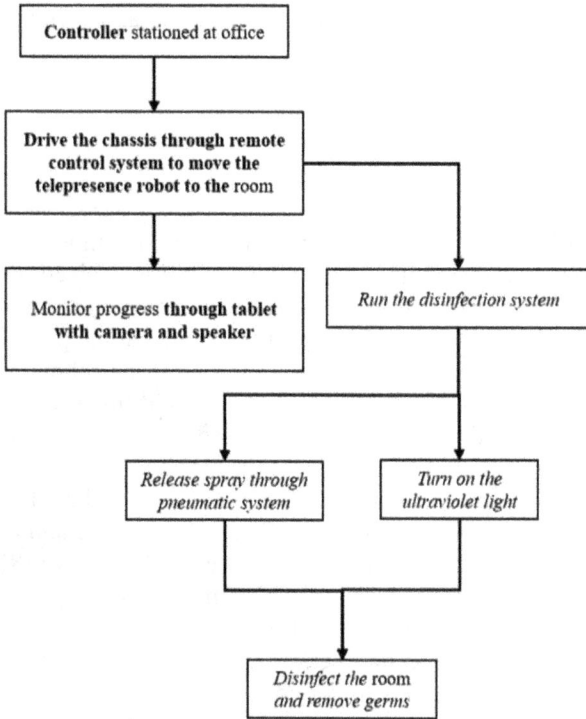

Figure 16.15   Flowchart for room disinfection scenario

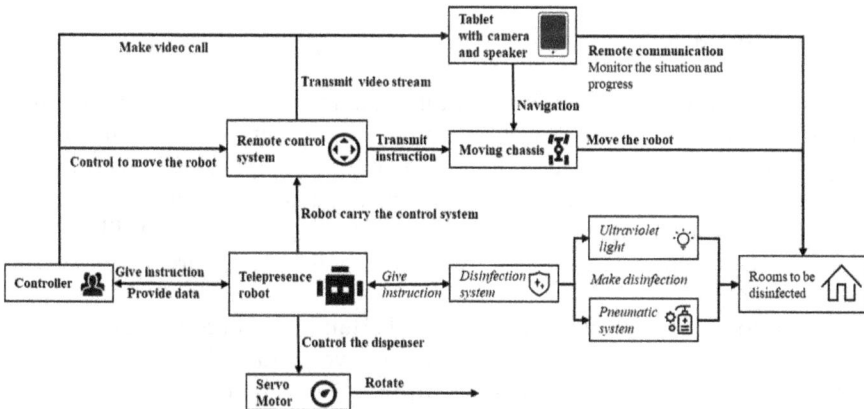

Figure 16.16   Architecture diagram for room disinfection scenario

Users can remotely monitor the progress via the camera as shown in Figures 16.15 and 16.16.

16.4   Discussion

Telepresence robots are still a relatively new technology in which a person can transmit his presence by controlling a robot with his projection on a screen, the idea is that someone can be present in the room even though they are located anywhere in the world. Telepresence robots can be particularly useful for elderly care, where family members can control the robot and give attention to the elderly on a more regular basis, with additional functions such as being able to monitor the medication intake and being alerted when a fall has been detected. However, current telepresence robots for the elderly are expensive according to the users [8], around 5 to 15 thousand dollars for a model, the persistent connectivity issues also make it hard to operate and control, causing a negative feedback from the elderly and caretakers alike [8]. We started with the telepresence robot specification used in EU VH project for aged care, and designed and implemented of FLEXTRA. In comparison with existing products, with the similar feature set, FLEXTRA costs approximately $500, which is far cheaper than the general cost of several thousands. In addition, FLEXTRA is extremely extensible with the use of off-the-shelf components and open standards.

The infectious nature of pandemics like COVID-19, makes it necessary for telepresence robots to be used (between patient and health professionals) to reduce the chances of infection. We have also discussed how this telepresence robot can be used for five types of COVID-19 application scenarios.

16.5   Limitations

This work has two major limitations. First, the feature analysis and the initial specification for FLEXTRA was based on the evaluations from the EU VH project, which was deployed mainly in the developed countries. Therefore, it remains unclear if FLEXTRA is suitable and applicable for the elderly care in developing countries, such as China. The second limitation is that FLEXTRA has not been deployed into real scenarios in the aged care facilities and hospitals.

Therefore, we plan to collaborate with Haiyang group, the largest aged care company in China, to carry out on-site evaluation of FLEXTRA as the next stage of work. This will help to resolve the aforementioned limitations and verify the capability and suitability of FLEXTRA in the elderly care in China as a comparison study.

16.6 Conclusion

In this chapter, a Flexible Telepresence Robot Assembly was proposed to address the requirements of flexibility, extensibility, and economy in the aged care applications. The main strategy has been to exploit recent advances in embedded computing, tablet-based low-cost robot display, and mechatronics dynamics for the robot. Therefore, FLEXTRA is built with off-the-shelf hardware components and open software standards and protocols at the cost of approximately $500, which is only a small fraction of most existing telepresence robots with the same features. It may serve as a basis for many applications of telepresence robots for the elderly, especially in the case of pandemics like COVID-19 applications. However, due to the resource limit, we have not done on-site evaluations to verify the capability and suitability of FLEXTRA in the elderly care and in the case of pandemics. Instead, we first experimented the functionality of FLEXTRA to prove that it can satisfy the proposed engineering specifications and functions. Thereafter, we simulated the application of FLEXTRA in four common operation scenarios of telepresence robots in COVID-19. The on-site evaluation of FLEXTRA is planned to be the next stage of work.

16.7 Acknowledgment

The project was partly supported by the capstone project team of the UM-SJTU Joint Institute in Shanghai, China. This is to acknowledge the support of the Leader of VictoryaHome project Prof Artur Serrano of NTNU, Norway for his support in the Robots for Elderly Project in mHBR. Authors would also like to thank A/Prof. Donald Kerr of the University of Sunshine Coast for his leadership role in mHBR Robots for Elderly Project.

References

[1] Becevic M., Clarke M.A., Alnijoumi M.M., *et al.* 'Robotic telepresence in a medical intensive care unit–clinicians' perceptions'. *Perspectives in Health Information Management*. 2015, vol. 12, p. 1c.

[2] Reynolds E.M., Grujovski A., Wright T., Foster M., Reynolds H.N. 'Utilization of robotic remote presence technology within North American intensive care units'. *Telemedicine and e-Health*. 2012, vol. 18(7), pp. 507–15.

[3] Hedge Z. *'Phil's stock world: Meet the global robot army that's been deployed To fight COVID-19'*. 2020. Available from https://www.zerohedge.com/technology/meet-global-robot-army-thats-been-deployed-fight-covid-19 [Accessed Feb 10, 2021].

[4] Loten A. Travel industry automates pandemic response with new digital tools: a fever-detecting camera that screens travelers and a hotel-room cleaning robot join the industry's front-line workers. 2020.The Wall Street Journal May.

Available from https://www.wsj.com/articles/travel-industry-automates-pandemic-response-with-new-digital-tools-11588361276 [Accessed February 10, 2021].

[5]　Shaaban A. *This robot can remotely detect Covid-19 patients*. Chicago: TCA Regional News; 2020.

[6]　Cesta A., Cortellessa G., Orlandini A., Tiberio L. 'Addressing the long-term evaluation of a telepresence robot for the elderly'. *ICAART*. 2012, pp. 652–63.

[7]　Gonzalez-Jimenez J., Galindo C., Gutierrez-Castaneda C. 'Evaluation of a telepresence robot for the elderly: a Spanish experience'. International Work-Conference on the Interplay Between Natural and Artificial Computation; 2013. pp. 141–50.

[8]　Kerr D., Serrano J.Artur., Ray P. 'The role of a disruptive digital technology for home-based healthcare of the elderly: telepresence robot'. *Digital Medicine*. 2018, vol. 4(4), pp. 173–9.

[9]　Niemela M., van Aerschot L., Tammela A., Aaltonen I. 'A telepresence robot in residential care: family increasingly present, personnel worried about privacy' in Kheddar A., Yoshida E., Ge S.S., Suzuki J.J., Eyssel C.F., He H. (eds.). *Social Robotics, ICSR 2017*. Cham: Springer; 2017. pp. 85–94.

[10]　Wang M., Pan C., Ray P.K. 'Technology entrepreneurship in developing countries: role of telepresence robots in healthcare'. *IEEE Engineering Management Review*. 2021, pp. 1–6.

[11]　Akao Y. *Quality Function Deployment: Integrating Customer Requirements into Product Design*. New York: SteinerBooks; 1990.

[12]　Berk J., Berk S. 'Quality function deployment: understanding and satisfying customer expectations' in Berk J., Berk S. (eds.). *Quality Management for the Technology Sector*. Woburn: Butterworth-Heinemann; 2000. pp. 124–34.

[13]　Kiran D.R. 'Quality function deployment' in Kiran D.R. (ed.). *Total Quality Management*. Oxford: Butterworth-Heinemann; 2017. pp. 425–37.

[14]　Kuppuraju N., Ittimakin P., Mistree F. 'Design through selection: a method that works'. *Design Studies*. 1985, vol. 6(2), pp. 91–106.

Chapter 17

Conclusion and future work

The book discussed some underlying principles and examples of the use of digital methods and tools for healthy ageing. It brings together major international projects supported by the global bodies, such as the WHO, EU, and other international agencies from researchers in Australia, Bangladesh, China, Europe, Japan, and the USA. Many of the projects involve collaboration between governments, universities, NGOs, and/or private enterprises. They are discussed from the multi-disciplinary perspective of economics and entrepreneurship, government and business policies, and digital health maturity [1] – *the information & communication technology (ICT) infrastructure, essential digital tools and apps, enterprise architecture to support sharing of high quality data, workforce development and regulations on data privacy and protection* – to implement and quality assure clinical, population, social and environmental health programs. The chapter authors have discussed the challenges presented to those seeking to deploy digital technologies that have become so important for healthcare and aged care as evidenced during the COVID-19 pandemic. The book should be of interest to governments and industry, researchers, and academics working in aged care. As well as sections on the use of digital technologies (e.g., IOT, robots, mobile applications) the book has also included case studies related to the development of public–private partnerships and the cooperation required to facilitate the deployment of digital methods and tools to care for the vulnerable and aged population.

The topic of this book has been quite popular given its applications in many parts of the world and hence many groups of researchers, industries, and global organizations (e.g., WHO and EU) are working on this topic. As stated earlier, this book has been an outcome of collaborative research led by the WHO Collaborating Centre on eHealth in UNSW and partners (including the EU) across many countries, especially in Asia Pacific. The book has brought together related research led by the editors; Siaw-Teng Liaw (through WHO-funded projects in the Indo-Pacific and globally), Pradeep Ray (Belt and Road Initiative led by China), and Artur Serrano (EU Framework Programmes). Ongoing research is discussed in the context of the three major sections of the book: Underpinning Principles, Digital Health Services, and Digital Technologies for Healthy Ageing. Each of these sections are then discussed in the context of various chapter topics in each section of the book.

17.1   Underpinning principles of healthy ageing

This section summarized the importance of a systematic approach to digital health maturity assessment to guide the development of essential foundations such as ICT infrastructure, essential digital tools, enterprise architecture to support information exchange and data quality, and facilitators of digital health adoption such as capacity building and regulatory protection of personal data.

17.1.1   Digital health maturity

Digital health maturity assessment is a systematic process to assess if a country or organization has the infrastructure, tools, resources, and workforce competencies to achieve and sustain a robust interoperable information system that creates, collects, curates, manages, and delivers high-quality data for practice and policy [1, 2]. More than that, it is an inter-professional and inter-sectoral knowledge-sharing and quality improvement exercise. These attributes and applications of digital health maturity assessment are illustrated by use cases in the rest of this section and, indeed, the rest of this book. Future research and development will focus on optimizing applica-tion of digital health maturity assessment in the development of roadmaps for the sustainable implementation and quality improvement of digital health programs [3].

17.1.2   Ageing population in the world

This chapter provides a context for international variation in digital health matu-rity to develop, implement, and maintain information-enhanced integrated care of the elderly and support age-friendly environments. Regardless of the COVID-19 pandemic, the transition from communicable to non-communicable diseases, espe-cially mental health and dementia, are significant challenges. The corresponding shift to integrated long-term care are significant challenges and opportunities for digital health. Future work will include research into the digital divide and variations in digital health maturity and strategies to harness digital technologies to improve integrated person-centered health services, access and equity, healthy ageing in age-friendly environments and "smart neighborhoods," and an age-friendly com-munitarian society that values its senior citizens. Interoperable information systems generating high quality data are essential to harness data to support and monitoring the safety and cost-effectiveness of digital health in aged care [2].

17.1.3   Geriatric care

The essential digital health foundations to consider in this scenario are digital clini-cal tools and information exchange to support integrated person-centered health services. The international digital divide between low- and high-resource countries needs to be addressed and is consistent with the WHO Global Strategy and Action plan on ageing and health (2016–2020) [4]. Future work will need to be global and examine individual senior citizens and their carers' ability to use digital health, usa-bility of digital tools aimed at the elderly, implementation strategies of digital health interventions and programs, ethical and legal challenges, policy implications, equity and access challenges, and contextual factors such as social, economic, religious, and cultural determinants of health beliefs and health.

17.1.4 Healthy ageing and climate change

The facilitators of digital health adoption have been illustrated by exploring the co-benefits of climate action policies, strategies, and actions for the physical and cultural environment, society, economy, and health, especially for senior citizens. Future work can include in-depth examination of the mechanisms of co-benefits and unintended consequences with sustainable development policies generally and within the framework of health impact assessment, policy development, and implementation by local, state, and national governments [5]. It includes capacity building programs through education from schools to technical and higher education. Contexts may include development projects in rural and urban settings, extreme weather changes, greenhouse gas emissions, climate and air pollution, and rising sea levels.

17.1.5 Privacy protection of ageing population in digital services

Cybersecurity and health data privacy are essential digital health foundations to facilitate adoption through engendering trust in digital health systems and tools. This is even more important in the increasing migration of data and data systems into the "cloud." However, implementation and evaluation of privacy protection systems and processes are not as widespread as desired as indicated by regular data breaches and hacking of systems. This need has been exacerbated by accelerated uptake of telehealth during COVID-19. The challenges with implementing health data privacy regulations and policy, as with all aspects of digital health, are dependent on the digital health maturity of the country, a topic of substantial international research, e.g., the EU project AU2EU (2014–2016) as discussed in chapter 22 of [6]. Future research and development will study the bio-psycho-socio-technical aspects of digital health development, implementation and evaluation as a complex adaptive system approach as applied to the individual, health professional, organization, and heath system. The contexts will be guided by the WHO Global Strategy and Action Plan (2016–2020) on ageing and health.

17.2 Digital services for healthy ageing

This section presents a discussion of the topic of Digital Health Services from the following several business perspectives as discussed next.

17.2.1 Human resource management

Human Resource Management (HRM) is probably the most important aspect of managing digital services for healthy ageing because we need to manage the capabilities (reservoir of great amount of experience that is hardly used by the society) and expectations of the elderly in terms to financial, emotional, and physical needs (that require an appreciation of ageing-related changes in human life, difficult for a young person to appreciate). This book discussed the global demographic changes in Chapter 3 and Chapter 7 discussed an innovative HRM model called *Silvercare* to address some of these needs. Pradeep Ray has been a part of the Centre for Excellence for Population and Ageing Research (CEPAR) and addresses some of these issues through multi-disciplinary, global research funded by the Australian Research Council [7]. Pradeep Ray led to completion of several research projects on digital health services for the elderly, partly funded by CEPAR and other agencies, such as the WHO and EU and the Australian industry [8, 9].

17.2.2   Government and business policies

Chapter 8 has illustrated the difficult problem of the development and manage-ment of government policies in public health during COVID-19 pandemic that has impacted all walks of our social and business life all over the world. The chapter highlighted the need for more research to develop more practical, granular lock-down policies that need to be customized for different countries and regions based on their needs, while maintaining a global standard to enable international activi-ties (e.g., trade and travel) across countries. Although the chapter has presented the results of a systematic survey conducted in 2020, this field is a fertile field of brisk research and another systematic survey can unravel substantial amount of knowl-edge related to the management of a pandemic. Pradeep Ray's research students at the Asia Pacific ubiquitous Healthcare Research Centre (APuHC-redesignated as a WHO Collaborating Centre of eHealth at UNSW since 2013) have developed a methodology called Policy Deviation Management to decide the extent to which a policy can be deviated without breaking it [10]. WHO has been working on health system policies in Asia Pacific countries [11].

17.2.3   Digital mental health services

Many publications and conferences during this pandemic of COVID-19 have illustrated the rapid uptake of digital health services, such as telehealth, mHealth, telemedicine, etc., all over the world to protect health professionals from COVID-19 infections though these technologies have existed for more than a dec-ade and there have been many successful trials without leading to the expected mass adoption. Some of these examples have been discussed in Chapters 8 and 16 and in [6]. Since mental illness management for the elderly (e.g., dementia) is a common and increasingly important health problem in aged care, digital mental health is used to illustrate digital health service in Chapter 9 of this book. This is a challenging field because of several reasons, such as social stigma, denial by patients and their families, and debilitating side effects of the medications. Also the field is multi-disciplinary involving psychology, social sciences, law, and aspects of medicine, making it rather complex. Nevertheless, mental health has been a major success of digital health in Australia where patients in remote rural regions are supported by psychiatrists through video consultations for many years [12]. After the success of telehealth during COVID-19, many insurance companies and primary care practices are now freely supporting digital mental health in many countries.

17.2.4   Supply chain management in digital health

Chapter 10 has discussed the problem of the operations management of digital health service from the perspective of medication management, an important aspect of supply chain management. However, the public is now daily reminded of medical supply chain management in the context of COVID-19 vaccine development, manufacture, and distribution. Once the process is completed in 2021–2022, there will be many publications on the successes and failures of current supply chain management practices to COVID-19 vaccination management in various countries. On the other hand, there is a growing practice of online delivery of medications and health equipment (e.g., oxymeters) to homes during COVID-19, immensely helping families and patients during the COVID-19 outbreak. However, the pandemic has accelerated geo-political tension in the management of global supply chains (especially the dependence on one particular country) in the context of security. Secure global supply chains require shared responsibility and trust among all supply chain partners. For example, developing countries may not trust vaccine manufacturers from developed countries to supply vaccines to them at low cost and with promptness. Interestingly, services to the elderly are supported by a chain of providers that share personal data of the elderly, and these services need to meet the evolving privacy laws in different countries discussed in Chapter 22 of [6].

17.2.5   Country case studies

Chapter 11 discussed a case study of digital health for the aged care in China. This was a part of the joint research led by Pradeep Ray across the University of Michigan-Shanghai Jiao Tong University Joint Institute and Haiyang Group, the largest private aged care group in China based in Shanghai. Chapter 16 discussed the development of the telepresence robot technology for this project called "Digital Health for the Elderly." Similar case studies on Digital Health Services for Aged Care are evolving from various countries, partly reported by the WHO [4].

17.3   Digital technologies for healthy ageing

This section presents today's innovations and future challenges in the context of the rapid advances in the digital technologies for Aged Care.

17.3.1   Exoskeletons for rehabilitation

Chapter 12 addressed the potential benefits of combining social features to powered exoskeletons in defining the next generation of robotic rehabilitation. The chapter has drawn on the efforts of the partners' network in the EU project "LIFEBOTS Exchange" [13]. Technical aspects were discussed in the light of social implications of the introduction of such technologies to the aged population. The concept of

Responsible Research and Innovation (RRI) proposed by the European Commission [14] was the starting point to discuss seven societal considerations targeting designers, developers, and deployers of technology, with the aim of facilitating the planning for the future of social exoskeletons.

17.3.2   Innovative digital care technology for the mental health of the elderly

Chapter 13 discussed the SENSE-GARDEN, an innovative care technology for the treatment of dementia. The method was designed to help preserve the identity and self-awareness in elderly people living with dementia [15]. The potential benefits for the person with dementia, relatives and professional caregivers resulting from the use of the SENSE-GARDEN were presented. Details of the technology, from the functional aspects and system architecture, to the creation of the space itself, were given and explained. Concrete examples of implemented SENSE-GARDEN rooms across Europe were shown. These immersive spaces have produced promising positive outcomes for the persons with dementia in several aspects, including emotional state, cognitive ability, and physical function.

17.3.3   IoT and smart home technologies for healthy ageing

In Chapter 14 three main themes were addressed in relation to IoT-based solutions for the elderly, namely the main areas of intervention, or use cases, such as fall detection; the most frequently reported adoption barriers, such as privacy and security; and future research directions including the users' perspective in design and personalized care. These themes emerged from a critical review [16] investigating the current status of the development and adoption of IoT, collecting data from 26 elderly specific review studies. The discussion under each theme was divided into two categories: wearables and smart homes. Given the lack of formal clinical studies and the reported contradictions in existing study findings, the authors suggest newer studies to find the best Quality Appraisal criteria and frameworks [17], and gathering more empirical evidence as a strong basis for a large-scale adoption of IoT technologies by the older population.

17.3.4   Designing mobile applications for the aged population

Targeting application designers and developers, Chapter 15 discussed the challenges associated with designing mobile healthcare applications for the elderly and offered a series of recommendations for the creation of this type of apps. Two examples of applications were used to illustrate the possibilities and opportunities offered in designing applications for seniors. The technology acceptance model (TAM) and the unified theory of the acceptance and usage of technology (UTAUT) [18] were used to guide the presentation of results from a literature review on applications targeting the elderly. Through a series of observations, the author arrives at a list of suggestions for the effective design of applications for seniors.

17.3.5 Robots for healthy ageing

The COVID-19 pandemic has renewed the interest in using robots for care. The reduction in infection risks in the aged population, together with the extended possibility of remotely monitoring health condition, among other advantages, has catalyzed research activity in this area. Chapter 16 focused specifically on telepresence robots able to perform remote healthcare operations, complying with current social distancing measures. The chapter reported on the developments on a previous collaboration between UNSW and University of Sunshine Coast in the scope of the European Union VictoryaHome (VH) project (2014–2016) involving Australia and the EU countries Norway, Sweden, the Netherlands, and Portugal [8]. These developments led to the creation of the project "Robots for Elderly" involving Australia, China, Bangladesh, and EU, in mHealth for Belt and Road (mHBR) Initiative led by the UM-SJTU Joint Institute in China from 2018. The chapter presented and discussed the design, implementation, and testing of a low-cost telepresence robot for healthcare, bringing a possibility of disrupting the market, still populated by expensive technologies in this area.

17.4 Summary

This book has provided a broad overview of the principles and application of "Digital Methods and Tools for Healthy Ageing" from a multi-disciplinary (economics, public health, information technology and systems, geriatrics, environment, and climate action) perspective. It also described the application of digital health maturity assessment in the development of roadmaps for the sustainable development, implementation, and quality improvement of digital health programs. The chapters used various types of methodologies, with examples and case studies from different countries, such as Australia, Bangladesh, China, European Union, and the USA. Some chapters have carried out systematic literature surveys based on keywords, one chapter is based on expert legal opinions, one chapter has used qualitative interview-based research, and some others have provided descriptions of ongoing digital systems design and applications for healthy ageing. However, this is a vast and fast evolving topic and the book is not intended to cover all aspects comprehensively. Therefore, some topics (e.g., extensive trials of digital methods and tools for aged care) have not been discussed in this book. Besides, the world is now learning about the impact of pandemics and climate change in healthy ageing, and we hope there will be many rigorous research publications on related topics in the future.

References

[1] Liaw S.-T., Zhou R., Ansari S., Gao J., *et al.* 'A digital health profile & maturity assessment toolkit: cocreation and testing in the Pacific Islands'. *Journal of the American Medical Informatics Association.* 2021, vol. 28(3), pp. 494–503.

[2]   Liaw S.-T., Guo J.G.N., Ansari S., *et al.* 'Quality assessment of real-world data repositories across the data life cycle: a literature review'. *Journal of the American Medical Informatics Association.* 202126 Jan 2021.

[3]   Liaw S.-T., Georgiou A., Marin H. 'Evaluation of digital health & information technology in primary care'. *International Journal of Medical Informatics.* 2020, vol. 144,p. 104285.

[4]   World Health Organization Department of Ageing and Life Course. *Global Strategy and Action Plan on Ageing and Health (2016–2020).* Geneva: WHO; 2017.

[5]   Rudnicka E., Napierała P., Podfigurna A., Męczekalski B., Smolarczyk R., Grymowicz M. 'The World Health Organization (WHO) approach to healthy ageing'. *Maturitas.* 2020, vol. 139, pp. 6–11.

[6]   Ray P.K., Nakashima N., Ahmed A., Ro S.-C., Soshino Y. (eds.). *Mobile Technologies for Delivering Healthcare in Remote, Rural or Developing Regions, IET Book Series on Health Technologies.* UK: IET Press; 2020. Available from https://shop.theiet.org/mobile-technologies-for-delivering-healthcare-in-remote-rural-or-developing-regions.

[7]   CEPAR. *ARC centre for excellence in population and ageing research (CEPAR) [online].* 2020. Available from https://www.cepar.edu.au/ [Accessed July 2021].

[8]   Kerr D., Serrano J.Artur., Ray P. 'The role of a disruptive digital technology for home-based healthcare of the elderly: telepresence robot'. *Digital Medicine.* 2018, vol. 4(4), pp. 173–9.

[9]   Ray P., Li J., Ariani A., Kapadia V, Shah V. 'Tablet-based well-being check for the elderly: development and evaluation of usability and acceptability'. *JMIR Human Factors.* 2017, vol. 4(2),e12.

[10] Bakshi A., Ray P. *Policy Deviation Management for Telehealth Services Paperback – April 30, 2020.* Republic of Moldova: Academic Book Publishing Company (lap-publishing.com); 2020.

[11] WHO. *Asia pacific observatory on health systems and policies [online].* 2021. Available from http://www.searo.who.int/entity/asia_pacific_observatory/about/en/ [Accessed July 2021].

[12] eMHprac. *E-nental health in practice, a guide to digital mental health resources [online].* 2021. Available from https://www.emhprac.org.au/wp-content/uploads/2019/12/eMHPrac-Resource-Guide-Feb21.pdf [Accessed July 2021].

[13] LIFEBOTS Project. 'LIFEBOTS exchange – creating a new reality of care and welfare through the inclusion of social robots, supported by the EU Horizon 2020 Programme Marie Skłodowska-Curie Research and Innovation Staff Exchange (MSCA-RISE), Grant Agreement ID: 824047'. 2020.

[14] European Commission. *Options for strengthening responsible research & innovation [online].* 2012. Available from https://ec.europa.eu/research/science-society/document_library/pdf_06/options-for-strengthening_en.pdf [Accessed July 2021].

[15] SENSE-GARDEN. 2018. Available from www.sense-garden.eu [Accessed June 2021].

[16] Kardas P., Lewek P., Matyjaszczyk M. 'Determinants of patient adherence: a review of systematic reviews'. *Frontiers in Pharmacology*. 2013, vol. 4, p. 91.

[17] Turjamaa R., Pehkonen A., Kangasniemi M. 'How smart homes are used to support older people: an integrative review'. *International Journal of Older People Nursing*. 2019, vol. 14(4), e12260.

[18] Davis F.D., Bagozzi R.P., Warshaw P.R. 'User acceptance of computer technology: a comparison of two theoretical models'. *Management Science*. 1989, vol. 35(8), pp. 982–1003.

Index

aged care services and providers
  Asia 185
  Australia 185–7
  Europe 187–8
  operations management 5
  service workflows
    drug request and delivery process
      189–90
    logistics activities 192
    medication management 189
    medication request and delivery
      191
    participants 190
    scenarios 190
    service integration 188
    sub-processes 190–2
  supply chain model, Jidoka
    information inaccuracy and
      inconsistency 193
    mechanism 192
    medical errors 192–3
    medication adherence 193–8
ageing population worldwide
  Germany 130–1
  Japan 128–9
  Netherlands 130
  Scotland 129–30
  Singapore 131
Alzheimer's disease 38, 251
Ambient Assisted Living (AAL)
    Programme 6
anxiety-related disorder 164
artificial intelligence (AI) 150, 263
Australian Digital Health Agency
    (ADHA) 103
Australian health data privacy 4

Electronic Health Records (EHRs)
    97–8
  legal framework
    actors and resources 107–8
    data processor 107
    data subject 107
    data types and assurance levels
      108
    resource 108
    rights and responsibilities
      108–10
    third party 108
  My Health Record for aged care
    access 111
    benefits 113
    health record registration process
      and upload 113
    legal actors 114
    legal analysis 114–15
    safety and convenience 112
    security 112
  online health data regulations
    Australian Privacy Principles 102
    Consumer Data Rights (CDR) 100
    contracts and blockchain 105–6
    Corporations Act 2001 99–100
    criminal law 101
    Data Breach scheme 102
    dementia patient, legal analysis
      115–18
    My Health Records Act 2012
      103–4
    The Privacy Act 1988 102
    Tort law 99
  Personal Health Records (PHRs)
    97–8

Australian Privacy Principles (APP)
    102–3, 120–1
authorised representatives 112

Bangla Montgomery Asberg Depression
    Rating Scale (MADRSB) 174
blockchain 105

caregiver-mediated digital health
    support 56, 59
Care Planning Assessment Tool (CPAT)
    187
Centre for Excellence for Population
    and Ageing Research (CEPAR)
    326
Chassis implementation, FLEXTRA
    309, 310
China's aged care
  COVID-19
    development prospect 214, 217
    existing digital technology
        214–17
    institution-based care 213–14
    situations of institutions 213
  digital technologies 215–17
  elderly care modes and percentage
    213
  elderly care services
    acceptance 209
    market 219, 222
    participation 208–9
    promotions of development 206–7
  Haiyang group
    industry 218–19
    technology 219–21
    venture 217–18
  internet penetration rate 204
  internet plus nursing services 207
  literature search methodology
    summary 205
  mobile devices and communication
    networks 203
  mobile medical industry 211–12

  network development summary 204
  new Chinese seniors 212
  opportunities 209
  policy documents 207, 208
  PRISMA methodology
    data extraction and analysis 206
    relevant articles selection 206
    resources and search strategy
        205–6
  silver economy
    iiMedia Research 210
    market size 210
  social participation 204
  study limitations 223
  technological innovation 203
  universal two-child policy 203
Cities for Climate Protection (CCP)
    programme 89–90
climate action policies, healthy ageing.
    see also health co-benefits
  co-benefits
    climate and air co-impacts 74
    'climate and other goal' approach
        76
    climate co-benefits 74
    'climate first' approach 76
    co-impact 74
    conceptual diagram 75
    development 73
    'development first' approach 75–6
    GHG emissions-reduction
        measures 73
    Health Impact Assessment (HIA)
        83–6
    health impacts 74
    identifying and considering 76–8
    impact assessment tools 82–3
    mapping pathways 79
    Paris Climate Agreement 72–3
    phases 77
    policy-decision-making 80–2
    quantifying and valuing
        78–80
    win-win strategy 73
  global policies 72

low-carbon measures and
technologies 71–72
'climate and other goal' approach 76
climate co-benefits 74
'climate first' approach 76
Clinical Dementia Rating (CDR) Scale
251
co-benefits concept. *See* climate action
policies, healthy ageing
co-creation approach 20
Consumer Data Rights (CDR)
100–1
contact-tracing wristband or wearable
156
Continuing Care Home-based
Community (CCHC) 218
continuous medication monitoring
(CoMM) 194
contracts 105–6
coronavirus (COVID-19) pandemic 5
China's aged care
development prospect 214, 217
existing digital technology
214–17
institution-based care 213–14
situations of institutions 213
comparison and provable outcome
158
data privacy 157
dynamic cycle lockdown 157
FLEXible Telepresence Robot
Assembly (FLEXTRA)
contactless delivery scenario
316–18
remote consultation and reception
315–16
remote temperature measurement
315, 316
room disinfection scenario 317,
319
lockdown approaches (*see* lockdown
approaches, Covid-19)
lockdown response stringency index
157
mental health care crisis

Bangladesh (*see* digital mental
health services, Bangladesh)
COVID-19 pandemic 165
mortality rate 157
Corporations Act 2001 99–100
criminal law 100
Cyberdyne 233

Daily Senior Fitness 292
data confidentiality 118
data-driven innovation 47
data protection and access 63
Data Subject 118
dementia 38–40, 164. *See also*
SENSE-GARDEN method
demographic dividend theory 44
development co-benefits 73
'development first' approach 75–6
diabetes 164
digital divide 54–5
digital health, definition 12
Digital Health for the Ageing
Population project 2
digital health maturity 3, 324
assessment
co-creation approach 20
DHP-MAT 18, 19
digital health profile co-creation
16, 18
WHO-endorsed document 20
WHO guideline 20
co-creation 16
digital tools 14
essential digital health foundations
14–15
examples 16, 17
health service-oriented conceptual
framework 14
ICT infrastructure 14
indicators 13, 15
levels 15–16
model 13
technical models and guides 13
work done related to 13

Digital Health Profile and Maturity
  Assessment Toolkit (DHP-
  MAT) 3, 18, 19
digital mental health services (DMHS),
  Bangladesh
  comparison 167–9
  government's total expenditure 166
  mobile network coverage 166
  MonerDaktar
    case example 173–4
    design 171–2
    evaluation and challenges 174–6
    intervention programs 170
    service delivery 170
    testing and assessment 172
  rapid digital transformation 166
  Telepsychiatry Research and
    Innovation Network (TRIN)
    166
  Union Digital Centers 166
drug-ordering process, logistics activity
  192

eHealth 12
elderly care
  developed countries 53–4
  low-and middle-income countries
    caregiver-mediated digital health
      support 54, 59
    digital divide 54–5
    digital tools 56–8
    eHealth/mHealth projects 54
    and healthcare provider
      communication 61
    informal caregiver 60
    institutional living 54
    mobile health (mHealth)
      technology 54
    non-communicable diseases 53
    policy implications 61–3
    primary care 54
    psychosocial support 60–71
    self-management 60
electronic contracts 106

Electronic Data Interchange (EDI) 106
Electronic Health Records (EHRs)
  97–8
Electronic Transfer of Prescription
  (ETP) 190
environmental impact assessment (EIA)
  82–3
ePrescription 194
ethics and consent 61–2
exoskeletons 327–8
Exowalk 235
ExternE Project 78

FLEXible Telepresence Robot
    Assembly (FLEXTRA) 303
  actuators and sensors 312
  camera 311–12
  Chassis implementation 309, 311
  components interactions 311
  control system 312
  COVID-19 pandemics
    contactless delivery scenario 316–18
    remote consultation and reception
      315–16
    remote temperature measurement
      315, 316
    room disinfection scenario 317,
      319
  design principles 303–4
  design processing
    components 306
    medicine dispenser 306–8
    mixed pill manual sorting 307
    Pill Blocks Automatic Sorting 307
    QFD matrices 305–6
  economy 304
  flexibility and extensibility 304
  functionality 304
  functionality test
    Chassis movement 314
    medicine dispenser 314
    remote video communication 315
  hardware 304–5
  limitations 320

operational functionality 308–9
overview 310
Raspberry Pi 312
safety and power 304
software implementation
control system 313–4
device management system 313
video streaming system 312, 313
specification 305
stability and usability 304
functional ability 2–3

gamification 294
General Data Protection Regulation
(GDPR) 99
general equilibrium models 77
geriatric care 324–5
global trend, population ageing
fertility rate 31, 32
life expectancy 28–30
median age projection 32
number of physicians 36
old-age dependency ratio 34
government-sponsored digital health
program 11

health-adjusted life expectancy 42
Healthcare Identifiers Act 2010 105
healthcare provider organisations 114
health co-benefits 3–4
air pollution 87
Australian perspective
background 90
CCP program 89–90
research methods 90
results 90
Sydney Greater Metropolitan
Region 90
categories 87
local climate action 88–9
Health Impact Assessment (HIA) 83
EIA methodology 83–4
generic case-study template 86

implementation process 85
securing city's (council's) mandate
85–6
WHO European Healthy Cities
Network (EHCN) 84
Health in All Policies (HiAP) 84
Health Information Systems
Interoperability Maturity Toolkit
(HISIMT) 13
Health Information System (HIS)
Stages of Continuous
Improvement Toolkit (HISSCIT)
13
health system adoption 15
healthy ageing 2
ageing population, world 324
and climate change 325
definition 71
determinants 71
digital health maturity 324
digital services
government and business policies
326
human resource management
325–26
IoT and smart home technologies
328
mental health services 326–7
mobile applications 328
robots 329
supply chain management 327
exoskeletons 327–8
geriatric care 324–5
privacy protection 325
SENSE-GARDEN 328
home-based health monitoring 47
Honda Walking Assist Device® 233
human resource management (HRM)
325–6
Hybrid Assistive Limb (HLA) 233, 235
hybrid blockchain solution 106

information and communication
technology (ICT) 12

information and computer technologies
      (ICTs) 48
informed consent process 62
integrated assessment modelling (IAM)
      77
Intended Nationally Determined
      Contributions (INDCs) 72
Internet of Things (IoT)
   barriers
      smart home adoption 280–1
      wearables 279–80
   interoperable networks 270
   literature review 271
   longevity 270
   smart homes cases 272–9
   systematic literature 271
   wearables 270–2, 281

lightweight- powered
      exoskeletons 235
lockdown approaches, Covid-19
   actions taken by different countries
      153, 154
   digital health and alternative
      approaches 156
   digital health and approaches
      154–5
   research context
      AI and big data 150–1
      contact tracing tools and services
         149–50
      digital health tools 149
      digital services and technologies
         149
      mobile applications 149
      social disconnection 148
      wearables 149
   research design
      article screening results 152–3
      database and keywords 151
      inclusion and exclusion criteria
         152
      limitations 152
   research questions 151

Lokomat treadmill- based robotic
      system 234
long-term care (LTC) 39–40

Mango Health 292
medication adherence-monitoring
      process 193–4
   defects 194
   medical errors 193–4
   non-adherence 193
   RFID technology
      access to information 195
      Continuous Medication
         Monitoring 194
      ePrescription 194
      five rights guidelines 195–6
      inpatient medication use 193
      Medication Adherence Intelligence
         System 194–5
      Medication Event- Monitoring
         System (MEMS) 194
      medication use-monitoring sub-
         process 195
      prescription information 194
      prescription regimen reading sub-
         process 195
      tagging system 196
medication errors 183
Medication Event-Monitoring System
      (MEMS) 194
medication management
   client's perspective 196
   supply chain management's
      perspective 196
mental health care crisis
   Bangladesh (*see* digital mental health
      services, Bangladesh)
   and chronic medical conditions 164
   COVID-19 pandemic 165
   South East Asia region 164
mental health disorders 5
Mercer Global Pension Index 43–4
mHealth for Belt and Road (mHBR)
      Initiative 329

mHealth for Belt and Road region 2
mixed pill manual sorting 307
mobile applications-based contact
        tracing 156
mobile healthcare applications 7
    designers
        accessibility 291–2
        customization feature 294–5
        gamification 294
        sample designs 292–3
        senior-considerate features 293
        senior demographics 295
        visual progress bar 294
    design trends 291, 292
    medical applications 287
    medical spending 287
    modern trends 287
    sample healthcare applications 291,
        292
    TAM and UTAUT theories
        casual observation 290–1
        desktop computing devices 290
        social influence 289–90
        younger demographics 290
MonerDaktar 5
multi-criteria analysis (MCA) 81–2
MyCentura Health 292
My Health Records Act 2012 103–5

National Transfer Accounts project 42
nominated representative 114
non-communicable diseases (NCDs)
        36–7, 53
non-repudiation, blockchain 106

old-age dependency ratio (OADR) 34, 35
overground robotic wearable
        exoskeletons 233, 234

Personal Health Records (PHRs) 97–8
Pill Blocks Automatic Sorting 307
policy-decision-making process 80–2

Political Declaration on the Madrid
        International Plan of Action on
        Ageing (MIPAA) 25
population ageing
    analysis and policy implications
        age-based discrimination 47
        economic participation 46
        fast ageing 45, 47
        health and autonomy 47–8
        information and computer
            technologies (ICTs) 48
        selected countries 44–5
        senior entrepreneurship 46
        social engagement 47
        sustainable economic growth
            45–6
    challenges 25–6
    economic challenges
        demographic dividend theory 44
        financial sustainability 43
        Mercer Global Pension Index 43
        National Transfer Accounts project
            42
        public health expenditure 43
        public pension system 42, 43
    global trend 28–34
    healthcare system challenges
        compression of morbidity 42
        dementia 38–40
        expansion of morbidity 42
        general practitioners (GPs) 37
        health-adjusted life expectancy 42
        healthcare expenditure burden
            40–41
        life expectancy 40
        long-term care (LTC) 39–40
        non-communicable diseases
            (NCDs) 36–7
        OECD 40
        primary care system (PHC) 37
    Sustainable Development Goals
        (SDGs) Regions 26
    and world population growth 27
powered exoskeleton
    back injuries 233

Exowalk 235
Hybrid Assistive Limb 233, 235
Indego Personal 235
lightweight-powered exoskeletons
    235
lower limb exoskeletons 232
mechatronics technology 232
minimalistic exoskeletons 235
overground robotic wearable
    exoskeletons 233
reduced mobility impacts 241
Responsible Research & Innovation
    (RRI) 237–41
search results 232
social interaction 233
social robots
    aging- related conditions 236
    AI-enabled exoskeleton 236
    rehabilitation device 237
    ROBIA 238, 242
spinal cord injury 232
treadmill-based robotic systems 233
Preferred Reporting Items for
    Systematic Reviews and Meta-
    Analyses (PRISMA) 205–6
prescription regimen reading sub-
    process 195
primary care system (PHC) 37
public health data 119
public pension system 43

Quality Function Deployment (QFD)
    matrices 305–306
quality improvement, measurement,
    monitoring and evaluation
    (QIMME) 15

residential aged care 184. *See also*
    aged care services and providers
Responsible Research & Innovation
    (RRI)
    accessibility considerations 239
    cultural considerations 240

definition 238
economic considerations 239
environmental considerations 240
ethical considerations 241
inclusivity considerations 240
legal considerations 240–1
RFID-based medication adherence-
    monitoring system 193–4
Roam Robotics Ascend[r] 233
Robot Impact Assessment (ROBIA)
    238
Robots for Elderly project 7

Senior Safety Phone 292
SENSE-GARDEN method 6
    Aan de Beverdijk care home,
        Hamont-Achel (Belgium) 260
    activities 260
    ALMA digital patient profile 248,
        264
    architectural concept 249
    artificial intelligence (AI) algorithm
        263
    Bokkotunet care home, Odda
        (Norway) 260
    dementia
        Alzheimer disease 251
        Clinical Dementia Rating (CDR)
            Scale 251
        cognitive decline symptoms 250
        major neurocognitive disorder 251
    digital playlists 248
    ELIAS Emergency University
        Hospital in Bucharest 260
    ethical concerns 263
    factual memories 248
    Google analytics results 259
    history 251–3
    language loss 249
    Lar Santa Joana Princesa care home,
        Lisbon (Portugal) 260
    logo of 253
    multidisciplinary team 253
    in Odda, Norway 257, 258

perspectives 254
pictures and videos 260
project team 247
qualitative impact studies 261–2
quantitative impact studies 262
resources 263
self-contained physical rooms 247
system architecture 265–7
user-centered design process 254–5
user requirements list 254
service providers 188
Silvercare model 4
  anxiety 142
  beneficiaries 132
  community-based care 131–2
    operations 139–40
    outcomes 140
    structure and organisation 139
    volunteering 139
  coordinators 132
  facilitating conditions 141
  intention to use 142
  KINSPARC
    active ageing 139
    awareness programmes 136–7
    celebrating birthdays 137–8
    information and communication
      technology 137
    Kalyani 136–8
    local background 134–5
    operations 136
    project outcomes 138
    recreational events 137
    structure and function 136–7
  performance expectancy 140
  primary aims 131
  self-efficacy 141–2
  service providers 132–3
  social influence 141
  support group 132
  tablet-based well-being project
    133–4
smart homes cases, Internet of Things
    (IoT) 272–9
reliability 282

theory-based studies 281–2
social cost-benefit analysis 81
software products 114
spinal cord injuries 236
strategic environmental assessment
    (SEA) 83
sustainability assessment (SA) 83
Sustainable Development Goals (SDGs)
    regions
  fertility rate 31
  life expectancy 30
  median age projection 32, 33
  number of physicians 36
  old-age dependency ratio 35

tablet-based well-being project
    132–3
technology acceptance model (TAM)
    288–91
telemedicine and mobile clinics 47
telepresence robots 7
  COVID-19 pandemics 302–3
  low-cost robots 302
  multi-disciplinary collaboration 301
Telepsychiatry Research and Innovation
    Network (TRIN) 166
test–trace–isolate strategy 156
The Privacy Act 1988 102
third-party logistics providers 190, 192
Tort law 99
treadmill-based robotic systems 233,
    234

Unified Theory of Acceptance and Use
    of Technology (UTAUT) model
    140, 282–5
Universal Health Coverage 11
user-centered design (UCD) process
    254–5

WHO European Healthy Cities
    Network (EHCN) 84